How to Use Evidence-Based Dental Practices to Improve Your

Clinical Decision-Making

Alonso Carrasco-Labra, D.D.S.
Romina Brignardello-Petersen, D.D.S.
Michael Glick, D.M.D.
Amir Azarpazhooh, D.D.S.
Gordon Guyatt, M.D.

ADA American Dental Association®
America's leading advocate for oral health

Book ISBN: 978-1-68447-061-7
E-book ISBN: 978-1-68447-062-4
ADA Product No.: J079BT

Acknowledgments

This book would not have been possible without the support of the following American Dental Association staff members:

- From the ADA Center for Evidence-Based Dentistry (EBD): Jeff Huber, M.B.A., Scientific Content Specialist, for production management and editing; Erica Colangelo, M.P.H., Senior Manager; and Tyharrie Woods, M.A., Coordinator, for logistics support.

- From ADA Publishing: Kathy Pulkrabek, Manager/Editor, Professional Products, Department of Product Development and Sales, and Pamela Woolf, Senior Manager, Department of Product Development and Sales, for production management and editing.

- From ADA Scientific Information: Anita M. Mark, Senior Scientific Content Specialist, for proofreading and copyediting.

- From the ADA Science Institute: Aaron Pinkston, Coordinator, for meetings coordination.

Thank you to Kimberly Ruona, D.D.S., Associate Dean for Patient Care, University of Texas School of Dentistry at Houston, for her input into the development of the cover for this book.

And a big thank you to the broad community of enthusiastic and forward-thinking EBD leaders who conceived the idea of, and wrote, this book. Their knowledge and hard work were essential in producing this compendium of the skills necessary to practice and teach EBD.

Table of Contents

Chapter 3. How to Appraise and Use an Article about Therapy 41

Romina Brignardello-Petersen, D.D.S., M.Sc., Ph.D.; Alonso Carrasco-Labra, D.D.S., M.Sc., Ph.D.;
Michael Glick, D.M.D.; Gordon H. Guyatt, M.D., M.Sc.; and Amir Azarpazhooh, D.D.S., M.Sc., Ph.D.

Chapter 4. How to Use an Article about Harm 57

Romina Brignardello-Petersen, D.D.S., M.Sc., Ph.D.; Alonso Carrasco-Labra, D.D.S., M.Sc., Ph.D.;
Michael Glick, D.M.D.; Gordon H. Guyatt, M.D., M.Sc.; and Amir Azarpazhooh, D.D.S., M.Sc., Ph.D.

Chapter 5. How to Appraise and Use an Article about Diagnosis

Romina Brignardello-Petersen, D.D.S., M.Sc., Ph.D.; Alonso Carrasco-Labra, D.D.S., M.Sc., Ph.D.; Michael Glick, D.M.D.; Gordon H. Guyatt, M.D., M.Sc.; and Amir Azarpazhooh, D.D.S., M.Sc., Ph.D.

Chapter 6. How to Use a Systematic Review and Meta-Analysis

Alonso Carrasco-Labra, D.D.S., M.Sc., Ph.D.; Romina Brignardello-Petersen, D.D.S., M.Sc., Ph.D.; Michael Glick, D.M.D.; Gordon H. Guyatt, M.D., M.Sc.; and Amir Azarpazhooh, D.D.S., M.Sc., Ph.D.

Chapter 7. How to Use Patient Management Recommendations from Clinical Practice Guidelines 111

Alonso Carrasco-Labra, D.D.S., M.Sc., Ph.D.; Romina Brignardello-Petersen, D.D.S., M.Sc., Ph.D.; Michael Glick, D.M.D.; Gordon H. Guyatt, M.D., M.Sc.; Ignacio Neumann, M.D., M.Sc., Ph.D.; and Amir Azarpazhooh, D.D.S., M.Sc., Ph.D.

Chapter 8. How to Appraise an Article Based on a Qualitative Study . . . 129

Joanna E.M. Sale, Ph.D.; Maryam Amin, D.M.D., M.Sc., Ph.D.; Alonso Carrasco-Labra, D.D.S., M.Sc., Ph.D.; Romina Brignardello-Petersen, D.D.S., M.Sc., Ph.D.; Michael Glick, D.M.D.; Gordon H. Guyatt, M.D., M.Sc.; and Amir Azarpazhooh, D.D.S., M.Sc., Ph.D.

Chapter 9. How to Appraise and Use an Article about Economic Analysis

Lusine Abrahamyan, M.D., M.P.H., Ph.D.; Petros Pechlivanoglou, Ph.D.; Murray Krahn, M.D., M.Sc.; Alonso Carrasco-Labra, D.D.S., M.Sc., Ph.D.; Romina Brignardello-Petersen, D.D.S., M.Sc., Ph.D.; Michael Glick, D.M.D.; Gordon H. Guyatt, M.D., M.Sc.; and Amir Azarpazhooh, D.D.S., M.Sc., Ph.D.

Chapter 10. How to Avoid Being Misled by Clinical Studies' Results in Dentistry

Alonso Carrasco-Labra, D.D.S., M.Sc., Ph.D.; Romina Brignardello-Petersen, D.D.S., M.Sc., Ph.D.; Amir Azarpazhooh, D.D.S., M.Sc., Ph.D.; Michael Glick, D.M.D.; and Gordon H. Guyatt, M.D., M.Sc.

Chapter 11. What Is the Difference between Clinical and Statistical Significance?

Romina Brignardello-Petersen, D.D.S., M.Sc., Ph.D.; Alonso Carrasco-Labra, D.D.S., M.Sc., Ph.D.;
Prakeshkumar Shah, M.Sc., M.B.B.S., M.D., D.C.H., M.R.C.P.; and Amir Azarpazhooh, D.D.S., M.Sc., Ph.D.

Chapter 12. A Primer to Biostatistics for Busy Clinicians

Michael Glick, D.M.D., and Barbara L. Greenberg, Ph.D., M.Sc.

Chapter 16. Implementing Evidence into Practice

Satish S. Kumar, D.M.D., M.D.Sc., M.S.; Ben Balevi, D.D.S., M.Sc.; Rebecca Schaffer, D.D.S.;
Romesh Nalliah, D.D.S., M.H.C.M.; Martha Ann Keels, D.D.S., Ph.D.; Norman Tinanoff, D.D.S., M.S.;
and Robert J. Weyant, D.M.D., Dr.P.H., M.S.

Preface

Evidence-based medicine was first articulated in the early 1990s[1], and by 1995[2], articles on evidence-based dentistry (EBD) were starting to appear in the dental literature. While the uptake of EBD approaches and improvements in the quality of dental research have been slower than early adopters of the concepts would have hoped for, this has not been for lack of support from the American Dental Association.

The establishment of the ADA Center for EBD and its development of a definition for EBD (that is, a patient-centered approach to treatment decisions, which provides personalized dental care based on the most current scientific knowledge[3]) have been important milestones along the road to a more evidence-based dental profession. The ADA has actively promoted EBD in its journal, *The Journal of the American Dental Association,* and organized EBD courses and workshops for a number of years. The ADA EBD website also provides a broad range of helpful EBD resources, including a number of evidence-based clinical practice guidelines, chairside guides, and videos.

Since 1995, Cochrane Oral Health has produced around 150 systematic reviews that have clarified not only what we know but also what is still uncertain in many areas of dentistry. In addition to Cochrane reviews, there has been a significant increase in dentistry's overall number of systematic reviews, which more often than not identify gaps in knowledge and limitations in the quality of our primary research.

All of this means that it is important to continue teaching the key skills of the evidence-based approach, including how to search for and critically appraise evidence as well as how to translate this evidence into the practice of dentists and the wider dental team. While courses and conferences can stimulate and excite interest in a subject, having a tangible resource that pulls short, informative, how-to articles together in a practical format is a great help for teachers and students alike. That is why I believe this book will prove invaluable to the dental community.

Derek Richards, M.Sc., D.D.P.H.
Centre for Evidence-Based Dentistry
School of Dentistry
University of Dundee
Dundee, Scotland, U.K.

References

1. Guyatt GH. "Evidence-based medicine." *ACP J Club* 1991;114(*ACP J Club,* suppl 2):A-16.
2. Richards D, Lawrence A. "Evidence based dentistry." *Br Dent J* 1995;179(7):270-273.
3. "About EBD." ADA Center for Evidence-Based Dentistry. *https://ebd.ADA.org/en/about.* Accessed March 5, 2019.

How to Use This Book

Evidence-based dentistry (EBD) relies on personalization. Dentists work with each of their patients to make a unique treatment decision that integrates the dentist's expertise, the patient's needs and preferences, and the most current, clinically relevant evidence. Melding all three of these elements ensures that the identified treatment decision appropriately addresses the clinical scenario in question. There is no one-size-fits-all approach to patient care.

As with EBD, there is no one way to use this book. Some may start at the very beginning and read to the very end, since each chapter builds on the one before it. Most will probably open the book when they're in need of a handy reference, turning to the section that is most relevant to them at that time. Others will test their ability to critically appraise evidence by reading the real-world examples that are highlighted in some chapters' call-out boxes and then go back to review sections that cover self-identified gaps in knowledge. Any strategy works. There is no one size fits all approach to reading this book.

Regardless of what tack you take, we hope that you find this book covers a wide breadth of EBD topics. Perusing the pages ahead should assist anyone who wants to learn about practicing EBD, teaching EBD, defining an EBD curriculum, conducting a journal/study club, or engaging in other activities that incorporate evidence into patient care. The overall goal is to provide you with the foundational knowledge you need to improve patient care through the application of EBD.

Although this wealth of information is often addressed toward clinicians throughout the book, readers from all walks of the dental community can use this book to better harness the latest scientific evidence in their clinical decision-making. That's what EBD is all about—empowering everyone to identify the best treatment for a particular clinical scenario.

Alonso Carrasco-Labra, D.D.S., M.Sc., Ph.D., and Jeff Huber, M.B.A.
Center for Evidence-Based Dentistry
Science Institute
American Dental Association
Chicago, Illinois, U.S.A.

Chapter 1. Understanding and Applying the Principles of Evidence-Based Dentistry (EBD)

Romina Brignardello-Petersen, D.D.S., M.Sc., Ph.D.; Alonso Carrasco-Labra, D.D.S., M.Sc., Ph.D.; Michael Glick, D.M.D.; Gordon H. Guyatt, M.D., M.Sc.; and Amir Azarpazhooh, D.D.S., M.Sc., Ph.D.

In This Chapter:

Definition and Principles of EBD

The Process of EBD

Introduction

Scientific evidence is a crucial underpinning of clinical practice. Nevertheless, the first series of articles aimed at providing clinicians with guidelines for critically appraising the evidence that informs clinical practices did not appear until 1981.[1] Ten years later, the term "evidence-based medicine"[2] first appeared in the medical literature. Subsequently, between 1993 and 2000, a group of evidence-based medicine enthusiasts[3] published a series of 25 articles aimed at assisting clinicians in understanding and applying the medical literature to their clinical decision-making in a clinical setting.[4]

The concept of evidence-based medicine soon expanded to other clinical areas. The first article to use the term "evidence-based dentistry" (EBD) was published in 1995 by Richards and Lawrence,[5] and since then other articles have been published on the topic.[6–11] There is, however, still no guide easily accessible for current and future dental practitioners that addresses the critical appraisal and use of evidence specifically aimed at clinicians and educators in oral health care fields.

This book aims to provide an overview of the basic concepts of EBD to assist oral health care professionals in making use of evidence to inform their clinical decisions. This book addresses the main topics in EBD, including how to formulate questions that are easy to answer using the scientific literature, effectively search for relevant evidence, identify the strengths and limitations of different study designs and interpret their findings, and apply findings to clinical decisions. Although this book mostly focuses on the application of research to clinical practice, it also provides a perspective at the health policy level.

Definition and Principles of EBD

The American Dental Association defines EBD as "an approach to oral healthcare that requires the judicious integration of systematic assessments of clinically relevant scientific evidence, relating to the patient's oral and medical condition and history, with the dentist's clinical expertise and the patient's treatment needs and preferences."[12] The definition of EBD has three main components:

- the best current research evidence;

- the clinician's expertise;

- the patient's values and preferences.[13]

Figure 1.1. The Components of Evidence-Based Dentistry

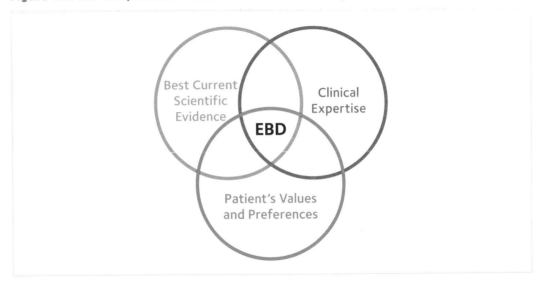

One definition of evidence is "any empirical observation whether systematically collected or not."[14] Evidence can be obtained from a range of sources, including clinical observation of the course of a single patient or a multicenter and multinational clinical study. Evidence to inform any clinical decision is abundant. However, as some evidence is more trustworthy than other evidence, it is both necessary and desirable to prioritize certain types of evidence.

Because unsystematic clinical observations of a small number of patients are more likely to introduce more bias than are appropriately designed and conducted clinical studies, for example, astute clinicians always should prefer the latter evidence to the former.[14] For each type of clinical question, there is a hierarchy of evidence that is based on degree of trustworthiness. For instance, to answer questions regarding the effectiveness of a particular intervention, the strongest evidence would come from randomized clinical trials with a low risk of bias and large sample sizes, as such evidence provides more precise estimates and more consistent results and is directly applicable to the patients at hand. If findings from such studies are not available for the specific question of interest, clinicians must rely on less trustworthy evidence, including well-designed and conducted observational studies, such as cohort and case-control studies. If no randomized trials, cohort and case-control studies, or case series/case reports are available, individual observations by a clinical expert may become a valuable source of evidence. In subsequent chapters, we discuss the hierarchy of evidence for each type of clinical question (that is, therapy and prevention, harm, prognosis, and diagnosis) and how to appraise the relevant literature critically.

As stated above, evidence alone is not enough to support clinical decision-making from an EBD perspective; decision-making should rely on the integration of evidence with clinical expertise and patients' needs and preferences. The success of an intervention that has proven to be effective in a clinical study depends on the ability of a clinician to use the intervention in an appropriate clinical setting. In other words, clinical expertise is key to determining whether and how the evidence can be applied to a specific patient's case.[14] Finally, because clinical procedures are associated with potential adverse effects, including the burden of the procedure and its costs, it is important to consider patients' values and preferences when making a decision regarding treatment.

The Process of EBD

The decisions clinicians must make in daily clinical practice are the most important source of questions for which we seek evidence-based solutions. Such questions constitute the starting point of the EBD process, which encompasses the following main steps:

- translating the clinical question into a well-formulated searchable question format;

- searching for the best available evidence to answer this question;

- critically appraising the evidence and applying it to the particular clinical scenario that motivated the question.

To translate a clinical question into a well-formulated searchable question, it is necessary to identify four main components of the question: the Patient or Population of interest, the Intervention (or exposure or new diagnostic test strategy, depending on the type of the clinical question), the Comparison (or reference standard, depending on the type of clinical question), and the Outcomes of interest according to a patient-centered approach—hence, PICO.[15] Examples of the PICO approach for the variety of types of clinical question are discussed in detail in subsequent chapters in this book.

The PICO components of the question at hand are used as the basis of searching for evidence in the literature by using electronic databases and other sources. There are a number of sources that provide clinicians with useful information. Depending on the degree of detail sought, information from primary studies, summaries and critical appraisals, and clinical practice guidelines may all provide evidence.[16] How to choose the most relevant source to search in any particular case is addressed in subsequent chapters in this book.

Once a clinician obtains the evidence to answer the clinical question at hand, it is necessary for him or her to conduct a critical appraisal of the evidence discovered. As described in detail in subsequent chapters, the critical appraisal of individual primary studies has three main domains: risk of bias assessment, results, and applicability.[17] The first domain explores whether the study was designed and conducted in a manner in which potential biases were minimized.[18] The second domain is an interpretation of the results of the study in terms of direction, magnitude, and precision. The third domain contextualizes the available evidence to determine implications for clinical practice.[19] Subsequent chapters in this book cover how to appraise and apply evidence in a critical fashion to different types of clinical questions.

Scientific evidence constitutes one of the fundamental tenets of dental practice. Evidence-based dental practice integrates the use of the best available evidence, clinicians' expertise, and patients' needs and preferences to inform decision-making in clinical practice. This book provides oral health care professionals with the fundamental concepts of EBD and guidance on how to use evidence in their clinical practices.

References

1. "How to read clinical journals, part I: why to read them and how to start reading them critically." *Can Med Assoc J* 1981;124(5):555-558.

2. Guyatt GH. "Evidence-based medicine." *ACP J Club* 1991;114(ACP J Club, suppl 2):A-16.

3. Evidence-Based Medicine Working Group. "Evidence-based medicine: a new approach to teaching the practice of medicine." *JAMA* 1992;268(17):2420-2425.

4. Guyatt GH, Rennie D. "Users' guides to the medical literature." *JAMA* 1993;270(17):2096-2097.

5. Richards D, Lawrence A. "Evidence based dentistry." *Br Dent J* 1995;179(7):270-273.

6. Azarpazhooh A, Mayhall JT, Leake JL. "Introducing dental students to evidence-based decisions in dental care." *J Dent Educ* 2008;72(1):87-109.

7. Cruz MA. "Evidence-based versus experience-based decision making in clinical dentistry." *J Am Coll Dent* 2000;67(1):11-14.

8. Faggion CM Jr, Tu YK. "Evidence-based dentistry: a model for clinical practice." *J Dent Educ* 2007;71(6):825-831.

9. Forrest JL, Miller SA. "Evidence-based decision making in dental hygiene education, practice, and research." *J Dent Hyg* 2001;75(1):50-63.

10. Laskin DM. "Finding the evidence for evidence-based dentistry." *J Am Coll Dent* 2000;67(1):7-10.

11. Scarbecz M. "Evidence-based dentistry resources for dental practitioners." *J Tenn Dent Assoc* 2008;88(2):9-13.

12. American Dental Association Center for Evidence-Based Dentistry. About EBD. *http://ebd.ADA.org/en/about*. Accessed Oct. 5, 2014.

13. Sackett DL, Rosenberg WM, Gray JA, Haynes RB, Richardson WS. "Evidence based medicine: what it is and what it isn't." *BMJ* 1996;312(7023):71-72.

14. Guyatt GH, Haynes B, Jaeschke R, et al. "The philosophy of evidence-based medicine." In: Guyatt GH, Rennie D, Meade MO, Cook DJ, eds. *Users' Guides to the Medical Literature: A Manual for Evidence-Based Clinical Practice*. 2nd ed. Columbus, Ohio: McGraw-Hill Education; 2008:9-16.

15. Guyatt GH, Meade MO, Richardson S, Jaeschke R. "What is the question." In: Guyatt GH, Rennie D, Meade MO, Cook DJ, eds. *Users' Guides to the Medical Literature: A Manual for Evidence-Based Clinical Practice*. 2nd ed. Columbus, Ohio: McGraw-Hill Education; 2008:17-28.

16. McKibbon A, Wyer P, Jaeschke R, Hunt D. "Finding the evidence." In: Guyatt GH, Rennie D, Meade MO, Cook DJ, eds. *Users' Guides to the Medical Literature: A Manual for Evidence-Based Clinical Practice*. 2nd ed. Columbus, Ohio: McGraw-Hill Education; 2008:29-58.

17. Guyatt GH, Rennie D, Meade MO, Cook DJ, eds. *Users' Guides to the Medical Literature: A Manual for Evidence-Based Clinical Practice*. 2nd ed. Columbus, Ohio: McGraw-Hill Education; 2008.

18. Guyatt GH, Jaeschke R, Meade MO. "Why study results mislead: bias and random error." In: Guyatt GH, Rennie D, Meade MO, Cook DJ, eds. *Users' Guides to the Medical Literature: A Manual for Evidence-Based Clinical Practice*. 2nd ed. Columbus, Ohio: McGraw-Hill Education; 2008:59-64.

19. Dans A, Dans L, Guyatt GH. "Applying results to individual patients." In: Guyatt GH, Rennie D, Meade MO, Cook DJ, eds. *Users' Guides to the Medical Literature: A Manual for Evidence-Based Clinical Practice*. 2nd ed. Columbus, Ohio: McGraw-Hill Education; 2008:273-289.

A version of this chapter originally appeared in the November 2014 edition of *JADA* (Volume 145, Issue 11, Pages 1105–1107). It has been reviewed and updated for accuracy and clarity by the editors of *How to Use Evidence-Based Dental Practices to Improve Your Clinical Decision-Making*.

Chapter 2. Searching for the Best Oral Health Evidence: Strategies, Tips, and Resources

Elizabeth Stellrecht, M.L.S., and H. Austin Booth, M.L.I.S., M.A.

Introduction

To find answers to clinical inquiries, it is necessary to conduct an evidence-based literature search. This chapter describes the most commonly used evidence-based resources, recommends search strategies that will help enable the oral health practitioner to retrieve the most useful clinical information, and suggests a workflow for navigating evidence-based information.

The practice of evidence-based dentistry includes articulating a clinical question, conducting a search for relevant literature, evaluating the retrieved evidence, applying that evidence to answer the clinical question at hand, and putting that answer into effect in a clinical setting.

The amount of health-related information available via the internet is staggering. Even just the published results of clinical trials and systematic reviews are impossible to keep up with. It is estimated, for example, that an average of 11 systematic reviews and 75 results of clinical trials are published in the medical literature daily.[1] In addition, health information found within the peer-reviewed literature can be contradictory. The exponential growth of complex health information is why it is essential to learn not only how to search for the best evidence-based literature, but also how to evaluate that literature.

Effective searching of medical databases is a very valuable skill these days. Below, we outline effective and efficient ways for busy clinicians to search the most important medical resources. For more complex searches and the development of expert searching skills, such as conducting systematic reviews, we recommend working with a librarian who has been trained in extensive searching of the scientific literature.

General Tips for Searching Electronic Resources

A general search tip is to keep things simple when first starting a search. Begin with a broad search and use only a few terms without applying any search filters; take a look at the results to determine if the search is too broad or too narrow and whether it's displaying relevant results. Try using nouns as search terms rather than adjectives, as adjectives are difficult to quantify and can muddy the results. Beginning a search with too many terms or multiple filters applied may result in the inadvertent exclusion of relevant literature (Table 2.1).

Table 2.1. General Searching Tips for Electronic Resources

Searching Tips to Remember
• Begin with a broad, simple search.
• Use nouns as search terms; avoid adjectives.
• Add additional terms using Boolean searching to narrow results.
• Still too many results? Consider using search filters to limit results according to study design type, age, publication date, language, and so on.
• Not getting the expected results? Use synonyms and variations in spelling for original search terms.

If the search is not yielding the expected results, consider using synonyms for search terms, including variations of spelling, such as U.S. versus U.K. spelling of terms. For instance, a synonym for "pregnant women" is "pregnancy." Searching different terms for the same concept can yield different results. Databases will often have a controlled vocabulary, which is preferred terminology that is found in the database's thesaurus and can be very helpful when searching for relevant literature, as database thesauri typically include all synonyms for a search term. A team of indexers is responsible for reading all included materials in any given database and identifying the main concepts represented in each individual work; once the main topics are identified, the indexer assigns subject headings to the work using the preferred terminology. Using the preferred terminology therefore standardizes the search process, making it easier and quicker to locate relevant literature. The searcher should consider looking up search terms in the database's thesaurus and using the suggested term, which will yield results in which the term is one of the main subjects of the retrieved literature. If a database does not use a controlled vocabulary, consider searching by a specific field such as title, abstract, or author to further limit results. Keyword searches will look for the terms to appear anywhere in the record, while searching in a specific field limits where the term will appear. The majority of the resources described below allow searching by phrase by placing the phrase within quotation marks. Most also recognize common misspellings and abbreviations, and will suggest alternative search terms when no results are found. In addition, most of the resources below search plurals automatically.

Boolean searching refers to connecting search terms with one of the following three terms: AND, OR, or NOT. When combining two terms with AND, search results will contain both terms, resulting in fewer results than searching using only one of the terms. Combining terms with OR will return results that contain at least one of the terms, resulting in a higher number of search results than if only one of the terms was searched. Combining two terms with NOT will yield results in which the first term appears but not the second term, narrowing the number of results (Figure 2.1).

Figure 2.1. Examples of Boolean Searching

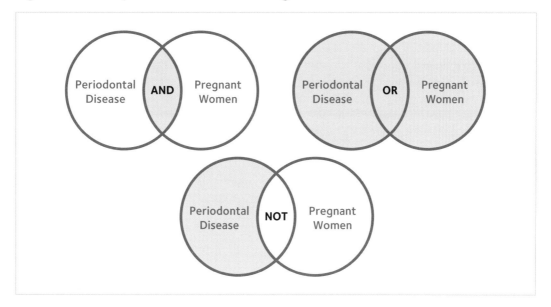

Searching Workflow

We suggest searching several databases; searching a combination of databases helps to ensure that information is not missed that might influence the answer to the clinical question at hand. While the exact databases searched will depend on the question/topic/need, the importance of finding results that contain high levels of evidence calls for, at a minimum, Cochrane, Trip, and PubMed to be searched. Information about many additional available databases are listed in the Resources section of this chapter. To avoid missing important results, use all three resources: there is less overlap among them than one would imagine, they cover different types of materials, and the content in each is updated on different cycles. Each resource has a unique architecture, vocabulary, and results algorithm and, therefore, will return unique results. Searching Cochrane, Trip, and PubMed is free, but the full text of results is not always available without a subscription to source material, which is typically provided when operating in an academic setting. For those in clinical practice outside academic settings, the American Dental Association (ADA) Library and Archives offers members access to full-text articles identified through these databases. All three resources are relatively easy to search and provide up-to-date information. By using these three databases, the oral health practitioner will have searched the gold standard for evidence-based information (Cochrane), the best "preappraised" resource (Trip), and the most comprehensive medical literature search engine (PubMed).

We recommend framing the search strategy using the PICO framework to articulate the clinical question. PICO assists clinicians in creating a clear, focused clinical question by breaking down the question into four components: population (Who is being treated? What specific characteristics does this population have?), intervention (What treatment or therapy is being considered?), comparison (What is the gold standard? The comparison can also be no comparison, or a placebo), and outcomes (What improvements or changes are hoped for?). Of course, PICO will not fit every clinical question as not all questions are ones of therapy; the framework can be modified depending on the type of question. For instance, if it is a question of harm, the clinician will frame the question by considering what exposure, rather than what intervention, to search for. We recommend that clinicians refer to the framework as a starting point and modify as necessary for individual research needs. Using the PICO framework is likely to result in the return of relevant results because the framework encourages clarity and specificity and it breaks down the clinical question into easily searchable components. Using the PICO framework to articulate the question will save the clinician time when conducting the search and better enable the clinician to review the results of the search for relevance and applicability to clinical practice (or to a particular patient) (Table 2.2).

 Searching a combination of databases helps to ensure that information is not missed that might influence the answer to the clinical question at hand.

Use keywords, indexing terms, and synonyms related to the components of the PICO question for the search. We suggest beginning with two PICO components as search terms rather than all four. Begin with search terms based on the population and intervention components of the PICO question, as the results will most likely include the comparison term or concept. Adding the outcome terms will further narrow the results, and these terms should be added if the initial search yields far too many results. Using all four components as search terms initially will narrow a search too early and will miss results that may be important. Use the Boolean operator OR to account for synonyms of the same concept. Conversely, use the Boolean operator AND to require different components to be present in the results. See Figure 2.1 for examples of Boolean searching.

Table 2.2. Main Components and Examples of Clinical Questions, According to Their Natures

Nature of the Question	Example	Population	Intervention (Exposure or Diagnostic Test)	Comparison (or Reference Standard)	Outcomes
Therapy or Prevention	What is the effectiveness of antibiotics in preventing complications such as postoperative infections after third-molar extractions?	Patients undergoing third-molar extractions	Antibiotic prophylaxis	No prophylaxis	Alveolar osteitis, surgical wound infection
Harm or Etiology	Does giving toddlers milk instead of water to drink at night cause caries?	Toddlers	Drinking milk at night	Drinking water at night	Caries
Diagnosis	How useful is a periapical radiograph in detecting interproximal caries?	Patients suspected of having interproximal caries	Periapical radiograph	Bitewing radiograph	Diagnostic accuracy (as assessed by means of true-positive, true-negative, false-positive and false-negative findings)
Prognosis	Are patients with diabetes at higher risk of experiencing complications after third-molar extractions than are patients without diabetes?	Patients undergoing third-molar extractions	Presence of diabetes	Absence of diabetes	Pain, swelling, trismus, postoperative infections

Source: Brignardello-Petersen R, Carrasco-Labra A, Booth HA, Glick M, Guyatt GH, Azarpazhooh A, Agoritsas T. "A practical approach to evidence-based dentistry: II: how to search for evidence to inform clinical decisions." *J Am Dent Assoc.* 2014 Dec;145(12):1262-7. doi: 10.14219/jada.2014.113. PubMed PMID: 25429040.

Most databases have a thesaurus that lists the preferred terminology or subject headings used to index articles as they are added to the database. Searching by subject headings is a simple way to retrieve a smaller pool of relevant results, as subject headings standardize the search process and return results where the search term is considered a main topic (that is, subject) of the manuscript. When not using subject headings to search, limit the search to the title and abstract. If the initial search retrieves too many results, limit the results to secondary and preappraised literature such as clinical practice guidelines, summaries, critical summaries, and systematic reviews. If secondary literature does not exist, it will be necessary to consult primary studies; we suggest initially limiting the search to randomized controlled trials as they are typically less prone to bias (Figure 2.2).

Figure 2.2. Hierarchy of Evidence for Primary Studies, Level of Processing, and Link to EBD Resources

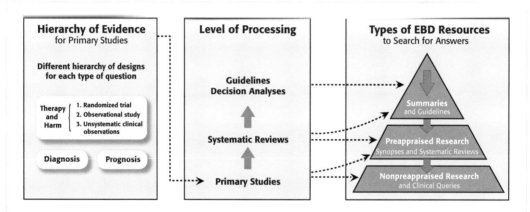

Types of evidence, according to their level of processing and resources to find them
The figure illustrates how to navigate across available types of evidence-based dentistry (EBD) resources. The left panel illustrates the hierarchy of evidence for primary studies, the middle panel helps determine the type of evidence for which to look, and the right panel illustrates where to search for such evidence. Depending on the nature of the question, primary studies follow a hierarchy of study designs from lower to higher risk of bias (left panel). They can be processed further into systematic reviews, where they are comprehensively synthesized, and then clinical guidelines, which move from evidence to recommendations (middle panel). Once the desired evidence has been determined, the pyramid of types of EBD resources (right panel) helps to choose the type of resource in which to search for the evidence. Efficient searches should start from the top—for example, with online summaries. These typically include more processed evidence, providing the gist and links to selected guidelines and systematic reviews. If no answer is found, sources of preappraised research provide synopses of selected and methodologically sound reviews and studies. Finally, large databases of nonpreappraised research contain all current studies, yet results are often are diluted with numerous citations irrelevant to the question. Reproduced with permission of the American Medical Association from Agoritsas and colleagues.[20]

Copyright © 2015 American Medical Association.

Initially, set aside results that are more than a decade old. If the search still retrieves too many items, do a search using all four PICO components, starting with adding the outcome terms to the search. If the results of the search include materials from the highest levels of evidence (for example, guidelines or systematic reviews), consider stopping the search and declaring it "good enough." To conduct a more comprehensive search, consult the additional databases listed below. Note that this workflow is intended to be used as a roadmap for an evidence-based search for a clinical question in order to decide action in a clinical setting—it is not a substitute for a search that would be used to conduct a systematic review or literature review.

There is always an element of creativity in developing a search strategy around a particular question and in determining the appropriate balance among relevance, breadth, and depth of results. Developing a search strategy is an iterative process; that is, as the oral health practitioner searches, he or she will modify, narrow, or expand the search terms used as well as the combinations of terms and the overall search strategy based on results. The effectiveness and efficiency of the search strategy will improve as the search progresses. If too few results are retrieved in a particular database, it may be necessary to modify the search by removing some search terms, search filters, or both. Please note that simply adding more terms to the search may not increase the number of relevant results as the terms may retrieve redundant results. Once a search is begun, there is a certain amount of trial and error in terms of refining the search terms to be used in the end. Adding and removing search terms and synonyms will allow the oral health practitioner to retrieve varying amounts, breadth, and quality of levels of evidence.

> There is always an element of creativity in developing a search strategy around a particular question and in determining the appropriate balance among relevance, breadth, and depth of results.

We suggest beginning the search process with Cochrane, then searching Trip if not enough relevant results are found, and then PubMed to fill in any remaining gaps in information. Since Cochrane is a database consisting solely of systematic reviews, the results presented are considered to be of a higher quality according to the evidence pyramid hierarchy. Due to the type of content, it is also a smaller database, so it is possible that the evidence needed might not be available in Cochrane. PubMed will almost always retrieve the most results from the search because of the breadth and scope of the resource. As noted below, even when using the Systematic Review filter or Clinical Queries search, which limits search results to clinical study categories, systematic reviews, and medical genetics, PubMed retrieves narrative reviews as well as descriptive articles. (For more information about Clinical Queries, please see the PubMed section of this chapter. Note that while Cochrane systematic reviews are indexed in PubMed, we recommend a separate search of the Cochrane Library because the results of a search of the Cochrane Library database and a search of Cochrane systematic reviews in PubMed will not retrieve identical results.)

We suggest conducting a search using both (that is, a combination of) keywords and subject headings. Note that Cochrane and PubMed share index terms—both databases use MeSH (Medical Subject Headings) as a controlled vocabulary or thesaurus for subject headings (see the PubMed section of this chapter for a detailed explanation of MeSH). Trip does not use a controlled vocabulary. Do not rely solely on index terms: many new articles and updates appear in databases before they are indexed, and these materials may prove to be the most useful. As the initial search is conducted, note related terms and at the end, go back and do a search using all relevant search terms. Including related terms or synonyms is crucial to conducting an effective search (Table 2.3).

Table 2.3. Workflow for Searching for Evidence

Type of Question/Situation	Resources to Consult	Level of Evidence Available
Consider first: Does a guideline for the question/ situation exist?	1. Epistemonikos 2. Trip 3. ECRI Guidelines Trust 4. Point-of-care resources	Guidelines, guideline summaries
Therapy/Prevention question (general)	1. Cochrane Database of Systematic Reviews 2. Trip 3. PubMed	Critical summaries, meta-analyses, systematic reviews, randomized controlled trials (RCTs)
Therapy/Prevention question (drug therapy)	1. Cochrane 2. Trip 3. Embase 4. PubMed	Critical summaries, meta-analyses, systematic reviews, RCTs
Harm/Etiology question	1. Cochrane 2. Trip 3. PubMed	Critical summaries, meta-analyses, systematic reviews, observational studies
Diagnosis question	1. Cochrane 2. Trip 3. PubMed	Critical summaries**, meta-analyses**, systematic reviews**, cross-sectional studies, case report/series
Prognosis question	1. Cochrane 2. Trip 3. PubMed	Critical summaries**, meta-analyses**, systematic reviews**, observational studies, case report/series
Situation: Can only find one or two articles on topic, need more	1. Web of Science or Scopus (cited reference searching) 2. Gray literature	Follow standard evidence pyramid

** Indicates that this type of evidence may not be available for this type of question.

For this chapter, our search examples will refer to the following PICO framework question: Are pregnant women with periodontal disease at greater risk of preterm birth or low birth weight than pregnant women without periodontal disease? In this instance, the population identified is pregnant women. Because this is not a question of therapy but of harm, the exposure is periodontal disease, with the comparison as the absence of periodontal disease. Outcomes of interest are preterm birth and low birth weight.

Resources

Comprehensive Resources

Epistemonikos

Website: *www.epistemonikos.org*
Cost: Free, with some limited full-text availability
Specialty of resource: Clinical practice guidelines, synopses, systematic reviews, primary studies, other

Epistemonikos is a publicly available resource whose objective is to "gather scientific information (i.e., evidence) that might be relevant for health decision-making and to provide rapid access to the best available evidence for real-life questions." It was created primarily for health professionals, researchers, and individuals who make decisions in health care.[2] Epistemonikos, which translated from Greek means "what is worth knowing," includes evidence-based policy briefs, systematic reviews, primary studies, and synopses of systematic reviews as well as primary studies; although all of these different levels of evidence are available in this resource, there is a heavy emphasis on primarily identifying systematic reviews. Epistemonikos acts as an aggregator and pulls information from 10 different databases: PubMed, the Cochrane Database of Systematic Reviews, Embase, CINAHL, PsycINFO, LILACS, the Database of Abstracts of Reviews of Effects (DARE), the Campbell Collaboration online library, the JBI Database of Systematic Reviews and Implementation Reports, and the EPPI-Centre Evidence Library. Individuals are able to search all of these resources simultaneously with one search, saving time, which may make this resource one of the best places to begin a search.

Individuals can perform a basic search from the main page or select the "advanced search" option. We recommend going straight to the advanced search option as the basic search is meant to search only one term at a time and does not support Boolean searching. For instance, entering our search terms "periodontal disease" and "pregnant women" into the basic search function returns fewer than 20 results, but entering those same terms into the advanced search returns more than 60 results. The advanced search builder allows for individuals to enter in PICO elements and combine them as needed. Filters are available on the main page of search results to further narrow down the original search results if needed.

Results are identified by level of evidence and include a basic citation, as well as an abstract, for each result. As previously mentioned, Epistemonikos is an aggregate database, so the full text of an identified article is available at the original resource (linked in the database). Availability of the full text depends on the individual's institutional subscriptions; ADA members may also check with the librarians at the ADA Library. A helpful feature of this database is the "related evidence" tab, which is available on the main search results page. When a primary study is selected, the related evidence tab includes citations of systematic reviews that include the primary study and links to these systematic reviews. When a systematic review is selected, the related evidence tab includes citations of the included primary studies of the review, as well as a statement that identifies the total number of systematic reviews that include the individual primary study. This feature provides a quick and easy way to find more evidence on a topic.

Epistemonikos allows for the option to create a free personal account. Oral health care practitioners can save searches as well as individual article citations, marking them as favorites. Creating a personal account also allows individuals to create and save matrices of evidence. Matrixes of evidence pull the included articles from a selected systematic review and then search for other systematic reviews that include the original review's primary studies; the end result is a grid that demonstrates what systematic reviews on the topic include which primary studies and where they overlap. The option to create a matrix is available within the record of a systematic review. The created matrix can then be saved to the personal account (Figure 2.3).

Figure 2.3. Example of an Epistemonikos Matrix of Evidence

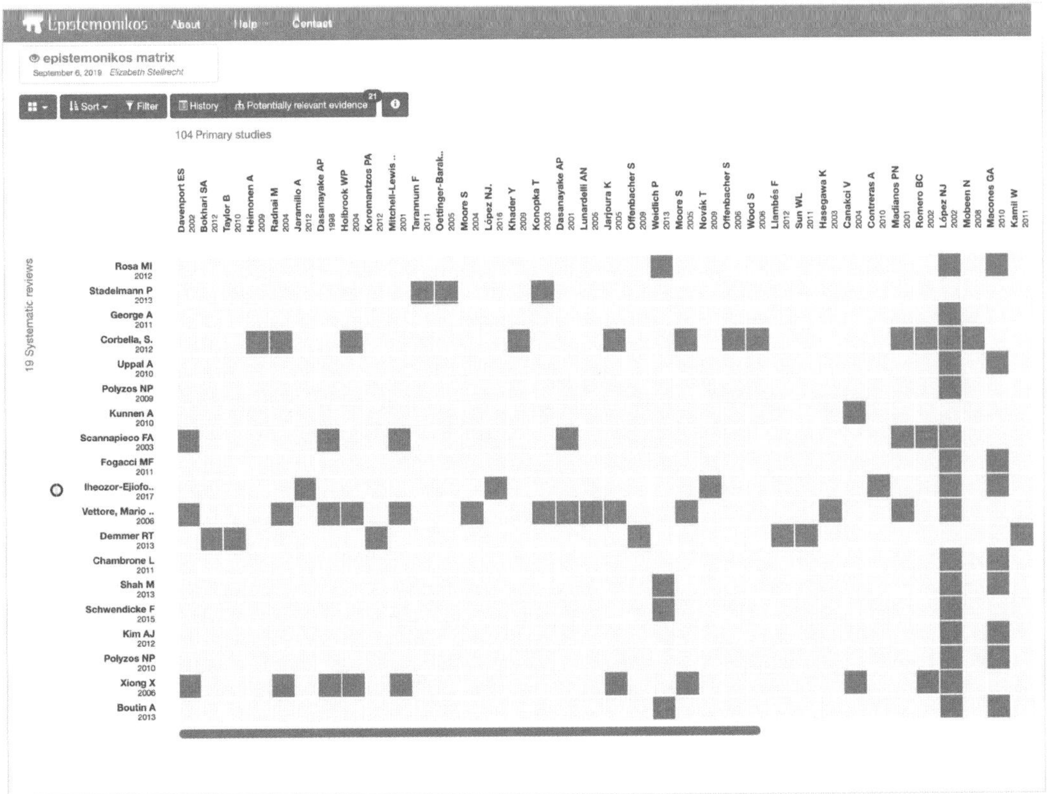

Source: Epistemonikos.org, accessed on March 18, 2019.

Trip

Website: *www.tripdatabase.com*
Cost: The Trip database, previously only available via a subscription, is now freely accessible. A premium version of Trip is available to individuals via a subscription.
Specialty of resource: Clinical practice guidelines, synopses, systematic reviews, primary studies, other

Trip (which originally stood for Translating Research into Practice) is a database/meta-search engine that covers a wide range of sources, including MEDLINE, the Cochrane Library, guidelines, and more. Trip is a useful resource to consult initially because it covers a wide range of material and its search technology allows individuals to find high-quality evidence quickly and easily. Trip results provide information from multiple sources and are color-coded by level of evidence as well as sorted by category. Results are displayed according to an algorithm that provides relevant, recent, and higher quality information first. "Higher quality" information in Trip means types of information that are more highly ranked in the hierarchy of evidence-based information represented in the evidence pyramid (Figure 2.4). Results can be filtered using the "refine by" function on the right-hand side of the screen to filter by level of evidence. Results may be refined by systematic reviews, evidence-based synopses, guidelines, primary research from a core set of more than 300 journals, controlled trials, electronic textbooks, and more. Each of these categories contains information from multiple resources. "Guidelines," for example, includes guidelines issued within North America, Europe, and other countries, while "evidence-based synopses" includes material from Bandolier, BestBets, POEMs (Patient-Oriented Evidence that Matters), Clinical Evidence, the journal *Evidence-Based Complementary and Alternative Medicine,* and more. The type of information being provided by any given result is indicated by an accompanying image locating the type of information on the evidence pyramid.

> Trip is a useful resource to consult initially because it covers a wide range of material and its search technology allows individuals to find high-quality evidence quickly and easily.

To retrieve the highest-level evidence from Trip, begin the search with just one or two terms and then move to more complex searches. Use the synonyms tab at the top of the search results if no results are retrieved. Special features of Trip include an ability to filter for evidence relevant to the developing world. A search using "pregnancy and periodontal disease," for instance, results in "Trip's best suggested answer": "Although periodontal disease treatment is recommended during pregnancy, the results of a systematic review of 13 randomized controlled clinical trials, for which a meta-analysis was conducted in 11 of the trials, do not indicate that there is a lower risk of preterm birth or low birth weight" and links to the 2014 critical summary "Periodontal Disease Treatment Does Not Affect Pregnancy Outcomes" in the *Journal of the American Dental Association*[3] as well as systematic reviews and more.

Trip also provides additional useful ways to search, including a "PICO search," which allows the oral health practitioner to search by PICO categories. All four categories of the PICO search do not need to be entered in order to use the tool. The more categories that are supplied, however, the more focused the search results will be. Trip also provides a useful image and video search and includes information leaflets for patients.

The full text of documents, when available, can be accessed by clicking on the title of the document. Citations from Trip may be exported to a citation manager. Trip allows individuals to share results via Facebook or Twitter. Trip's awareness tool, My Trip, allows individuals to select and register keywords that are automatically searched whenever the database is updated. If material is retrieved, results may be sent to the oral health practitioner's e-mail address (Figure 2.4).

Tutorials:

- The Trip site provides useful how to videos for new users (www.tripdatabase.com/how-to-use-trip).

Figure 2.4. Trip Database

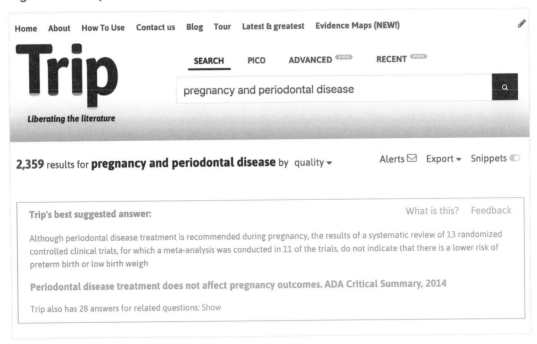

Source: Tripdatabase.com, accessed on March 18, 2019.

Summaries and Guidelines: Point-of-Care Resources

Point-of-care resources aim to deliver the best available evidence to support decisions made by health care providers in clinical settings. These tools are also excellent resources for gathering information on both foreground and background questions. Although we highlight several resources below, there is a wide variety of point-of-care tools available.

UpToDate

Website: *www.uptodate.com*
Cost: Only available via a subscription. Access to the patient content of UpToDate is free.
Specialty of resource: Summaries

UpToDate is a peer-reviewed database of point-of-care information that provides a summary of research on a range of medical topics. The database is aimed at clinicians: It is very useful not only for staying current with the latest research, but also for providing information to patients. It includes access to more than 10,000 topics that are divided into more than 20 specialties (for example, drug information and pediatrics). The information included in UpToDate is provided by more than 4,000 expert clinicians who review content from more than 460 medical journals. It includes information focused on specific clinical issues (diagnosis and treatment), descriptions of diseases and conditions, and analysis of medical treatments and recommendations. It is important to note that UptoDate is not a general literature database like PubMed. (One cannot search by author name or the title of an article or journal.) Information in UptoDate that is judged to be of pressing importance is updated promptly after the peer review process (these are marked as "practice changing updates"); all topics are updated every four months. Each recommendation is graded for strength using a modified GRADE (Grading of Recommendations, Assessment, Development and Evaluations) classification scheme. Grades 1 and 2 are based on the strength of the recommendation, and grades A through C are based on the certainty in the evidence (see Chapter 14).

UpToDate includes the drug information database Lexicomp, so it is particularly helpful in looking for information concerning drug dosing, interactions, and adverse effects. It is possible to conduct a search for a drug name just like any other search. UpToDate also includes medical calculators, accessible via browsing or by medical specialty. UpToDate contains a great deal of patient-oriented information, written in plain language, divided by topic and then further subdivided into two categories: "The Basics" and "Beyond the Basics." "Basics" information is generally one to three pages long, while "Beyond the Basics" information is generally five to 10 pages long.

Searching UpToDate is quite easy. Searches are automatically conducted across all specialties. Searches can be narrowed using the drop-down menu to the right of the search box by selecting one of the following facets: all topics, adult, pediatric, patient, or graphics (that is, pictures, algorithms, graphs, tables, movies, and figures). All results are displayed, but the results more closely associated with the chosen facet are displayed first.

Hovering over a topic title provides a preview of the topic outline for that topic, allowing the individual to jump to specific parts of the topic when necessary.

A "What's New" section, organized by specialty, lists important updates in each field from the past three to six months, and a separate section, "Practice Changing Updates," notes updates that may significantly change clinical practice.

Tutorials:

- Video tutorials: *www.uptodate.com/home/help-demo*

ClinicalKey

Website: *www.clinicalkey.com*
Cost: Only available via subscription
Specialty of resource: Summaries

ClinicalKey includes content from Procedures Consult, more than 800 point-of-care monographs from First Consult (highly respected drug monographs), and material from a variety of sources including Elsevier's Medical and Surgical Clinics of North America content, clinical trials, clinical practice guidelines, select third-party journals, and more than 22 million MEDLINE citations.

ClinicalKey has a simple search interface (similar to an internet search engine search box), while filtering features allow for more complex searches by expert users. Resource types are listed along the right side of the results page: journal articles, systematic reviews, meta-analyses, randomized control trials, narrative reviews, books, images, clinical trials, First Consult, and patient education. When entering a search term, ClinicalKey will suggest topics, keywords, procedures, and/or drugs related to the search terms. Filtering by category may be done after the initial search; categories include clinical summary, etiology, diagnosis, treatment, prevention, and prognosis. Results can also be limited to study type (for example, systematic review or narrative review), date, specialty, and content type (for example, journals and books). A search for "pregnancy and periodontal disease," for example, retrieves more than 1,500 results, including journal articles, as well as more 30 systematic reviews, 17 meta-analyses, nine guidelines, and 90 randomized control trials. ClinicalKey uses a taxonomy called EMMeT (Elsevier Merged Medical Taxonomy) that helps the oral health practitioner discover the most clinically relevant information. ClinicalKey also includes very useful drug information and patient education material.

It is possible to create a free ClinicalKey account, called My ClinicalKey, to save searches and create reading lists and presentations. The presentations feature of ClinicalKey is particularly useful: It allows any of the more than four million images in ClinicalKey to be directly exported to a presentation slide deck.

Tutorials:

- How to search: *https://help.elsevier.com/app/answers/list/p/9702/c/7956*

- How-to videos: *www.youtube.com/user/ClinicalKey*

Lexicomp

Website: *www.wolterskluwercdi.com/lexicomp-online*
Cost: Only available via a subscription
Specialty of resource: Summaries

Lexicomp is a point-of-care resource that provides up-to-date comprehensive drug information for both prescription and over-the-counter drugs. It includes several drug information databases, toxicology databases, drug medical safety sheets (including information on antidotes), a database of natural products, and several patient-education databases. It also includes an infectious disease database, information on laboratory tests and diagnostic procedures, and brief information regarding select drugs available outside North America. The drug databases are useful for searching for information on adverse reactions, contraindications, dosing, alerts from the U.S. Food and Drug Administration (FDA), safety issues, pregnancy and lactation guidelines, pharmacodynamics, pharmacogenomics, and international trade names. Lexicomp includes databases for pediatric/neonatal and geriatric populations that feature guidelines (including dosage recommendations) for those populations. Special features of Lexicomp include audio pronunciation guides, lists of drug shortages with references to alternative therapeutics, common off-label uses, and prices. Lexicomp includes links to relevant PubMed journal articles and evidence-based guidelines. In addition to drug databases, Lexicomp includes clinical decision tools such as a drug interaction database, clinical calculators, a pill identifier, and an intravenous-drug interaction tool.

 Lexicomp is a point-of-care resource that provides up-to-date comprehensive drug information for both prescription and over-the-counter drugs.

Lexicomp is very easy to search; a single search box searches all of the databases, although it is possible to limit a search to a specific category (for example, patient education or international drugs). Individuals can choose from numerous optional filters in order to limit the search; searches can be limited, for example, to "contraindications." Of particular use is the interaction module, which provides information regarding potential drug–drug interactions, drug–allergy interactions, and drug–food interactions. Each of these interactions is assigned a risk rating, and Lexicomp provides suggestions regarding therapy modification. All drug monographs include a section called "Dental Information," which lists any possible dental treatment complications from the drug in question, including effects on bleeding.

Tutorials:

- *www.wolterskluwercdi.com/lexicomp-online/training-videos*

ECRI Guidelines Trust

Website: *https://guidelines.ecri.org*
Cost: Free; must sign up for free account to use
Specialty of resource: Clinical practice guidelines, guideline summaries

With the sunset of the National Guideline Clearinghouse (NGC) in 2018, the ECRI Guidelines Trust was created by the ECRI Institute. The ECRI Guidelines Trust is a freely available resource that provides access to guideline summaries of evidence-based clinical practice guidelines.[4] Funded by the Gordon and Betty Moore Foundation, the ECRI Guidelines Trust has detailed inclusion criteria that a guideline must meet before being accepted to the site: The guideline must be in English, be online, and have been published in the past five years; include a recommendation that provides guidance for patient care; be produced by a known clinical practice guideline organization such as a medical specialty association or professional society; and be based upon a systematic review that includes a transparent search strategy, detailed information about study selection, and evidence analysis. Once a guideline is accepted, the summary or guideline brief is created, as well as a TRUST (Transparency and Rigor Using Standards of Trustworthiness) Scorecard that has a rating of how well the guideline fulfills the National Academy of Medicine standards for developing trustworthy clinical practice guidelines.[4] If a guideline only meets the first three criteria mentioned, ECRI will not provide a summary and will only link to the original guideline. ECRI also requires permission from the original guideline creator before creating the guideline summary. While the ECRI Guidelines Trust was created to try to fill the void left by the NGC, it should be noted that it does not have the exact same content, but it hopes to become the equivalent of the NGC in the near future.

To search and access the ECRI Guidelines Trust's information, it is necessary to create a free account first. Once an account has been created, it is possible to search via keyword term as well as Boolean searching. Because this database is quite small, we recommend beginning the search with one term and then adding more if the amount of results is too high. Once the results are displayed, it is possible to limit by publication year, organization, patient age, clinical area, and intervention. The full text of all guideline briefs and TRUST Scorecards are available. When trying to view the original guideline, the ECRI Guidelines Trust will link to the association or organization that created the guideline; depending on the individual association or organization, the full text of the guideline may or may not be available.

It is also possible to browse all guidelines and guideline summaries by entering an asterisk (*) into the search bar. This will return the entire database's content; then, on the left side of the screen, select the clinical area(s) to browse all guidelines and summaries specific to those areas of practice. At the time of writing this chapter, there are 15 dentistry guidelines indexed in the database, only five of which have guideline briefs.

Tutorials:

- ECRI Guideline Trust Searching FAQ, *https://guidelines.ecri.org/search-tips*

ADA Center for Evidence-Based Dentistry

Website: *https://ebd.ADA.org/en/evidence/guidelines*
Cost: Free, with some limited full-text availability
Specialty of resource: Clinical practice guidelines

The ADA Center for Evidence-Based Dentistry (Center for EBD) is a publicly available resource that operates under the mission "to assist dental practitioners and improve the oral health of the public by appraising and disseminating the best available scientific evidence on oral health care and helping practitioners understand and apply the best available evidence in their clinical decision-making."[5] The Center for EBD is an excellent resource for clinical practice guidelines supported by the ADA. Links are provided to the individual guidelines, as well as to the systematic reviews that are the basis of the guidelines. These guidelines and systematic reviews are open access and freely available to all. The Center for EBD also has a robust list of evidence-based resources, including critical appraisal tools, a glossary of terms, and a list of related organizations.

Tutorials:

- EBD Education Tutorials: *http://ebd.ADA.org/en/education/tutorials*

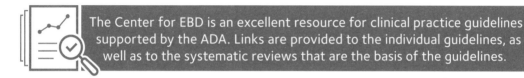

The Center for EBD is an excellent resource for clinical practice guidelines supported by the ADA. Links are provided to the individual guidelines, as well as to the systematic reviews that are the basis of the guidelines.

Preappraised Resources

Cochrane Library

Website: *www.thecochranelibrary.com*
Cost: Only available via subscription; ADA members have free access via the ADA Library
Specialty of resource: Systematic reviews, primary studies

The Cochrane Library provides access to the Cochrane systematic reviews, one of the highest levels of evidence in evidence-based health care. The Cochrane Library is produced by the Cochrane Collaboration, a group of contributors from around the globe, including Cochrane Oral Health. Cochrane review groups consist of more than 50 groups, each of which focuses on a particular topic area and is led by a coordinating editor and an editorial team.

The Cochrane Library has an especially strong focus on the effectiveness of interventions. It consists of six separate databases that can be searched together or individually. Out of those six, the first three—Cochrane Database of Systematic Reviews, Other Reviews, and Cochrane Central Register of Controlled Trials—are the most useful and are often a "must" when doing evidence-based work. Not only is Cochrane the database for searching for systematic reviews, but results found under "Other Reviews" and "Trials" are worth exploring as not all of these results would be discoverable through a PubMed search. The seven databases within Cochrane include the following:

- *Cochrane Database of Systematic Reviews* provides full-text systematic reviews of health care interventions. Cochrane reviews are highly structured and include evidence from clinical trials based on explicit quality criteria, thereby minimizing bias. The database also includes "protocol reviews," which are systematic reviews that are in progress. Protocol reviews summarize the background, rationale, and proposed methods of the review and are open to comment.

  Cochrane reviews are available in full text (HTML or PDF), but protocol reviews are only available in brief format because they are unfinished reviews. Cochrane reviews may be lengthy, but their structure is standardized, and a table of contents on the menu bar to the left of each review allows the quick location of any needed section. Three sections of each review summarize the evidence: The abstract summarizes the background, objectives, methods (search strategy, selection criteria, and data collection and analysis), results, and conclusions of the review; the synopsis provides a 100-word plain-language summary of the review; and the reviewer's conclusions provide an overview of the most important findings of the review as well as a discussion of the implications of the findings for clinical practice and further research. Unique to Cochrane, the "Add/View Feedback" feature allows comments and criticism to be submitted to the reviewers. Both the comments and the reviewers' responses appear in subsequent updates of the review in question.

  If the oral health practitioner is interested in a particular review group or would like to speak to someone concerning reviews in a particular subject, he or she should go to the About Menu, and choose Cochrane Review Groups, which will give the full listing of review groups.

- *Other Reviews* presents structured abstracts of systematic reviews on topics not yet addressed by Cochrane reviews, but only references systematic reviews that have met minimum quality criteria.

- *Cochrane Central Register of Controlled Trials (CENTRAL)* is an index of published clinical trials. CENTRAL includes details from published articles (found in MEDLINE and Embase) reporting on controlled trials, as well as other published and unpublished sources reporting on controlled trials. CENTRAL frequently provides summaries of original articles, but it does not contain the full text of the articles in question.

- *Methods Studies* provides full-text systematic reviews of methodological studies. Cochrane Methodology Reviews are full text, while, again, protocols are reviews in progress and provide the background and rationale for the review.

- *Methodology Register* is a bibliography of publications that report on methods used in controlled trials. Publications include journal articles, books, and conference proceedings. In some cases, a summary of the original article is given; however, full text of the article is not provided.

- *Technology Assessment* provides access to completed and ongoing projects from health technology assessment organizations. Structured abstracts are frequently given, but full text of the reports is not given. Full bibliographic information is provided, however.

- *Economic Evaluations* provides structured abstracts of articles that describe economic evaluations of health care interventions. For articles to be included in *Economic Evaluations,* articles must provide a comparison of treatments and must explore both the costs and outcomes of the treatments discussed. Articles covered come from key medical journals, other databases, and gray literature. Full text of the articles is not given; however, full bibliographic information is provided.

Cochrane search results are displayed in the order of databases listed above. The oral health practitioner can limit the search to one of the databases by clicking on the left of the screen, where a count of results in each database is given. The first three databases in the Cochrane Library are listed in order of the hierarchy of levels of evidence: Cochrane reviews, other systematic reviews, and, finally, trials. For example, a search using "pregnancy and periodontal disease" resulted in a 2017 Cochrane systematic review, "Treating Periodontal Disease for Preventing Adverse Birth Outcomes in Pregnant Women."[6] The same search in the trials database retrieved 12,197 results. Every entry is annotated to indicate whether it is new (since the last update), withdrawn, or has reached a new conclusion. A more advanced search of the Cochrane Database can be done using MeSH. When conducting a MeSH search, be aware that the newest materials may not have been indexed with MeSH at the time of the search, so for the most up-to-date information as well as for comprehensive coverage, it is best to perform both simple keyword searches and MeSH searches.

The Cochrane Library can also be browsed by topic, new reviews, updated reviews, an A–Z list, or review group. Oral health practitioners may be interested in browsing systematic reviews produced by Cochrane Oral Health.

The Cochrane Library contains a great deal of information—if the oral health practitioner is looking for information regarding a specific treatment for a particular condition, it is useful to use the Boolean AND to combine treatment and condition terms in the same search. If, however, the search does not retrieve any results, or retrieves too few results, try changing the search limit from title, abstract, and keyword (the default) to "all text."

To save an article or a search, it is necessary to register (registration is free) and log on to Cochrane Library. On the saved searches screen, click on the "alerts" box in order to receive e-mail messages whenever new articles matching the search are loaded into the database.

For individuals interested in contributing a systematic review, go to the Help menu and choose "How to Prepare a Cochrane Review."

Tutorials:

- *www.cochranelibrary.com/help/how-to-use-cochrane-library.html*

Journals

Evidence-based journals publish articles, abstracts, and reviews of the literature, using articulated criteria to appraise and assess the methodologies of studies. Many EBD journals offer free registration for tables-of-contents e-mail alerts that will notify the oral health practitioner when a new issue is published and provide the table of contents. We encourage the oral health practitioner to sign up for tables-of-contents alerts from the journals listed in this section; by receiving these alerts, practitioners will be able to quickly browse what is newly available. We also encourage clinicians in specialty areas to sign up for table-of-contents alerts from the major specialty-specific journals. Full access to the entire issue/archive of a particular journal usually requires either a personal subscription or an institutional subscription.

The majority of EBD journals offer "export citation" or "export references" links that automatically download bibliographic information for the article in question or its reference list into citation management software.

Evidence-Based Dentistry (EBD)

EBD is produced by the British Dental Association. Each issue contains 10-plus "summary reviews" that cover specific questions (for example, "Does toothbrushing frequently reduce caries?" or "Is orthodontic treatment under 11 years of age effective?") and are divided into broad categories such as caries and orthodontics. Each summary provides an evaluation of the relevant evidence and the conclusions reached by the studies mentioned. In addition to the summaries, each issue contains a toolbox and a listing of events—evidence-based conferences and courses that may be of interest to the reader. Please note that *EBD's* "see more articles like this" box links to other articles, but only articles published by Springer Nature, which is the publisher of *EBD*. It is not, in other words, a substitute for a literature search.

Journal of Evidence-Based Dental Practice (JEBDP)

JEBDP includes original articles and reviews of articles that discuss clinical procedures and treatments. The reviews evaluate a given article's relevance to clinical practice and differentiate between clinical value and statistical significance. *JEBDP* uses strength of recommendation taxonomy (SORT) grading to evaluate guidelines and the results of systematic reviews.

The Journal of the American Dental Association (JADA)

JADA is produced by the ADA. *JADA* regularly includes systematic reviews and meta-analyses as well as journal scans and specialty scans. Journal scans provide very useful brief summaries of the background, methods, and results found in selected articles from the recent oral health literature as well as a brief discussion of why the article in question is important. Specialty scans consist of quarterly e-mails that gather articles from the dental specialty literature that may be of interest to the general dentist. In the spring of 2017, *JADA* launched JADA+ Clinical Scans, a special (online) section that provides evidence-based assessment of selected published journal articles covering a wide range of subdisciplines. These short scans offer a summary of the article in question, including a description of the type of study conducted, findings, whether the findings were statistically significant, and the strength and limitations of the study design and data analysis.

Nonpreappraised Resources

PubMed

Website: *www.ncbi.nlm.nih.gov/pubmed*
Cost: Free, with limited full-text availability
Specialty of resource: Primary studies, systematic reviews

PubMed is a publicly available biomedical database that contains more than 29 million citations for biomedical literature from MEDLINE, life sciences journals, and online books.[7] Developed and maintained by the National Center for Biotechnology Information (NCBI) at the U.S. National Library of Medicine, PubMed provides access to citations and abstracts from biomedical and health literature. Specific subjects include but are not limited to dentistry, medicine, nursing, bioinformatics, and epidemiology. Although access to the resource is free, there is limited availability of full text. Freely available full-text content includes open access publications from PubMed Central, a free archive or repository of biomedical and life sciences journal literature that is maintained by NCBI.[8] Currently, there are more than five million freely available full-text articles available within PubMed Central. Individuals with academic or hospital affiliations may have further access to full text as it is possible for such institutions to have PubMed link to institutional journal subscriptions. ADA members can contact the ADA Library for more information about available electronic journal subscriptions.

There are a variety of ways to search for evidence within PubMed. An easy option is the basic search function, which is available from PubMed's homepage. For example, typing "pregnant women and periodontal disease" into the basic search field yields more than 500 citations. Adding "and preterm birth" to the search will yield fewer results, totaling about 190 citations. When an individual performs a basic search, PubMed will return results that have the search terms appear anywhere in the citation's record. Note that a basic search may also result in citations that are not relevant to the topic as the terms used may not be main subjects of the results, but only mentioned in passing in the article.

One way to perform a more focused search is to use MeSH (Medical Subject Headings) to search for relevant articles in PubMed. Most databases have a thesaurus that lists the preferred terminology or subject headings used to index articles as they are added to the database; PubMed's thesaurus is MeSH. Most citations in PubMed are indexed with MeSH; exceptions include prepublication articles (articles available electronically, but not yet in print), in-process articles, and some articles within PubMed Central. The basic search function will also try to automatically map keyword terms to MeSH terms and will search both; this can be seen in the Search Details box on the results page. Using only MeSH terms in a search returns articles that have the selected terms listed as subject headings, indicating that the term is likely a main topic or subject of the resulting articles.

To search using MeSH terms, select the MeSH Database *(www.ncbi.nlm.nih.gov/mesh)* from PubMed's homepage. After typing in one of the search terms, the database will return potential MeSH matches. The best match for the search term can be determined by reading the scope note or definition of the MeSH term. For example, although there is a MeSH term for "pregnant women," the term is to be used in cultural, psychological, or sociological instances; the MeSH term "pregnancy" is much more appropriate for our search. On occasion, MeSH will return an exact match; for instance, when searching for the MeSH term for periodontal disease, "periodontal disease" is returned as an exact match. Once in the MeSH record of a term, it is also possible to add subheadings to a MeSH term to further narrow a search. Subheadings will return results that focus on a specific aspect of a term, such as therapy or prevention and control. If a subheading is not selected, all subheadings are automatically searched. The MeSH tree for the term can also be viewed in the MeSH record, as MeSH terms are arranged in a hierarchy that is arranged from broader term to narrower term. When searching by MeSH, all narrower terms beneath the term are automatically included unless otherwise specified. Searching the MeSH term "periodontal disease," for instance, will return results that include articles indexed with "gingival diseases," periodontitis," or any other term included under "periodontal disease."

The PubMed Search Builder on the right side of the page allows individuals to add MeSH terms to a search by selecting the "add to search builder" button below the search builder. When adding terms to the search builder, it is possible to choose if AND or OR should appear between terms. When viewing results of any search, we suggest viewing the list of MeSH terms assigned to articles that are relevant, as these terms could also be used as possible later search terms.

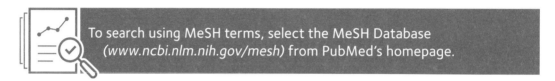
To search using MeSH terms, select the MeSH Database (www.ncbi.nlm.nih.gov/mesh) from PubMed's homepage.

Another way to search PubMed is using the Advanced Search Builder option. The Advanced Search option can be found directly below the basic search bar. Using the Advanced Search Builder has several advantages. It is possible to create sophisticated searches using Boolean logic that search specific parts of the citation record, resulting in focused searches that yield relevant results. Although the basic search function automatically searches all fields of a record, the Advanced Search Builder allows the individual to specifically determine which fields to search, such as title, abstract, or author. The Advanced Search Builder also saves the last eight hours of searches, allowing individuals to rerun searches with the click of a button. It is also possible to tweak previous searches by combining them with new terms or other previously run searches saved in the builder. In addition, MeSH terms may be used in the Advanced Search Builder by either searching the terms one at a time from the MeSH database in PubMed and combining them in the builder or by selecting MeSH Terms from the field drop-down menu. If the latter option is chosen, it will be necessary to look up the MeSH terms prior to the search as the MeSH terms will not automatically load unless they are known items.

The Advanced Search Builder allows the oral health practitioner to easily combine PICO elements. Figure 2.5 provides an example of putting PICO elements together to create an effective search strategy. In this instance, the terms are restricted to searching the title/abstract fields only; the reason for creating such restrictions is that if a term appears in the title or abstract of the article, it is most likely a main component of the article. Searching by "Title/Abstract" rather than "All Fields" will result in fewer results and is also a strategy for those who prefer not to use the MeSH database. Because we are interested in retrieving articles concerning the risk for preterm birth and low birth weight in pregnant women with periodontal disease, it is important that at least preterm birth or low birth weight is present in the results. It is also possible that there are studies that focus on one or the other, and not necessarily both; because of this, our example search has paired the two outcomes with an OR between the terms. This search string was created first and then combined with a search for periodontal disease and pregnant women (both terms also limited to title/abstract). When all parts are combined, the final search string is as follows: (((periodontal disease[Title/Abstract]) AND pregnant women[Title/Abstract])) AND ((low birth weight[Title/Abstract]) OR preterm birth[Title/Abstract]). This search returns 113 results.

Figure 2.5. PubMed Advanced Search Builder

PubMed Advanced Search Builder YouTube Tutorial

((periodontal disease[Title/Abstract]) AND pregnant women[Title/Abstract]) AND ((low birth weight[Title/Abstract]) OR preterm birth[Title/Abstract])

Edit   Clear

Builder

	All Fields	periodontal disease[Title/Abstract]	⊖	Show index list
AND	All Fields	pregnant women[Title/Abstract]	⊖	Show index list
AND	All Fields	(low birth weight[Title/Abstract]) OR preterm birth[Title/Abstract]	⊖	Show index list
AND	All Fields		⊖ ⊕	Show index list

Search or Add to history

History   Download history Clear history

Search	Add to builder	Query	Items found	Time
#13	Add	Search (low birth weight[Title/Abstract]) OR preterm birth[Title/Abstract]	37981	16:54:51
#12	Add	Search preterm birth[Title/Abstract]	14563	16:54:31
#11	Add	Search low birth weight[Title/Abstract]	25527	16:54:20
#10	Add	Search pregnant women[Title/Abstract]	82416	16:54:09
#9	Add	Search periodontal disease[Title/Abstract]	17218	16:53:57

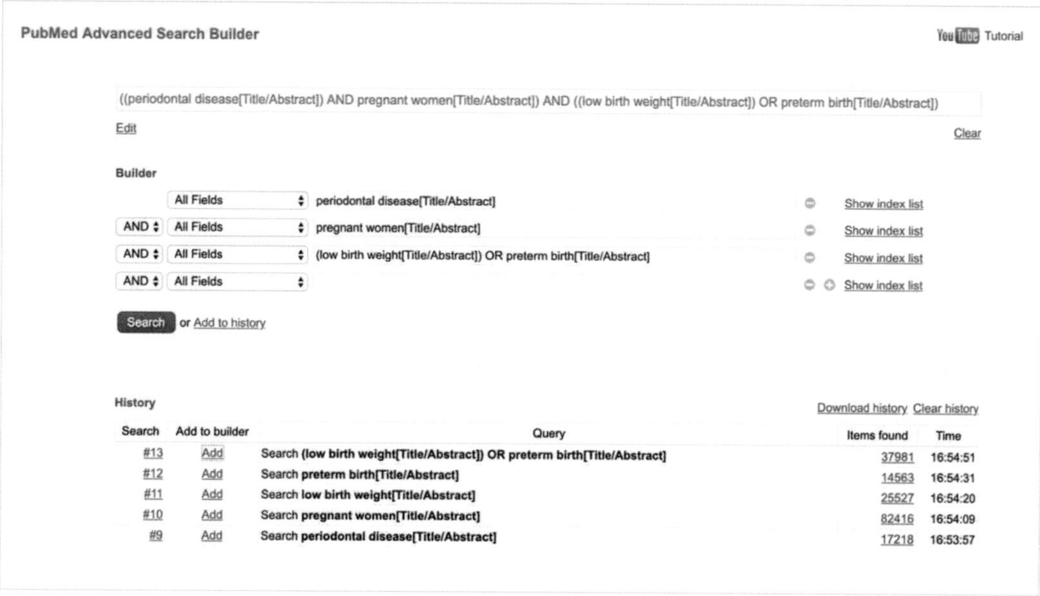

Source: www.ncbi.nlm.nih.gov/pubmed, accessed on March 18, 2019.

Although 113 results are much fewer than 190 results, most individuals will probably not want to comb through all 113 results because of time restrictions. It is possible to further limit the amount of results by using search filters, which appear on the left side of the search results page. Available search filters include limiting by type of article, publication dates, language, age of study participants, and text availability, as well as several other options. Limiting to free full text will result in freely available articles. Use this limit with caution—if the dentist is affiliated with an institution, PubMed can link to full text available through the institution's subscriptions; using the free full text can filter out important relevant articles that are available elsewhere. It is important to note that once a limit is applied to a search, it will be applied to all following searches unless the individual removes the limit. Because systematic reviews summarize available evidence on a focused topic, we will select the limit of "systematic reviews"; this limited search now returns eight articles, a much more reasonable number to review.

Clinical Queries also presents another way to search PubMed for evidence. Clinical Queries (*www.ncbi.nlm.nih.gov/pubmed/clinical*) can be found on the homepage of PubMed under PubMed Tools. Clinical Queries automatically limits the amount of search hits by dividing results into three categories: clinical study categories, systematic reviews, and medical genetics. Oral health care practitioners can search by keyword terms; for example, a search for "periodontal disease AND pregnant women AND (preterm birth OR low birth weight)" yields 72 clinical study categories results, 13 systematic reviews, and seven medical genetics results. It is possible to further limit the clinical study categories results by selecting a specific category (therapy, etiology, diagnosis, prognosis, or clinical prediction guides) or scope (broad or narrow). Clinical Queries is especially useful for clinicians who are pressed for time and need results quickly, as the results are already limited to results that are generally higher up on the evidence pyramid.

PubMed also allows for saving searches and setting up search alerts by creating a free My NCBI account *(www.ncbi.nlm.nih.gov/account).* To save a search and set up search alerts, from the search results page select "Create Alert" under the search bar. Once the alert is created, it is possible to further customize the frequency of updates, the number of items to be sent at a time, and more. It is also possible to save a search without setting up search alerts by selecting "no" when prompted for choosing e-mail alerts. All saved searches will appear on the individual's My NCBI page and will list the last time the search was run as well as how many new results have been added to PubMed since then. My NCBI also allows for citations to be saved to collections to read later and saves the past six months of searches run while the dentist is logged into My NCBI.

Tutorials:

- PubMed Quick Start: *www.ncbi.nlm.nih.gov/books/NBK3827/#pubmedhelp.PubMed_ Quick_Start*

- PubMed Simple Search: *www.nlm.nih.gov/bsd/viewlet/search/subject/subject.html*

- Use MeSH to Build a Better PubMed Query: *https://youtu.be/uyF8uQY9wys*

- Advanced Search Builder: *https://youtu.be/dncRQ1cobdc*

MEDLINE

Website: *www.ncbi.nlm.nih.gov/pubmed* or *www.ovid.com/site/catalog/databases/901.jsp*
Cost: MEDLINE records are available within PubMed for free with limited full-text availability or available via subscription on several different platforms. ADA members have access through the ADA Library.
Specialty of resource: Primary research, systematic reviews

Produced by the U.S. National Library of Medicine, MEDLINE is considered the premier bibliographic database for life sciences and biomedicine.[9] MEDLINE makes up the primary subset of citations in PubMed; at this time, MEDLINE contains 24 million citations. The oral health practitioner can easily identify a MEDLINE record within PubMed as all MEDLINE records are indexed with MeSH. Records that do not contain MeSH are not available in MEDLINE and are unique to PubMed, such as in-process articles that are awaiting indexing and "Ahead of Print" articles.[10] To limit results to only MEDLINE records within PubMed, it is necessary for the oral health practitioner to search using MeSH terms only rather than keyword or natural language searches; for more information on searching with MeSH, please refer to this chapter's previous section on PubMed. Although searching for MEDLINE records within PubMed is free, access to the full text of individual journal articles can vary depending on individual or institutional journal subscriptions.

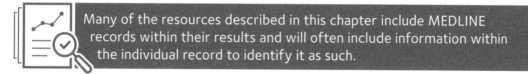

Many of the resources described in this chapter include MEDLINE records within their results and will often include information within the individual record to identify it as such.

Many of the resources described in this chapter include MEDLINE records within their results and will often include information within the individual record to identify it as such. For instance, Embase provides individuals with the option to limit results to MEDLINE records only. Several third-party organizations, such as Wolters Kluwer/Ovid, also provide subscription-based access to MEDLINE (referred to as Ovid MEDLINE) as a stand-alone database. When searching Ovid MEDLINE, we suggest searching each term individually as Ovid MEDLINE will automatically try to map individual terms to the most likely MeSH term. Because all MEDLINE records are indexed with MeSH, we suggest searching with MeSH terms to yield relevant, concentrated results. After entering a term, a list of possible MeSH terms will appear on the following page. Scope notes can be viewed to verify that the term is the most appropriate for the search. It is possible to explode or focus the term as well. Exploding a term will search for articles that include the MeSH term as well as all of its narrower terms, while choosing the focus option will return articles in which the MeSH term is a major component of the article. Once a term is selected, the next page provides a list of available subheadings to further narrow the search. If the individual does not select a subheading, all subheadings are searched as a default. Results are displayed on the following page. Once each term is individually searched, the individual can combine the terms using Boolean logic within the search history displayed on Ovid MEDLINE's homepage. The image below demonstrates how to combine searches.

Figure 2.6. Ovid MEDLINE

# ▲ Searches	Results	Type	Actions	Annotations
1 Periodontal Diseases/	25378	Advanced	Display Results More ⏷	🗨 Contract
2 Pregnant Women/	7252	Advanced	Display Results More ⏷	🗨
3 Infant, Low Birth Weight/	17622	Advanced	Display Results More ⏷	🗨
4 Premature Birth/	11832	Advanced	Display Results More ⏷	🗨
5 3 or 4	27901	Advanced	Display Results More ⏷	🗨

Source: www.ovid.com/product-details.901.html, accessed on March 18, 2019.

Ovid MEDLINE provides the oral health practitioner with multiple limits and filters to further narrow a search. We suggest using the limits available under the search bar rather than the filters available on the side of the search results, as the limits provide more robust options. For instance, possible available limits include publication types, journal subsets, age groups, languages, publication year, and more. To apply limits, select the search strategy from the search history, select the limits needed, and select "Limit a Search."

If searching MEDLINE records from within PubMed, it is possible to set up search alerts following the instructions detailed within the PubMed section of this chapter. Ovid MEDLINE allows searches to be saved by creating a free account within the database. After saving a search, the oral health practitioner can choose to receive e-mail alerts as new items are added to Ovid MEDLINE. It is also possible to create journal table-of-contents e-mail alerts for any journal indexed by MEDLINE by selecting the individual journal(s) from a list.

Tutorials:

- Searching PubMed Using MeSH Tags: *www.nlm.nih.gov/bsd/disted/meshtutorial/ searchingpubmedusingmeshtags*
- Ovid Online Training: *http://ovid.com/site/support/training.jsp*

Embase

Website: *www.embase.com*
Cost: Subscription-based
Specialty of resource: Primary research, systematic reviews

Embase is a biomedical database that provides access to international biomedical literature and specializes in drug, medical device, and disease information.[11] Embase is a useful resource for conducting research on an intervention question. This database contains more than 32,000 records and includes all journals indexed by MEDLINE, plus an additional 2,900 journals that are not available in MEDLINE. Embase also indexes conference abstracts from more than 7,000 international conferences, including multiple dentistry conferences. A complete list of included conferences is available from Embase's website.

Embase defaults to the quick search interface. Oral health professionals can perform a simple search by entering one or two terms, and the number of results will appear in the search box before displaying the resulting records. This results display is very convenient as the oral health professional will be able to get a sense of whether the search is too broad or too narrow from the number of results and can edit the search without having to leave the search page. The quick search page also allows for building complex searches, since multiple fields can be combined with Boolean searching. It is possible to determine which fields the search terms should appear in (for example: all fields, author name, journal name, title, or abstract). The quick search page also has search limits for evidence-based medicine (EBM), including limits for systematic reviews, randomized control trials, meta-analysis, Cochrane reviews, or controlled clinical trials.

When using the quick search, keyword terms will be automatically mapped to Emtree, the controlled vocabulary and subject headings of Embase. Similar to PubMed's MeSH, Emtree is the thesaurus of Embase and allows for more concentrated searching as almost all articles are indexed with Emtree terms. It is possible to build a search using Emtree terms under the Browse function. Like MeSH, Emtree will return terms that are possible matches for the search terms. For instance, the Emtree term for preterm birth is "premature labor." Selecting the term will then provide background on it—such as synonyms and a definition from Dorland's medical dictionary—so the oral health practitioner can verify that s/he has selected the right term for the search. The oral health practitioner can then choose either to search the database with the term or add the term to the query builder, where more terms can be added to further narrow the search. Embase also offers an advanced search option that allows for a variety of search filters to be selected to further narrow the search. The advanced search can be accessed from the query builder within Emtree, or it can be directly accessed from the search menu. Available filters or limits include the previously mentioned EBM limits, age, gender, language, field, date, and mapping of the search term. Mapping options include selecting the term to be a major focus of the article or having the term searched both as an Emtree term and a keyword term.

Embase also offers several specialized searching options. For instance, performing a drug search provides specialized limits to the search, such as using drug manufacturer names and drug trade names as searchable fields. There are also drug subheadings such as drug comparison, drug development, drug toxicity, and pharmacology available to further narrow the search. It is also possible to search only specific routes of drug administration. Similarly, there are disease and device search options that have subheading options specific to the search type.

Embase also has a PICO search interface, allowing individuals to enter search terms in the PICO format. As terms are added to the PICO search, the search will provide the option to add all known synonyms, creating an even more comprehensive search. Possible synonyms will appear to the left of the search box, with the option to select specific synonyms. All synonyms will otherwise be added by default. It is possible to determine which fields will be searched by selecting the caret next to the synonym option. Entering multiple terms in one of the PICO elements will prompt the individual to select which Boolean operator is to be used. The oral health practitioner can also set limits to the type of study design from the PICO search.

Once the results are displayed, it is possible to apply any of the previously mentioned limits available. For example, limiting our search to systematic reviews reduces the amount of results from more than 250 to 13. The results page also displays the search history and allows for combining previous searches using "and" or "or."

Embase allows oral health practitioners to set up a free account to save searches and receive e-mail alerts on these searches. The results page of Embase has an option to save any search, and once a search is saved, the search strings can be accessed via a practitioner's account. Saved searches can be rerun at any time. Embase automatically saves a search's creation date as well as the date the search was last run. E-mail alerts can be set up from the saved search page by selecting the search and choosing "Set E-mail Alert." E-mail alerts can be customized as far as frequency and information included in the alert.

Tutorials:

- Embase-created tutorials are only available from the help section from within the product. Once a subscription has been purchased, there are a wide variety of video tutorials available for the different search interfaces.

Web of Science/Scopus

Website: *https://apps.webofknowledge.com (Web of Science); www.scopus.com (Scopus)*
Cost: Subscription-based
Specialty of resource: Primary research, systematic reviews

Provided by Clarivate Analytics via subscription, Web of Science is a large multidiscipline database that contains more than 100,000 records from the sciences, social sciences, and arts and humanities fields. Web of Science was created as a direct result of Dr. Eugene Garfield's idea of citation indexing.[12] Citation indexing allows the oral health practitioner to view not only the bibliography of a manuscript, but also other works that have cited the manuscript since it was published. This allows individuals to find relevant literature by identifying an article on a topic and using citation indexing to find similar articles, in addition to typical literature searching with search terms. Although reference searching allows the reader of an article to trace the development of an idea chronologically backward through the literature, citation searching allows the reader to trace the development of an idea going forward chronologically. Searchers can use citation indexing in this database, but it is possible to conduct standard literature searches as well. Publication types included are articles of all study design, conference proceedings, and book chapters.

Web of Science offers a variety of ways to search for research literature. The basic search option allows the oral health practitioner to build simple or complex searches, depending on the research topic. Web of Science does not have a thesaurus or controlled vocabulary, so the oral health practitioner can search using natural language. The oral health practitioner can add as many search fields as appropriate and combine the terms with a Boolean operator. The basic search function also allows the oral health practitioner to select which fields to search, such as topic, title, author, or publication name. It is important to note that the field selection will remain the same between searches unless it is changed, which can affect subsequent searches; if receiving unexpected results, check which fields are currently selected.

Web of Science's results page offers a variety of search filters to further reduce the number of results. Possible filters include research areas, publication titles, year of publication, and author names. For instance, limiting to "dentistry" will eliminate about half of the displayed results. Web of Science sorts results by publication date as a default, but one option we recommend is to sort results by the number of times cited. Each result displayed will have the number of times cited available to the right of the record, allowing individuals to see how the publication of the article has impacted the research community. For instance, a 2008 article titled "Epidemiology and Causes of Preterm Birth" from the Lancet is the most-cited article in our results pool: it has been cited more than 2,000 times in about a decade.[13] This is a very good indication that this is an important article that has high impact in the research community and, as a result, is likely worth reviewing. When viewing the detailed record of a publication, the citation network will appear on the right side of the page. The citation network links to articles that have cited the article since publication, the article's bibliography, and articles related to the article in question. Using the citation network from the results of a literature search is one way to go about performing cited reference searching.

Oral health practitioners can also perform cited reference searching by inputting a known reference either into Web of Science's basic search interface or the Cited Reference Search interface. When using the Cited Reference Search interface, the default is entering the cited author, journal name, and year of publication. This search works best when using both the available author and journal name abbreviation index to input the correct information. Although Web of Science is a very large database, it does not index all journals. If a cited reference search yields no results, this does not necessarily mean the article in question has not been cited; it could just mean that Web of Science does not index the article's journal. If a journal is indexed by the database, it is listed in the journal name abbreviation index. Cited reference searches can also be performed from the basic search interface by entering a few words from the title of the article and the last name of the first author.

Web of Science allows individuals to create a free account to save searches and set up alerts. Search strings can be saved from the Search History page, and once a search is saved, it is possible to have regular alerts sent via e-mail for a predetermined amount of time. It is also possible to rerun searches from the saved search page. Alerts can also be set up for journals; the table of contents of a journal will be sent whenever a new issue is available. It is possible to set up citation alerts as well; the individual will be notified whenever a saved citation has been cited by a new publication. Dentists can set up alerts for selected citations or can set up alerts for their own publications.

Elsevier's Scopus is a similar database to Web of Science; Scopus also specializes in cited reference searching. Like Web of Science, it is only available via subscription. Scopus contains articles, books, and conference proceedings from the fields of medicine, science, technology, social sciences, and arts and humanities.[14] While both databases specialize in cited reference searching, Scopus is a much larger database that includes an estimated 60 million records. If the oral health practitioner cannot find a citation in Web of Science, he or she will most likely be able to locate the citation within Scopus because of the size of the database. Both databases are excellent tools, and depending on availability due to institutional subscription, either one should be consulted for cited reference searching.

Tutorials:

- General training page: *http://wokinfo.com/training_support/training/web-of-knowledge*
- Web of Science: Search Tips
  https://youtu.be/11gqkzXyj0w
- Web of Science: Saving Search Histories and Creating E-mail Alerts
  https://youtu.be/tSeXzwEn1ZE
- Scopus Tutorial Center: *https://service.elsevier.com/app/answers/detail/a_id/14799/supporthub/scopus*

Google and Google Scholar

Website: *www.google.com (Google); https://scholar.google.com (Google Scholar)*
Cost: Free, with limited full-text availability
Specialty of resource: Primary research, systematic reviews

Although there are many specialized resources and databases available to locate evidence, Google is an additional search engine option. Even though Google is freely available, access to any articles located via Google will depend on whether the article is available freely through open access or via a personal or institutional subscription to the journal in question. Most people use search engines like Google on a daily basis whether searching for evidence or not, so almost all oral health practitioners are already familiar with how to use it. When using Google, the number of search results can be overwhelming, with results typically numbering in the millions, and results are only displayed 10 at a time by default. For instance, searching for "pregnancy periodontal disease low birth weight OR preterm birth" results in more than 972,000 results. Fortunately, there are several ways to narrow down the search so relevant results appear in the first 10 results.[15] A few of these tips are outlined below.

- Putting quotes around a phrase will search for results in which the words appear next to one another. For example, "low birth weight" will return results that have the three words next to one another.

- Placing a "-" symbol in front of a term will remove extraneous results associated with that term. For instance, if we were interested in seeing articles about how periodontal disease in pregnant women affects low birth weight but not preterm birth, we would search the following: "pregnancy periodontal disease low birth weight -preterm birth."

- Using "site:" in front of a site domain type will only return results of that domain type. For example, "pregnancy periodontal disease low birth weight OR preterm birth site:. gov" will return results only from the .gov domain.

Using a few of these tips, if we now search for "pregnancy periodontal disease 'low birth weight' OR 'preterm birth' site:.gov" our search returns about 11,000 results with the first 10 results displayed being articles from PubMed.

Other internet search engines, such as *Bing.com* and *DuckDuckGo.com*, have similar searching capabilities; the above-mentioned searching tips can also be used on other search engines, but results vary.

Google Scholar works similarly to Google in that natural language can be used to search for information, but Google Scholar limits results to journal articles, books, book chapters, theses, dissertations, or conference papers.[16] The previously mentioned Google search tips work in Google Scholar. It is also possible to do an advanced search in Google Scholar by selecting the caret in the Google Scholar search bar. Search options such as author, publication name, or publication date range will then appear. Although our original search in Google without quotes or site limiting returned more than 972,000 results, the same search returns about 25,000 results in Google Scholar, demonstrating the difference between scholarly content and the nonscholarly content that results from a typical Google search.

It is also possible to update Google Scholar settings to work with a home institution's journal subscriptions to locate the full text of articles and other scholarly works. This is available under Google Scholar's settings, under Library Links. Search for the home institution's library, and once the library is selected, save the settings. When viewing results in Google Scholar, a link to the right of each result will appear to connect the oral health practitioner to his or her home institution's subscriptions and provide a link to the full text. If this link does not appear on the right, it may be also available under the record by selecting "Check Library Holdings" via the "More" link. Scholarly works available via open access or institutional repositories will also have links to the full text to the right of each record.

Tutorials:

- How to refine a Google search: *https://support.google.com/websearch/answer/2466433*

- Google Scholar Search Tips: *https://scholar.google.com/intl/en/scholar/help.html*

Citation Managers

Citation managers are excellent tools to assist in keeping research materials organized. Most databases are compatible with a variety of citation managers and allow citations to be saved by downloading the information from the database into the citation manager. Most citation managers enable full-text articles to be attached to individual citations, with the possibility of annotating the PDF within the citation manager itself, keeping notes and saved publications all in one location. Citation managers are compatible with most word-processing programs and can format in-text references as well as the bibliography of a manuscript. Cost, citation style availability, and features vary from product to product. Some examples of free citation managers are Mendeley (*www.mendeley.com*), RefWorks (*https://refworks.proquest.com*), Zotero (*www.zotero.org*), and EndNote Basic, often referred to as EndNote Web or EndNote Online (*www.myendnoteweb.com*). There is a version of EndNote called EndNote Desktop (*http://endnote.com*) that is available for purchase and is a more robust version of the tool. The desktop version of EndNote allows for unlimited storage space of references, for instance, and has more than 6,000 bibliographic styles available, while the online version limits to 50,000 references and has 21 bibliographic styles. Before purchasing EndNote Desktop, the oral health practitioner should check with their home institution as many of them have institution-wide subscriptions to the product or offer discounts for their constituents. Faculty of 1000 (*https://f1000.com*) is another popular for-fee citation manger. Most access this product via institutional subscription, but individual subscriptions are available.

 This is only a sample of available citation managers; there are multiple others available. Oral health practitioners who wish to organize saved research literature should find the citation manager that best suits their needs.

Gray Literature

When reading a systematic review, the dentist may come across the term "gray literature." Gray literature is defined as "the production, distribution, and access to multiple document types produced on all levels of government, academics, business, and organization in electronic and print formats not controlled by commercial publishing"—that is, "where publishing is not the primary activity of the producing body."[17] Examples of gray literature include conference abstracts, dissertations and theses, trial registries, white papers, and websites.[18] Gray literature is often searched when conducting systematic reviews in order to reduce publication bias, since gray literature may provide insight, such as negative trial results, not available in published literature. Because most gray literature documents do not go through the publication process, results from gray literature do not face the same delays as published literature results and may be more recent. Gray literature can also be very informative when there is little to no published information available on a topic. However, it is important to remember that most gray literature does not go through the peer review process. Although gray literature can reduce publication bias, it can also come with its own biases; like any other type of research literature, it is important to critically appraise the information before drawing any conclusions from gray literature.

Searching for gray literature can be very time-consuming as most databases do not index gray literature. Although some databases, such as Embase and Web of Science, index conference abstracts, most gray literature resources require the clinician to visit conference, government, or organizational websites to access the information. Some journals publish special issues of conference abstracts prior to annual meetings as well. Other gray literature resources include, but are not limited to, ClinicalTrials.gov *(https://clinicaltrials.gov)*, OpenGrey *(http://opengrey.eu)*, All Trials *(www.alltrials.net)*, the FDA *(www.fda.gov)*, and ProQuest's Dissertations and Theses Global *(www.proquest.com/products-services/pqdtglobal.html)*. Performing a site search in an internet search engine (site:) is also an easy way to find gray literature. Although gray literature can provide new and different perspectives on a topic, the oral health practitioner should consider the time commitment needed to find the information before initiating a search of gray literature.

 Examples of gray literature include conference abstracts, dissertations and theses, trial registries, white papers, and websites.[18]

Patient Information Resources

The patient is the most important part of EBD, as EBD begins and ends with the patient. Although biomedical literature can inform the oral health care practitioner when creating the treatment plan, the literature is often full of medical terminology that may be difficult for some patients to understand. It is important to share trustworthy information that patients can understand so they are not confused about what a treatment can entail. Using an internet search engine for information about health symptoms or treatments on the internet can lead to untrustworthy resources, misinforming the patient and further confusing things for both the patient and dental professional. Luckily, there are many reliable resources available in which patients can find unbiased health information written without medical jargon.

- MedlinePlus *(https://medlineplus.gov)* was created by the National Institutes of Health as a resource for patients as well as their family and friends.[19] It is a free resource that is provided by the National Library of Medicine where patients can go to find out information about medical conditions, drug information, and more that is written without medical jargon. The site also links to other government and organization websites for further information.

- MouthHealthy *(http://mouthhealthy.org),* provided by the ADA, has a comprehensive list of oral health care topics written specifically for the patient.

Many evidence-based resources mentioned above provide patient information sheets as well. For instance, Trip, UpToDate, Lexicomp, and ClinicalKey all provide patient information summaries of topics. Journals such as *JADA* and *JAMA: the Journal of the American Medical Association* also have patient information pages designed to inform the patient on health topics.

Conclusion

Finding available evidence is a vital part of EBD practice. There is an overwhelming amount of information available online today, which can make it difficult to locate reliable research. This chapter has outlined a sample of resources that contain all levels of evidence to assist the oral health practitioner in discovering quality evidence-based literature. Although it is not necessary for the oral health practitioner to become an expert in searching all of these resources, we suggest becoming familiar with a variety of these tools and using a combination of resources to find the information needed. It is ultimately up to the oral health practitioner to decide which resources to search and to decide when enough information has been located to answer a specific clinical question. If the individual is having difficulty locating quality research to answer a clinical question, we suggest consulting with a librarian to assist in locating high-quality evidence.

References

1. Bastian H, Glasziou P, Chalmers I. "Seventy-five trials and eleven systematic reviews a day: how will we ever keep up?" *PLoS medicine.* 2010;7(9):e1000326.

2. Epistemonikos Foundation. About Epistemonikos database. 2019; *https://www.epistemonikos.org/en/about_us/who_we_are#.* Accessed March 1, 2019.

3. Leader D. "Periodontal disease treatment does not affect pregnancy outcomes." *Journal of the American Dental Association* (1939). 2014;145(7):757-759.

4. ECRI Institute. About ECRI Guidelines Trust. 2019; *https://guidelines.ecri.org/about.* Accessed March 1, 2019.

5. American Dental Association. Center for Evidence-Based Dentistry; About EBD. 2017; *http://ebd.ADA.org/en/about.* Accessed March 31, 2017.

6. Iheozor-Ejiofor Z, Middleton P, Esposito M, Glenny AM. "Treating periodontal disease for preventing adverse birth outcomes in pregnant women." *Cochrane Database Syst Rev.* 2017;6:CD005297.

7. National Center for Biotechnology Information (US). PubMed Help. In: *NCBI Help Manual.* Last update: January 27, 2017 ed. Bethesda, MD: National Center for Biotechnology Information (US); 2005-: *https://www.ncbi.nlm.nih.gov/books/NBK3830/.* Accessed February 22, 2017.

8. National Center for Biotechnology Information (US). PMC Overview. 2011; *https://www.ncbi.nlm.nih.gov/pmc/about/intro/.* Accessed February 22, 2017.

9. U.S. National Library of Medicine. MEDLINE Fact Sheet. 2017; *https://www.nlm.nih.gov/pubs/factsheets/medline.html.* Accessed July 19, 2017.

10. U.S. National Library of Medicine. MEDLINE, PubMed, and PMC (PubMed Central): How are they different? 2017; *https://www.nlm.nih.gov/pubs/factsheets/dif_med_pub.html.* Accessed July 19, 2017.

11. Elsevier R&D Solutions. Embase Fact Sheet. 2016; *https://www.elsevier.com/__data/assets/pdf_file/0016/59011/R_D_Solutions_Embase_Fact_Sheet-Web.pdf.* Accessed May 10, 2017.

12. Clarivate Analytics. Web of Science. 2017; *http://clarivate.com/?product=web-of-science.* Accessed May 14, 2017.

13. Goldenberg RL, Culhane JF, Iams JD, Romero R. "Preterm birth 1 – Epidemiology and causes of preterm birth." *Lancet.* 2008;371(9606):75-84.

14. Elsevier. About Scopus. 2017; *https://www.elsevier.com/solutions/scopus.* Accessed May 14, 2017.

15. Google Search Help. Refine Web Searches. 2017; *https://support.google.com/websearch/answer/2466433?hl=en.* Accessed June 1, 2017.

16. Google Scholar. Inclusion Guidelines for Webmasters. 2017; *https://scholar.google.com/intl/en/scholar/inclusion.html#content.* Accessed June 1, 2017.

17. GrayNet International. About GrayNet. 2017; *http://www.graynet.org/home/aboutgraynet.html.* Accessed June 1, 2017.

18. GrayNet International. Document types in Gray Literature. 2017; *http://www.graynet.org/graysourceindex/documenttypes.html.* Accessed June 1, 2017.

19. National Institute of Health. About MedlinePlus. 2017; *https://medlineplus.gov/aboutmedlineplus.html.* Accessed June 1, 2017.

20. Agoritsas T, Vandvik P, Neumann I, et al. "Finding current best evidence." In: Guyatt G, Rennie D, Meade MO, Cook DJ, eds. *Users' Guides to the Medical Literature: A Manual for Evidence-Based Clinical Practice.* 3rd ed. New York City: McGraw-Hill; 2015.

Chapter 3. How to Appraise and Use an Article about Therapy

Romina Brignardello-Petersen, D.D.S., M.Sc., Ph.D.; Alonso Carrasco-Labra, D.D.S., M.Sc., Ph.D.;
Michael Glick, D.M.D.; Gordon H. Guyatt, M.D., M.Sc.; and Amir Azarpazhooh, D.D.S., M.Sc., Ph.D.

In This Chapter:

Introduction

In the two previous chapters in this book, we introduced the process of evidence-based dentistry[1] and explained how to search for evidence to inform clinical practice.[2] In this chapter, we explain how to use a research report to inform clinical decisions pertaining to questions of therapy. We will introduce and describe the basic concepts for understanding randomized controlled trials (RCTs), and we explain how to critically appraise such studies. In subsequent chapters in this book, we describe how to use other types of study designs.

Clinical Questions of Therapy

Dental practitioners spend most of their time administering treatments to their patients. A therapy or treatment can be defined as "any intervention, which may include prescribing drugs, performing surgery, or counseling, that is intended to improve the course of disease once it is established."[3] Many of the clinical questions that arise in clinical practice have to do with the effectiveness of treatments or interventions.

Box 3.1. Clinical Scenario

You referred a patient to an oral and maxillofacial surgeon for surgical extraction of an impacted mandibular third molar that has been causing the patient to have repeated episodes of pericoronitis. Your patient returned from the surgery consultation session and told you that the surgeon explained the risk of a postoperative infection and how to avoid it. The surgeon gave your patient the option to use either chlorhexidine gel or chlorhexidine mouth rinse. Your patient now is asking for your opinion regarding which of these two options may be more effective. You are not sure, so you decide to search for evidence from a clinical study to answer this question.

As described by the authors of Chapter 2 of this book, therapy questions can be stated using the population, intervention, comparison, outcomes (PICO) framework.[4] The population is the patients who are to receive the intervention, the intervention is the treatment of interest, the comparison is the reference to which we are comparing the intervention, and the outcomes are the health consequences that depend on the intervention. The comparison can be a different treatment or no treatment at all. Table 3.1 shows two examples of therapy questions and their corresponding questions in the PICO framework: one of them has no treatment as the comparison and the other has an alternative treatment.

Table 3.1. Examples of Therapy Questions and the PICO* Framework

Clinical Question	Population	Intervention	Comparison	Outcomes
Should I prescribe chlorhexidine gel or chlorhexidine mouth rinse to a patient undergoing third-molar extractions to avoid postoperative infection?	Patients undergoing third-molar extractions	Chlorhexidine gel	Chlorhexidine mouth rinse	Postoperative infections (alveolar osteitis, surgical site infection)
Should I prescribe antibiotic prophylaxis for patients with diabetes undergoing endodontic treatment?	Patients with diabetes who will receive endodontic treatment	Antibiotic prophylaxis	No treatment (that is, no administration of antibiotic prophylaxis)	Postoperative infection, other postoperative complications
What analgesic should I prescribe to my patients to manage pain after dental extractions?	Patients undergoing dental extractions	Ibuprofen	Acetaminophen	Postoperative pain

* PICO = population, intervention, comparison, outcomes.

What Study Design Best Addresses Questions of Therapy?

At the level of primary studies, RCTs represent the optimal study design to address questions of therapy. An RCT is an experiment assessing a medical treatment in patients.[5] In an RCT, participants are allocated randomly into two or more groups that are treated equally except for the intervention the participants receive. After the intervention is applied, investigators follow patients over a specified time and measure outcomes, ideally those that are important to patients. If the study has been well designed and implemented, we can attribute differences that arise to the treatment under investigation (Figure 3.1).[3]

Figure 3.1. Randomized Clinical Trial

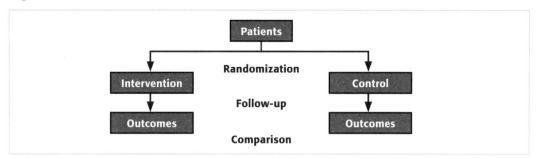

One RCT in dentistry, conducted by Hita-Iglesias and colleagues,[6] addressed whether chlorhexidine gel or chlorhexidine rinse was more effective in preventing alveolar osteitis following third-molar extraction. After the surgery was performed, the investigators randomly allocated patients to receive either the gel or the rinse for one week, and evaluated patients on the third and seventh days postextraction to determine the presence of alveolar osteitis.

RCTs are the best type of study design to determine the effectiveness of an intervention because they minimize bias—a systematic deviation from the underlying truth[7]—by ensuring that patients in the intervention and control groups are similar with respect to factors that determine whether the outcome of interest will occur. If well designed, RCTs also control events that occur after randomization and most aspects of the course of events, such as how the outcomes are measured.[8] Therefore, clinicians should aim to inform their clinical decisions regarding therapy using individual RCTs or, even better, systematic reviews of RCTs. In this chapter, we will focus on how to use stand-alone RCTs, and in subsequent chapters in this book, we will describe how to use systematic reviews.

> **Box 3.2. The Study You Found**
>
> During your search, you did not identify any summary or systematic review; however, you did find a randomized controlled trial (RCT) that seems to answer your question. The investigators of this RCT addressed whether postoperative chlorhexidine gel or chlorhexidine rinse was effective for preventing alveolar osteitis after extracting mandibular third molars.[6] You read the abstract of this RCT, which indicated that the researchers recruited 73 patients and followed them for one week after the third-molar extraction, and it seemed as though chlorhexidine gel was more effective than the mouth rinse. However, you decide that you need to read the entire article to review more details before accepting its results and deciding whether the results are applicable to your patient.

Critically Appraising an RCT to Inform Clinical Decisions

The process of using an article from the dental literature to inform clinical decisions involves assessing the risk of bias, the results, and the applicability of the results.[9] Below, we describe each of these three steps.

How Serious Is the Risk of Bias?

The extent to which a study's results are likely to be correct for the sample of patients enrolled[10] depends on how well the study was designed and conducted. Investigators of RCTs strive to ensure that determinants of the outcome of interest (factors such as age, sex, and disease severity, which we call prognostic factors) other than the treatment under investigation are similar between the groups being compared at the start of the study, and that these determinants remain similar throughout the study.[8] Only if investigators achieve and maintain prognostic balance can we be sure that any differences in outcomes are owing to the intervention (and not to bias introduced by the prognostic factors). Table 3.2[11-16] presents the aspects to consider when assessing the risk of bias of an RCT addressing a question of therapy.

Table 3.2. Critically Appraising the Risk of Bias in an Article About Therapy*

Aspect	Example	Explanation
1. Did intervention and control groups start with the same prognosis?		
1a. Were patients randomized?	"The sites presenting class II furcation lesions were randomly assigned, by a computer-generated list, to receive PDT [photodynamic therapy] or non-activated laser/only photo- sensitizer, both following [scaling and root planing]."[11]	Authors described that the sites were allocated randomly to the treatment groups and how the randomization sequence was generated. Examples of appropriate methods for generating the randomization sequence are random number tables, computer generators, and coin tossing. Inappropriate methods are those that do not produce true randomization, such as assigning patients to the groups on the basis of their date of birth or admission, or according to their record numbers.[12]
1b. Was randomization concealed?	"For each center, 16 consecutively numbered, opaque, sealed envelopes containing a note with the treatment (eight for each treatment) were made and placed in a larger envelope. For each patient, an independent person at each center randomly drew an envelope and handed it to Dentist B. This was repeated until 16 patients at each center were included."[13]	Authors described using consecutively numbered, opaque, sealed envelopes, which were handed to the clinician by an independent person. This is an appropriate method for concealing the allocation. Other adequate methods include the use of sequentially numbered drug containers, and—by far the best of all—central allocation (telephone, web based, or pharmacy controlled). Allocation schedules or lists, envelopes without safeguards, or alternation are not appropriate for concealing allocation.[12]

Aspect	Example	Explanation
1c. Were patients in the study groups similar with respect to known prognostic factors?	"There were no significant differences between groups for age, gender, duration of DM, glycemic status and category of DM regimen."[14][†]	The authors presented a table with the baseline characteristics (potential prognostic factors) of the patients per group. When assessing this aspect, it is important to determine whether all relevant prognostic factors were considered.
2. Was prognostic balance maintained as the study progressed?		
2a. To what extent was the study blinded?	"The entire study was blinded. The prophylaxis paste cups used had silver/blank lidstock and were only identified by a letter on the lidstock. The groups were not known by the examiners or patients. The examiner was in a different section of the building and the study coordinator gave the paste to the hygienist in yet another location of the building."[15]	Authors described that their study was blinded. They also mentioned that the patients, the person administering the treatment (hygienist), and the examiners (outcome assessors) were blinded, and they described how this was achieved. Ideally, the authors should have mentioned that the data analyst was blinded as well. If blinding was not possible, it is necessary to judge the extent that this could have influenced the outcome measurement.[12]
3. Were the groups prognostically balanced at the study's completion?		
3a. Was follow-up complete?	"Analyses of the dropouts revealed no differences in TMJ pain, physical functioning, emotional functioning, or demographic data compared to the patients who completed the study."[‡] The information provided in the study flowchart shows that the number of patients lost to follow-up was one in one group (patients refused participation) and three in the other (one patient refused participation and two moved from the area) at 10 weeks after the intervention.[13]	Authors described the number and reasons for losing patients to follow-up. They also assessed whether these patients were different from those who continued in the study and found no differences. This showed that the risk of bias owing to incomplete follow-up was low. Other methods to assess this are to check whether the number of patients lost to follow-up and the reasons are similar between groups, whether the proportion of patients lost to follow-up is high enough to change the results if they were not missing, or to perform data imputation and draw conclusions on the basis of the results.[12]
3b. Were patients analyzed in the groups to which they were randomized?	"Trial outcomes were analysed by intention to treat. Per-treatment and per-protocol analyses of trial outcomes were also done for comparison."[16]	Authors mentioned that they performed an intention-to-treat analysis. They described that they also did a per-protocol analysis to compare the results of both.
3c. Was the trial stopped early?	"[I]t was determined that 16 subjects per group would be necessary to provide an 80% power with an alpha of 0.05. . . . Thirty-eight subjects. . . . were selected from the population referred to the Periodontal Clinic of Guarulhos University."[14]	Authors described the calculation of the target sample size, and later they mentioned the number of patients recruited, from which it can be inferred that they did not stop the trial early. The authors of the trials that have been stopped early owing to some data-dependent process usually mention this.

* *Sources:* Luchesi and colleagues,[11] Higgins and colleagues,[12] Christidis and colleagues,[13] Santos and colleagues,[14] Neuhaus and colleagues,[15] and Kelleher and colleagues.[16]

† DM = diabetes mellitus.

‡ TMJ = temporomandibular joint.

▸ *Did the intervention and control groups start with the same prognosis?*

One key aspect of a study that can help answer a question regarding therapy is whether the groups were balanced with regard to prognostic factors at the beginning of the study. Investigators can achieve this balance through their control of how the patients are allocated to the intervention and control groups.

Randomization assigns patients to the intervention or control groups by chance.[8] The goal is to ensure that both known and unknown prognostic factors are distributed similarly in the intervention and control groups and, thus, avoid bias.[9, 17] This is why, when therapy questions are to be answered, the use of RCTs is superior to the use of observational studies: when the decision of what treatment to provide to a given patient is left to the dentist (as is done in observational studies), it is likely that patient characteristics may influence the choice of therapy. For instance, because of its ease of use, dentists may prefer to use chlorhexidine mouth rinse rather than gel in older patients who have a greater risk of experiencing subsequent infection, and to use the chlorhexidine gel in younger patients who have a lower risk of experiencing subsequent infection.

Even a well-prepared (typically, computer-generated) randomization schedule does not ensure random allocation. If those enrolling patients are aware of the treatment (intervention or control) to which the next patient will be allocated, they may make choices that undermine randomization.[18] For example, if the next scheduled patient is an older person, and a member of the research staff who is responsible for allocation believes that the assigned treatment of gel is not optimal for the patient, the staff member may manipulate the allocation to ensure that the patient receives the mouth rinse.

To prevent this manipulation of the randomization schedule, those recruiting patients should not be informed about which group the next patient will be allocated to. This strategy is called "allocation concealment."[19] The authors of one study found that the investigators of trials in which allocation concealment was either inadequate or unclear reported treatment effects approximately 40% larger than those reported by studies with adequate allocation concealment.[20]

Particularly if the sample size is small, even concealed randomization may fail to do its job of ensuring prognostic balance. It is important, therefore, to check whether the baseline characteristics of the patients in both groups are similar.[9]

In summary, concealed random allocation with evidence that patients in the intervention and control groups started with the same prognosis reassures us that we are likely to obtain unbiased estimates of treatment effect.

▸ *Was prognostic balance maintained as the study progressed?*

Awareness on the part of dentists administering the intervention, patients who receive the care, or those measuring the outcomes in the study of whether patients are receiving intervention or control treatment can influence their behavior. For instance, the judgment of whether osteitis occurs involves some subjectivity, and it is possible that an outcome assessor who favors using gel over wash will be more likely to diagnose osteitis in those receiving the wash.[21] Blinding (also known as masking) refers to investigators ensuring that patients, clinicians, and those collecting data and adjudicating whether an outcome has occurred are unaware of whether patients are receiving the intervention or the control.[9] Typically, trials are described as double-blinded, which may mean that none of the patients, clinicians, data collectors, or outcome assessors are aware of what treatment the patient was receiving.[21] The term "double-blind" does not leave us confident that all four groups are unaware of allocation, and optimal reporting will inform us whether this is the case.[9]

The method to achieve blinding in RCTs is the use of a placebo. A placebo is a treatment that resembles the intervention of interest but has no biological effect.[8] Most placebos are pills and are administered in the same way as the real drug. Many of the treatments administered in dentistry, however, are procedures. In this case, although doing so is ethically arguable, investigators of the most rigorously designed trials could use a sham procedure to blind patients.[22]

Many times, however, it is not possible to blind patients or clinicians. Fortunately, lack of blinding will not always result in bias. For instance, it may not be possible to blind the clinician because two materials with different appearance and techniques of use are being compared. If, however, patients and outcome assessors are blinded, and there are no other treatments that affect the outcome that the dentists may administer differentially to intervention and control patients (known as cointervention), not blinding the dentist may not affect the results. Therefore, when evaluating whether prognostic balance was maintained as the study progresses, not only do we have to assess whether the groups of interest were blinded, but also we must consider whether any lack of blinding may have caused any bias.[21]

▸ *Were the groups prognostically balanced at the completion of the study?*

Strategies to maintain the prognostic balance as the study proceeds include following up on all patients, analyzing them in the group to which they were allocated, and completing the trial as planned.[9]

There are circumstances in which researchers are not able to follow up and measure the outcome for some patients (referred to as "lost to follow-up"). Patients lost to follow-up may well have different prognoses from those who remain until the end of the study,[9] and hence, the similarity of prognosis in intervention and control groups may be compromised. Ideally researchers should know the outcomes of all participants in a trial (or at least know the reasons why some patients were lost to follow-up).

If the proportion of patients lost to follow-up is so small that including their results in the data analysis would not change the overall results even if all of them had the best or worst outcome, and if the reasons for losing those patients are reported in the trial and are not potentially related to the outcome (for example, a patient moved to another city and could not attend the follow-up visits), then the risk of bias does not increase materially.

Sometimes patients do not receive the intervention as intended because they do not adhere to instructions. Patients may even receive the treatment meant for the patients allocated to the other group. If nonadherence to a treatment is related to a prognostic factor, excluding these patients from the analysis and using data only from patients who adhered to the treatment (that is, doing a per-protocol analysis) will destroy the prognostic balance achieved and maintained through all the previous strategies. To avoid this, researchers use the "intention-to-treat" principle; that is, they analyze the data from each patient in the group to which the patient was allocated. In this way, they get an unbiased estimate of the effect of the intervention at the level of adherence observed in the trial.[23]

Randomization only can ensure prognostic balance when the sample size is large; when the sample size is small, chance can result in large prognostic imbalance. As a result, early in an RCT when sample sizes are small, results may not be indicators of the future overall results even if the RCT otherwise is designed meticulously.[24] Therefore, it can be misleading if investigators stop a trial early on the basis that they have seen a large effect.[9] Both simulations and empirical data show that, on average, the results of trials that were stopped early because of a perceived benefit overestimate treatment effects, and the smaller the number of patients randomized as well as the number of outcome events observed at the time the trial is stopped, the larger the overestimate of effect.[25] Thus, a final criterion to determine whether the intervention and control groups were balanced prognostically at the end of the study is to assess whether the trial was stopped early.

In summary, prognostic balance is maintained up to the completion of the study if there are few participants who are lost to follow-up, if the authors performed an intention-to-treat analysis, and if the trial was completed as planned.

Box 3.3. Your Assessment of the Risk of Bias of the Randomized Controlled Trial You Identified

With respect to initial prognostic balance, you find that patients were randomized adequately and that the randomization schedule was likely to be concealed in an appropriate way. Nevertheless, there were some differences between groups in the distribution of men and women and in the distribution of smokers. With respect to maintaining prognostic balance as the study progressed, only the surgeons were blinded to the interventions the participants received. With respect to prognostic balance at the study completion, the authors did not describe how many, if any, patients were lost to follow-up in each treatment group. Your judgment leads you to consider that the lack of blinding of some participants and the lack of information regarding the losses to follow-up may have biased the results, so you decide to keep reading this study with caution (see the Supplemental Table[6] at the end of this chapter for more details).

Randomization only can ensure prognostic balance when the sample size is large; when the sample size is small, chance can result in large prognostic imbalance.

What Are the Results?

After assessing the magnitude of the risk of bias, clinicians must consider the results—in particular, the magnitude and the precision of the treatment effects—and the implications for their patient care. Table 3.3[26-28] presents examples of the assessment of the results of an article about therapy.

Table 3.3. Critically Appraising the Results of an Article About Therapy

Example	How Large Was the Treatment Effect?	How Precise Was the Estimate of Treatment Effect?
"Compared to controls, the number of decayed teeth was significantly less in both the Xyl-2X* condition (relative risk [RR], 0.30; 95% confidence interval [CI] 0.13 to 0.66; P = 0.003) and the Xyl-3X† condition (RR, 0.50; 95% CI 0.26 to 0.96; P = 0.037)."[26]	The relative risk of the intervention groups compared with the control group was 0.3 and 0.5. This means that patients receiving the interventions had 0.3 times or 0.5 times the risk of caries than patients in the control group, which corresponds to a relative risk reduction of 70% and 50%, respectively. For both groups, this seems to be a large enough effect to consider administering this treatment in practice.	The confidence interval (CI) in one intervention group was 0.13 to 0.66. Because it is likely that both extremes of the CI would lead to a similar clinical action, this CI could be considered to be precise or narrow enough. On the other hand, the CI in the other intervention group was 0.26 to 0.96. The upper limit reflects only a 4% relative risk reduction in the risk of experiencing caries when using the intervention, which may not be an effect large enough so that a dentist would administer it. Because the extremes of the CI would lead to different clinical decisions, this CI is wide or not precise.
"There was, however, a statistical difference in mean attachment loss between the operated and unoperated (contralateral) canines (mean difference, 0.5 mm; 96% CI, 0.4-0.7; P < 0.001)."[27]	The difference in clinical attachment loss between the groups was 0.5 millimeters. A 0.5 mm of difference in attachment level seems to be very small, especially considering that the measurement error for this outcome has shown to be around 1 mm.[28] Therefore, the magnitude of these results does not seem to be big enough to support the administration of the intervention.	The CI of the mean difference was 0.4 to 0.7 mm. Both extremes represented values of differences of attachment loss that had a small magnitude; therefore, this was a precise CI that provided the reader with more confidence in the small effect of the intervention, even accounting for the uncertainty of the results.

* Xyl-2X: 2 xylitol [4.00-g] doses and 1 sorbitol dose twice a day.
† Xyl-3X: 3 xylitol [2.67-g] doses 3 times per day.

▸ *How large was the treatment effect?*

The researchers may analyze and present results of their RCTs in different ways, depending on the type of outcome of interest. When the outcome of interest is measured on a continuous scale (or numeric scale), such as probing depth and degree of trismus in millimeters, results usually are presented as differences in means between two groups. In this way, the mean of the outcome in the intervention group is subtracted from the mean of the outcome in the control group, and the numerical difference then would be attributed to the intervention. In this case, a value of 0 means that there is no difference between the intervention and control groups. Thus, the further the estimate of effect is from 0, the bigger the magnitude of the treatment effect.

On the other hand, the outcome of interest may be dichotomous (that is, the presence or absence or a condition or event), such as the presence of periodontal disease or trismus. With binary outcomes, investigators can present their results as the difference between the proportions in two groups. Imagine a trial comparing two drugs that prevent pain after dental extractions, and the outcome of interest is the presence or absence of pain. If 25% of the patients in the intervention group and 50% of the patients in the control group experience pain, the risk difference is 25%. This also is referred to as absolute risk reduction. As for the mean difference, a value of 0 for the risk difference means that there is no difference between the intervention and control groups, and the further the estimate of effect is from 0, the bigger the magnitude of the treatment effect.

Another way to compare these proportions is to express one effect relative to the other—as the proportion of events in one group divided by the proportion of events in the other. In the example described previously, the relative effect (or relative risk) is 0.25 / 0.50 = 0.50; patients receiving the intervention are at one-half of the risk of having pain as patients in the control group. From the relative risk we can derive the relative risk reduction, which reflects how much the risk of the outcome increased or decreased in the intervention group relative to the control group. Because relative risk is best expressed as a percentage, in this example, the relative risk reduction would be 50%. When using relative measures of effect, a value of 1 means that the proportion of events is the same in both groups; the further the estimate of effect is from 1, the larger the treatment effect.

How large the effect is depends on the clinical context. For example, a difference of 2 mm in clinical attachment level gain when comparing an intervention with a control would be interpreted as a large magnitude by most clinicians. When considering another outcome, such as the difference in pain reduction using a visual analog scale of 100 mm, a difference of 2 mm between the groups would be interpreted as a small effect. Therefore, the magnitude of the effect reflects its importance to patients.[29]

▸ *How precise was the estimate of the treatment effect?*

Because of the influence of chance on results, researchers never can be completely sure of the true effect estimate. This is why they not only use point estimates such as the mean difference and the absolute and relative risks, but also complement them with estimates that express the degree of uncertainty in this point estimate. The estimate most commonly used to assess the precision of the results is the confidence interval (CI). A CI is a plausible range of values within which the true value actually is likely to lie, given the data observed in a study.[30] A 95% CI range means that if the study was performed 100 times, the result would be within this range 95 times. The narrower the confidence interval, the more confident the researchers are of the estimate of effect. The interpretation of how wide or narrow a CI is depends—as it does in the case of the magnitude effect—on the clinical context.[30]

> **Box 3.4. Your Assessment of the Results of the Randomized Controlled Trial You Identified**
>
> You find that patients who received chlorhexidine gel have 0.3 times the risk of developing alveolar osteitis than patients who received chlorhexidine mouth rinse. The 95% confidence interval of this relative risk ranged from 0.08 to 1.02. After looking at these numbers, you conclude that even though the magnitude of the treatment effect shows a large reduction in the risk of alveolar osteitis when using the gel, these results are not precise enough to claim that the gel is more effective than the mouth rinse (see the Supplemental Table[6] at the end of this chapter for more details).

How Can I Apply the Results to Patient Care?

Finally, clinicians should consider the extent to which the results of a study are applicable to their particular context. Factors clinicians should consider include whether the patients in the study have the same characteristics as the patients to whom they will apply the results, how important the outcomes measured in the study are to their patients, whether the study investigators have measured all outcomes that are important to patients, and whether administering the intervention will result in more benefits than harms, costs, or both.

▶ *Were the study patients similar to my patients?*

In reading through a study, clinicians should evaluate the extent to which the patients studied are similar to the patients in their own practice and, hence, the extent to which results are applicable to their own patients (in other words, how generalizable are the results). When informing their clinical decisions with evidence from RCTs, clinicians should look at the selection criteria used for recruiting patients into a study and the description of the patients in the results. If the characteristics of the included patients are similar to the patients in their practice, clinicians could apply the results of the study in their practice. If there are characteristics that differ, such as age or severity of disease, clinicians should consider the likelihood that the effect of the intervention could be different if applied in their practice.[9]

▶ *Were all patient-important outcomes considered?*

Ideally, the investigators of a study whose results can inform a clinical decision should have considered all patient-important outcomes. A patient-important outcome is any outcome that may alter a patient's inclination to choose a particular treatment, such as a reduction in symptoms, improvement in quality of life, treatment effect duration, or adverse effects.[29] Examples of patient-important outcomes in dentistry are tooth loss, pain, swelling, and the longevity of a restoration.

▸ *Are the likely treatment benefits worth the potential harms and costs?*

Finally, when considering whether to administer a treatment to patients, clinicians should consider its benefits, harms, and costs.[31] There is no treatment that has no undesirable consequence, even if the only downside is the time required for administration.[32] Therefore, when considering using a treatment that seems to be beneficial, clinicians should put in the balance both the benefits and all potential downsides. The more inclined the balance is to one side, the easier it will be to make a decision.

> ### Box 3.5. Your Assessment of the Applicability of the Randomized Controlled Trial You Identified
>
> After assessing the applicability of the results, you conclude that even though the patients in the study were similar to your patient and there seem to be few harms associated with the use of either chlorhexidine gel or mouth rinse, the researchers did not consider all the infectious complications that could develop after the surgery. However, the authors did consider the most frequent infectious complication (see the Supplemental Table[6] at the end of this chapter for more details). Thus, you decide that this evidence is still applicable to inform the choice your patient has to make.

Conclusion

Because of their design, RCTs are the best type of study to inform clinical decisions about therapy. However, clinicians should know how to appraise these studies to inform their decisions adequately. The critical appraisal of an RCT focuses on aspects of validity, results, and applicability. Clinicians should apply these guidelines to achieve the best possible results for their own practices.

> ### Box 3.6. What You Say to Your Patient
>
> Despite the fact that the abstract of the study suggests that chlorhexidine gel may be more effective for preventing infectious complications after third-molar extractions than chlorhexidine mouth rinse, you inform your patient that there is no reason to believe that one of the options is better than the other, and you suggest that the patient should consider other aspects, such as the patient's preferences regarding the mode of administration and costs, when making a decision.

References

1. Brignardello-Petersen R, Carrasco-Labra A, Glick M, Guyatt GH, Azarpazhooh A. "A practical approach to evidence-based dentistry: understanding and applying the principles of EBD." *JADA* 2014;145(11):1105–1107.

2. Chapter 2 of this book was based on Brignardello-Petersen R, Carrasco-Labra A, Booth HA, et al. "A practical approach to evidence-based dentistry: II: how to search for evidence to inform clinical decisions." *JADA* 2014;145(12):1262–1267.

3. Fletcher R, Fletcher S. Treatment. In: Fletcher R, Fletcher S, eds. *Clinical Epidemiology: The Essentials.* 4th ed. Baltimore, MD: Lippincott Williams & Wilkins; 2005:125-146.

4. Guyatt GH, Meade MO, Richardson S, Jaeschke R. "What is the question?" In: Guyatt GH, Rennie D, Meade MO, Cook DJ, eds. *Users' Guides to the Medical Literature: A Manual for Evidence-Based Clinical Practice.* 2nd ed. New York, NY: McGraw-Hill; 2008:17-28.

5. Piantadosi S. "Clinical trials as research." In: Piantadosi S. *Clinical Trials: A Methodologic Perspective.* 2nd ed. Hoboken, NJ: Wiley; 2005:9-28.

6. Hita-Iglesias P, Torres-Lagares D, Flores-Ruiz R, et al. "Effectiveness of chlorhexidine gel versus chlorhexidine rinse in reducing alveolar osteitis in mandibular third molar surgery." *J Oral Maxillofac Surg.* 2008;66(3):441-445.

7. "Glossary." In: Guyatt GH, Rennie D, Meade MO, Cook DJ, eds. *Users' Guide to the Medical Literature: A Manual for Evidence-Based Clinical Practice.* 2nd ed. New York, NY: McGraw-Hill; 2008:769-808.

8. Piantadosi S. "Notation and terminology." In: Piantadosi S. *Clinical Trials: A Methodologic Perspective.* 2nd ed. Hoboken, NJ: Wiley; 2005:569-585.

9. Guyatt GH, Straus S, Meade MO, et al. "Therapy." In: Guyatt GH, Rennie D, Meade MO, Cook DJ, eds. *Users' Guide to the Medical Literature: A Manual for Evidence-Based Clinical Practice.* 2nd ed. New York, NY: McGraw-Hill; 2008:67-86.

10. Fletcher R, Fletcher S. "Introduction." In: Fletcher R, Fletcher S, eds. *Clinical Epidemiology: The Essentials.* 4th ed. Baltimore, MD: Lippincott Williams & Wilkins; 2005:1-16.

11. Luchesi VH, Pimentel SP, Kolbe MF, et al. "Photodynamic therapy in the treatment of class II furcation: a randomized controlled clinical trial." *J Clin Periodontol.* 2013;40(8):781-788.

12. Higgins J, Altman D, Sterne J. "Assessing risk of bias in included studies." In: Higgins J, Green S, eds. *Cochrane Handbook for Systematic Reviews of Interventions,* Version 5.1.0 (updated March 2011). The Cochrane Collaboration; 2011. Available at: *www.cochrane-handbook.org.* Accessed November 19, 2014.

13. Christidis N, Doepel M, Ekberg E, et al. "Effectiveness of a prefabricated occlusal appliance in patients with temporomandibular joint pain: a randomized controlled multicenter study." *J Oral Facial Pain Headache.* 2014;28(2):128-137.

14. Santos VR, Lima JA, Miranda TS, et al. "Full-mouth disinfection as a therapeutic protocol for type-2 diabetic subjects with chronic periodontitis: twelve-month clinical outcomes: a randomized controlled clinical trial." *J Clin Periodontol.* 2013;40(2):155-162.

15. Neuhaus KW, Milleman JL, Milleman KR, et al. "Effectiveness of a calcium sodium phosphosilicate-containing prophylaxis paste in reducing dentine hypersensitivity immediately and 4 weeks after a single application: a double-blind randomized controlled trial." *J Clin Periodontol.* 2013;40(4):349-357.

16. Kelleher J, Bhat R, Salas AA, et al. "Oronasopharyngeal suction versus wiping of the mouth and nose at birth: a randomised equivalency trial." *Lancet.* 2013;382(9889):326-330.

17. Roberts C, Torgerson D. "Randomisation methods in controlled trials." *BMJ.* 1998;317(7168):1301.

18. Torgerson DJ, Roberts C. "Understanding controlled trials. Randomisation methods: concealment." *BMJ.* 1999;319(7206):375-376.

19. Schulz KF, Grimes DA. "Allocation concealment in randomised trials: defending against deciphering." *Lancet.* 2002;359(9306):614-618.

20. Schulz KF, Chalmers I, Hayes RJ, Altman DG. "Empirical evidence of bias: dimensions of methodological quality associated with estimates of treatment effects in controlled trials." *JAMA.* 1995;273(5):408-412.

21. Day SJ, Altman DG. "Statistics notes: blinding in clinical trials and other studies." *BMJ.* 2000;321(7259):504-504.

22. Piantadosi S. "Contexts for clinical trials." In: Piantadosi S. *Clinical Trials: A Methodologic Perspective.* 2nd ed. Hoboken, NJ: Wiley; 2005:65-106.

23. Montori V, Guyatt GH. "Intention-to-treat principle." *Can Med Assoc J.* 2001;165(10):1339-1341.

24. Weatley K, Clayton D. "Be skeptical about unexpected large apparent treatment effects." Control Clin Trials. 2003;24(1):66-70.

25. Bassler D, Briel M, Montori VM, et al. "Stopping randomized trials early for benefit and estimation of treatment effects: systematic review and meta-regression analysis." *JAMA.* 2010;303(12):1180-1187.

26. Milgrom P, Ly KA, Tut OK, et al. "Xylitol pediatric topical oral syrup to prevent dental caries: a double-blind randomized clinical trial of efficacy." *Arch Pediatr Adolesc Med.* 2009;163(7):601-607.

27. Parkin NA, Milner RS, Deery C, et al. "Periodontal health of palatally displaced canines treated with open or closed surgical technique: a multicenter, randomized controlled trial." *Am J Orthod Dentofacial Orthop.* 2013;144(2):176-184.

28. Espeland MA, Zappa UE, Hogan PE, Simona C, Graf H. "Cross-sectional and longitudinal reliability for clinical measurement of attachment loss." *J Clin Periodontol.* 1991;18(2):126-133.

29. Brignardello-Petersen R, Carrasco-Labra A, Sash P, Azarpazhooh A. "A practitioner's guide to developing critical appraisal skills: what is the difference between clinical and statistical significance?" *JADA.* 2013;144(7):780-786.

30. Guyatt GH, Walter S, Cook D, Wyer P, Jaeschke R. "Confidence intervals." In: Guyatt GH, Rennie D, Meade MO, Cook D, eds. *Users' Guides to the Medical Literature: A Manual for Evidence-Based Clinical Practice.* 2nd ed. New York, NY: McGraw-Hill; 2008:99-107.

31. Andrews JC, Schunemann HJ, Oxman AD, et al. "GRADE guidelines, XV. going from evidence to recommendation determinants of a recommendation's direction and strength." *J Clin Epidemiol.* 2013;66(7):726-735.

32. Schunemann HJ. "Guidelines 2.0: do no net harm—the future of practice guideline development in asthma and other diseases." *Curr Allergy Asthma Rep.* 2011;11(3):261-268.

A version of this chapter originally appeared in the January 2015 edition of *JADA* (Volume 146, Issue 1, Pages 42–49. e1). It has been reviewed and updated for accuracy and clarity by the editors of *How to Use Evidence-Based Dental Practices to Improve Your Clinical Decision-Making.*

Supplemental Table. Example of Critically Appraising an Article About Therapy*

Hita-Iglesias P, Torres-Lagares D, Flores-Ruiz R, et al. "Effectiveness of chlorhexidine gel versus chlorhexidine rinse in reducing alveolar osteitis in mandibular third molar surgery." *J Oral Maxillofac Surg.* 2008;66(3):441–445.

1. How Serious Is the Risk of Bias?	
1a. Did the experimental and control groups begin the study with a similar prognosis?	
Were the patients randomized?	Yes. The study is described as a randomized clinical trial. The authors also described that they used a computer program to generate the allocation sequence.
Was randomization concealed?	Probably yes. The authors mentioned they used envelopes that indicated where the allocation assignment was recorded. These were opened right after the surgery. Ideally, they would have used opaque envelopes or the allocation sequence would have been kept in a different place such as a telephone central to prevent any misbehavior from researchers.
Were patients similar at baseline with respect to known prognostic factors?	Probably yes. The authors presented a comparison of the factors that they considered to be prognostically important in Table 3.1 of this chapter. These factors were fairly balanced between the gel and rinse group. The proportion of women and nonsmokers differed somewhat between the groups; however, it was thought that these differences were unlikely to bias the results.
1b. Was prognostic balance maintained as the study progressed?	
To what extent was the study blinded?	Surgeons were blinded because the allocation was done right after the surgery. Patients were not blinded because both antiseptics were administered in a different way and there was no mention of using placebos. There was no description of blinding of any of the other groups. Because the outcome had an explicit definition and the outcome assessor was trained, it was not very likely that the lack of blinding could have seriously biased the results.
1c. Were groups prognostically balanced at the study's completion?	
Was the follow-up complete?	Unclear. There was not enough information to make a judgment. The authors only reported the final number of participants in each group and did not mention whether this corresponded to all patients who were enrolled or whether some were lost to follow-up.
Were patients analyzed in the groups to which they were randomized?	Yes. The authors mentioned that they performed an intention-to-treat analysis. They also mentioned that there were no protocol violations as reported by patients, which would have made the results of both the intention-to-treat and the per-protocol analysis yield the same results.

Was the trial stopped early?	Probably not. There was no mention of stopping the trial early (which authors usually report). However, there were insufficient details to corroborate this, because there was no reporting of sample size calculation to assess whether the target sample size was reached.

2. What Are the Results?

2a. How large was the treatment effect?	7.5% of the patients in the gel group and 25% of the patients in the rinse group developed alveolar osteitis. The relative risk was 0.3, indicating that patients who received chlorhexidine gel had 0.3 times the probability of developing alveolar osteitis than patients who received chlorhexidine rinse. The risk difference was 17.5%. Based on both measures of effect, the reduction in risk when using gel seemed to be of large magnitude.
2b. How precise was the estimate of the treatment effect?	Not precise. The authors did not include the confidence intervals, but with the numbers reported, it was possible to calculate the 95% confidence intervals for the relative risk. The confidence interval ranged between 0.08 and 1.02. Because this confidence interval suggested a very large benefit in one extreme, and a very small harm in the other, we considered the results to be imprecise (from a 92% reduction to a 2% increase in the incidence of alveolar osteitis).

3. How Can I Apply the Results to My Patient Care?

3a. Were the study patients similar to my patients?	Probably yes. The selection criteria described by the authors seemed to match the characteristics of most of the patients undergoing third-molar extraction who would be eligible to receive this intervention. However, depending on the particular context, the clinician should reassess this.
3b. Were all patient-important outcomes considered?	Probably not. The authors only measured alveolar osteitis and adverse effects. If they wanted to inform dental practice with the aim of preventing infectious complications like surgical site infection and other types of complications, then the study investigators did not provide information regarding all the relevant outcomes.
3c. Are the likely benefits worth the potential harms and costs?	Probably yes. The gel seemed to reduce the risk of developing alveolar osteitis, and it had similar tolerance and adverse effects (no adverse effects in both groups), thus the benefit-harm balances inclined toward the benefits. However, other potential issues such as burden of treatment and costs should be considered.

Conclusion: The results of the study are likely to be correct; however, even though the magnitude of the treatment effect showed a large reduction in the risk of developing alveolar osteitis when using the gel, these results were not precise enough to reach a sound conclusion. Aspects regarding applicability should be assessed further before making a decision regarding the administration of chlorhexidine gel over chlorhexidine rinse.

* *Source:* Hita-Iglesias and colleagues.[6]

Chapter 4. How to Use an Article About Harm

Romina Brignardello-Petersen, D.D.S., M.Sc., Ph.D.; Alonso Carrasco-Labra, D.D.S., M.Sc., Ph.D.; Michael Glick, D.M.D.; Gordon H. Guyatt, M.D., M.Sc.; and Amir Azarpazhooh, D.D.S., M.Sc., Ph.D.

In This Chapter:

Introduction

In the three previous chapters in this book, we introduced the process of evidence-based dentistry (EBD)[1] and explained how to search for evidence to inform clinical practice[2] and how to use an article about therapy.[3] In this chapter, we explain how to use an article to inform clinical decisions regarding questions of harm. We introduce and describe the basic concepts needed to understand observational studies, and we explain how to use these concepts to critically appraise such studies. In subsequent chapters in this book, we describe how to use other types of study designs.

Box 4.1. Clinical Scenario

You met with a new patient who was referred to you by his family doctor. The patient explained to you that he had been having many physical problems, such as muscular pain in his shoulders, back, arms, and legs, and that his physician told him that one of the causes might be his oral health status. While examining the patient, you noticed that he has lost many teeth. The patient asks you if this tooth loss might be related to his general health problems. You are not sure, so you decide to search for evidence from a clinical study to answer this question.

Clinical Questions of Harm

Questions regarding potentially harmful exposures, either to dental treatments or external agents, are common in dental practice. Some examples of these questions are the following: Do people who live in areas where the water is fluoridated have a higher risk of having enamel defects? Does smoking increase the risk of having oral cancer? Does the dentist's use of rubber dams when placing a dental restoration increase the patient's risk of allergic reactions if the patient has a latex allergy?

The classic Population-Intervention-Comparison-Outcome (PICO) framework requires only minor modifications to address questions related to harm. The population is the patients of interest. In cases that address questions related to harm, the population is those patients who may face the potentially harmful agent. The intervention becomes the exposure, which corresponds to the harmful agent. The comparison is the reference, which is the absence of the exposure to the harmful agent. The outcome is the potential negative consequence of the exposure. Table 4.1 shows examples of questions related to harm and the corresponding PICO components.

What Study Design Best Addresses Questions of Harm?

Owing to the hierarchy of evidence used to answer questions about harm, even though investigators might identify randomized controlled trials as being the best type of study design to answer these types of questions, they generally cannot use this type of study design because of ethical reasons. Therefore, at the level of a primary study, an observational study is usually the most appropriate study design to answer questions regarding harm. This is not always true, however. Note, for example, that investigators could address the question listed in Table 4.1 about rubber dams by using a randomized controlled trial design.

Table 4.1. Examples of Questions Related to Harm and the Corresponding PICO* Framework

Clinical Question	Population	Exposure	Comparison	Outcome
Do people who live in areas where the water is fluoridated have a higher risk of having enamel defects?	Children and adults	Fluoride in water	No fluoride in water	Dental fluorosis
Does the dentist's use of rubber dams when placing a dental restoration increase the patient's risk of having an allergic reaction if the patient has a latex allergy?	Patients with allergy to latex	Rubber dams	No rubber dams	Allergic reactions

* PICO = population, intervention, comparison, outcomes.

An observational study is one in which the investigator does not assign an exposure or intervention; rather, these exposures or interventions occur naturally in the study setting. Although investigators have conducted descriptive observational studies in which they recruit only one group of patients and do not compare them with any other group of patients, in this chapter we describe the type of observational studies in which investigators use a comparison group (which can happen either because two groups of patients are recruited and followed, or one large group of patients is divided into two or more, on the basis of the presence of an exposure).

Observational studies can be classified according to the direction in which the exposure or outcomes are measured.[4] The intuitive design is one in which investigators enroll participants who either are exposed or are not exposed (for example, patients living in a community that has fluoride in the water or patients living in a community that does not have fluoridated water) and follow them over a period, recording whether the outcome of interest (that is, fluorosis) does or does not occur. We call these cohort studies (Figure 4.1, Table 4.2[5-7]).[8]

Figure 4.1. The Designs of Analytical Observational Studies

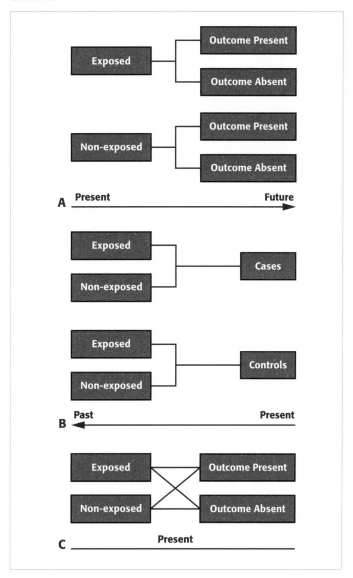

A. Cohort study: investigators recruit participants on the basis of the patients' exposure, and they follow up with patients over time to determine the presence of outcomes in the future. **B.** Case-control studies: investigators recruit participants on the basis of the presence or absence of an outcome, and investigators assess participants' histories to determine the presence of exposures in the past. **C.** Cross-sectional studies: investigators measure the presence of the exposure and the outcome at the same time point.

Table 4.2. Examples of Analytical Observational Studies

Design	Example
Cohort Study	Levin and colleagues[5] aimed to evaluate the effect of periodontal status (exposure) on implant failure (outcome). They recruited a group of patients who were undergoing implant placement surgery (population) and assessed their periodontal status (prognostic factor). Then, they followed up with these patients for an average of 12 years to determine how many of them had suffered implant failure, and the investigators compared the proportions among periodontal status categories.
Case-Control Study	The objective of the study conducted by Claus and colleagues[6] was to assess whether there was an association between having had dental radiographs (exposure) and having intracranial meningioma (outcome). To assess this association, the investigators recruited patients with diagnosed intracranial meningioma (cases) and healthy patients (controls). Then they interviewed the patients to determine their level of exposure to dental radiographs in the past and compared these levels between groups.
Cross-Sectional Study	Okada and colleagues[7] aimed to assess the relationship between periodontal disease (exposure) and issues with food acceptability (outcome) in older adults (population). The investigators recruited older adults and measured, at the same time, their periodontal status and their difficulty chewing different foods. Then they compared these difficulty levels among patients in groups with differing periodontal status.

A less intuitive design is one that involves investigators recruiting samples of study participants in whom the outcome has occurred (for example, they have had fluorosis [we call these participants "cases"]) and comparing them with similar study participants who have not had the outcome of interest (that is, no fluorosis [we call these participants "controls"]). Investigators then determine—by asking questions to participants or by looking at medical records or other information sources—whether participants in either group experienced the exposure of interest (that is, water fluoridation). We call these case-control studies (Figure 4.1, Table 4.2[5-7]).[9]

Investigators can use another type of design only when they can assess the exposure and the outcome at the same time. Here, the investigator looks simultaneously at the exposure (for example, the current exposure to fluoridated water) and the outcome (for example, fluorosis). We call such designs cross-sectional studies.[4]

In general, cohort studies are less susceptible to bias than are case-control studies, and case-control studies are less susceptible to bias than cross-sectional studies. Thus, if available, we would choose cohort studies as our source of evidence.

Why, then, would investigators bother conducting case-control studies? The reason is that if an outcome is rare or if the outcome occurs over a long period, conducting a cohort study may be challenging or not feasible at all and choosing the case-control design might be a better option.

Consider the question of whether smoking increases the risk of oral cancer. Because oral cancer is (fortunately) rare and because it develops over a long period, addressing the smoking issue would involve enrolling thousands of patients and following them for many years. Indeed, the initial studies demonstrating the association between smoking and cancer used a case-control design. Only later did investigators undertake the large cohort studies that definitively reported the association.

Sometimes, it might be completely infeasible to conduct cohort studies. Consider the question of whether pacifier use as an infant is associated with having temporomandibular disorders in adulthood. Following people from infancy to adulthood is likely to be impossible, and thus the only way to address the issue is by using a case-control design. Thus, these study designs may provide the best available evidence.

Box 4.2. The Study You Found

During your search, you did not identify any summary or systematic review; however, you did find an observational study with results that seem to answer your question.[10] The study investigators addressed whether there was an association between functional tooth number and physical complaints (using a cross-sectional design) and whether the functional tooth number was associated with mortality (using a prospective cohort design). The researchers recruited 5,584 people, measured the study participants' number of functional teeth and physical complaints at baseline (the cross-sectional design), and followed their cases for 15 years (the cohort design). The authors reported that "physical complaints were significantly associated with functional tooth number." You wonder about the trustworthiness of the results and the applicability of the results to your patient, and you proceed to find a more detailed appraisal.

Critically Appraising Observational Studies to Inform Clinical Decisions

The process of using an article from the dental literature consists of three steps: assessing the risk of bias (that is, determining whether the results are systematically different from the truth), assessing the results (that is, determining the magnitude and precision of the estimates of the association between exposure and outcome), and assessing the applicability of the results (that is, determining the degree to which the results of the study can be applied to the patients who generated the clinical question).[11] We describe each of these steps in the sections that follow.

How Serious Is the Risk of Bias?

The extent to which a study's results are likely to be correct for the sample of patients enrolled depends on how well the study was designed and conducted.[12,13]

▸ *Are exposed and unexposed study participants sufficiently similar?*

Bias—systematic difference from the truth—will occur if exposed and unexposed study participants differ with respect to an important determinant of outcome (which we call a prognostic factor).[14] For example, if we ask whether patients with dental crowding (exposed group) are more likely to have caries than patients without dental crowding (unexposed group), misleading results caused by bias could occur if patients with dental crowding brush their teeth less frequently (the extraneous prognostic factor).

Or consider the question of whether drinking milk at night (the exposure) causes dental caries (the outcome) in children. Parents who are less aware of appropriate oral health care practices for babies may be more likely to give their babies milk at night, and they might be less likely to brush their children's teeth (the extraneous prognostic factor). As a result, the imbalance in the extraneous prognostic factor (toothbrushing) may create a spurious association between milk at night and caries. We sometimes refer to prognostic imbalance (that is, the extraneous prognostic factor being distributed differently in exposed and unexposed) as selection bias or a confounding factor.

In both cohort and case-control studies, prognostic imbalance is likely to occur. What can investigators do when faced with these situations? Fortunately, there are statistical strategies to deal with the problem that involve comparing like with like. For instance, in the example previously described, investigators could focus first on children whose parents brushed their teeth and, among these children, compare those who did and who did not receive milk at night. Then, the investigators could focus on the children whose parents did not brush their teeth and, among those children, compare those who did and who did not receive milk at night. Finally, the investigators could combine the results across these two comparisons. In this way, they could avoid inadvertently causing the bias that could otherwise result from prognostic imbalance. We call this analytical strategy an adjusted or stratified analysis.[15]

▶ *Is information collected in the same way in exposed and unexposed study participants?*

Biased results will arise when investigators gather data in different ways regarding the presence of an exposure, a prognostic factor, or an outcome in the exposed and unexposed study participants, or the cases and the controls.[16] For example, in a case-control study, researchers may search more thoroughly for the presence of a past exposure if they know that the patient belongs to the group of cases rather than the group of controls. Even if the method of information collection is similar, bias will intrude if patients who are cases are more likely to remember a past exposure than patients who are controls.

Asking the following three questions can help clinicians assess the extent of the risk of bias in an article about harm: Were patients similar for prognostic factors known to be associated with the outcome, or did investigators conduct an adjusted analysis that considered all such factors? Were the circumstances and methods for detecting the exposure, prognostic factors, or outcome similar in both groups? In a cohort study, was the follow-up sufficiently complete? Table 4.3[6,17–20] lists these questions, provides some strategies to reduce bias to consider when answering them, and offers examples from the dental literature.

Box 4.3. Your Assessment of the Risk of Bias of the Observational Study You Identified

With respect to balance of prognostic factors, you find that there is not much information in the article. You can think of the main factors that may cause prognostic imbalance, which according to your experience and knowledge are the age of the patient, the presence of comorbidities, and the use of removable prosthesis. When you look more closely, you realize that the authors considered these factors when assessing the relationship between functional tooth number and physical complaints and mortality. With respect to exposure and outcome measurement, it seems like the same methods were used in all patients. With respect to the follow-up, the numbers reported in the article do not add up and make you doubt whether the authors were careful enough. Although your judgment leads you to believe that the prognostic balance may be in question and that the issues with follow-up are likely to bias the results, you decide to keep reading this study with caution (see the Supplemental Table[10] at the end of this chapter for more details).

Even if the method of information collection is similar, bias will intrude if patients who are cases are more likely to remember a past exposure than patients who are controls.

Table 4.3. Critically Appraising the Risk of Bias of an Article about Harm

Question	Strategies to Address the Bias	Examples
Were patients similar for prognostic factors known to be associated with the outcome? (Selection Bias and Confounding)	• Define explicit and appropriate selection criteria for entry to study, considering these prognostic factors • Conduct matching according to prognostic factors • Measure the prognostic factors and potential confounders to account for them in the analysis	"These randomly selected 41,346 comparison subjects were matched with the study subjects on sex, age group. . . . , urbanization level."[17] "Controls were selected by random-digit-dialing by an outside consulting firm (Krieder Research) and were matched to cases by five-year age interval, sex, and state of residence. . . . To assess the odds of meningioma associated with risk factors, conditional logistic regression was used to provide. . . . estimates of the odds ratios (OR) (adjusted for age, sex, race. . . . , education. . . . , and history of head CT)."[6]
Were the circumstances and methods for detecting the exposure or outcome similar in both groups? (Information Bias)	• Use outcomes that are objective or have explicit definitions • Verify self-reported information using external data • Standardize interviews • Mask outcome assessors to exposure status, or exposure assessors to outcome status	"All radiographs were taken with the same model x-ray machine with a long-cone, paralleling technique and standard settings of 70 kVp and 15 mA. . . . Preoperative, obturation, and follow-up radiographs were taken with a collimator to ensure standardized evaluation of the periradicular region . . . . all radiographs were viewed by 2 endodontists under standardized conditions."[18] "Clinical oral examinations were conducted identically at baseline and follow-up and independent (blinded) of participants' completion of questionnaires. . . . A tooth was recorded as decayed if there was evidence of a carious lesion clearly extending into dentine on any coronal or root surface. The carious lesion had to be cavitated, to have penetrated the fissure and undermined the enamel, or the dentine walls to be clearly softened."[19]
In a cohort-study, was the follow-up sufficiently complete? (Selection Bias)	• Ensure complete follow-up in exposed and nonexposed group • Record reasons for losses to follow-up and do sensitivity analyses	"For each model, missing variables and missing or incomplete breastfeeding histories were multiply imputed. . . . Losses to follow-up were relatively high but not unusual among cohort studies in low-resource settings, where participants frequently change address and contact information."[20]

What Are the Results?

After assessing the magnitude of the risk of bias, clinicians must consider the results—in particular, the magnitude and the precision of the estimates of association between exposure and outcome—and the implications for their patient care.[21] Table 4.4[6,19] provides examples of the critical appraisal of the results of an article about harm.

Table 4.4. Critically Appraising the Results of an Article About Harm

Example	How Strong Is the Association Between Exposure and Outcome?	How Precise Is the Estimate of the Risk?
"[A]dults drinking 1-2 . . . . SSB* daily had. . . . a rate 1.31 (95% CI† 1.02-1.67). . . . times greater for the 4-year net DMFT‡ increments than those drinking no SSB at baseline."[19]	The relative risk is 1.31, which means that adults who drink SSB are 1.31 times more likely to have DMFT than adults who do not drink SSB. It seems like there is moderate increase in the risk of increasing the DMFT number over a 4-year period. Therefore, the magnitude of the effect is moderate.	The 95% CI of the relative risk is 1.02 to 1.67. The lower limit reflects almost no increase in the risk of increasing the number of DMFT, whereas the upper limit suggests a moderate to high risk, and we cannot be completely confident about the harmful effect of SSB. Thus, the estimate of the harm is not precise.
"Significant increases in the risk of meningioma was associated with a young age at receipt of screening as well as more frequent screening, and individuals who were aged < 10 years at the time of screening had an almost 5-fold increase in risk (OR,§ 4.9; 95% CI, 1.8-13.2)."[6]	The OR measuring the association between screening with dental radiographs at a young age (exposure) and meningioma (outcome) is 4.9. That is, when patients receive radiographs at a young age, they are 4.9 times more likely to develop meningioma than when they do not. This represents a large increase in the magnitude of effect.¶	The CI of the OR is 1.8 to 13.2. This seems to be a wide range, both 1.8 and 13.2 in which an OR of 1.8 represents a small magnitude of effect (especially considering the low prevalence of meningioma). Thus, we can be confident that there is an association between the exposure and outcome. This estimate of the harm is not precise.¶

* SSB = sugar-sweetened beverages.
† CI = confidence interval.
‡ DMFT = decayed, missing, filled teeth.
§ OR = odds ratio.
¶ The aim of this example is to illustrate how to appraise the results by appraising their magnitude and precision. Authors should assess the risk of bias of the study first to determine whether these numbers are likely to be correct or the result of bias.

▸ *How strong is the association between exposure and outcome?*

As in randomized controlled trials, the authors of an observational study can present their results as mean differences when the outcome of interest is continuous (for example, probing depth) and as absolute and relative measures of effect when the outcome is dichotomous (for example, the absence or presence of some feature, such as having or not having a periapical abscess). When mean differences (that is, the differences in the mean of the outcome between the exposed and nonexposed groups) and risk differences (that is, the difference in the proportion of patients with the outcome present between the groups) are used, larger numbers represent big magnitudes of effect. The clinical significance of this magnitude depends on the specific context and outcome.[22]

The relative risk, which expresses how many times more likely is one group to have the outcome with respect to another group, is the preferred relative measure for cohort studies. For example, when comparing populations exposed to fluoride in water or not exposed to fluoride in water to determine if this exposure increases the risk of dental fluorosis, finding a relative risk of 1.5 means that people exposed to fluoride in water are 1.5 times more likely to develop dental fluorosis than people who are not exposed to fluoride in water.

Two other relative measures of effect that are particularly relevant to observational studies are the odds ratio (OR) and the hazard ratio (HR). The OR is the ratio of odds of the event or outcome comparing the exposed and control group.[23] This measure of effect can be interpreted similarly to a relative risk (for example, as how many times more likely to have the outcome is the exposed group with respect to the control group) when the frequency of the outcome is low (approximately 10% or less), whereas it should be interpreted as a shift in odds when it is not (for example, as how many times the exposed group has the odds of the control group of having the outcome).[24] Although the OR can be used as the measure of association in all study designs, it is the only measure of effect that can be used in case-control studies.

The HR is a measure of effect that investigators use when they are interested not only in whether an event occurs but also when it occurs. For example, patients with bruxism (exposed group) and healthy patients (control group) can be followed because an implant is placed to determine the time to failure of such implant (outcome). The HR is the risk of the outcome in one group compared with the risk of the outcome in the other group at any specific time during the follow-up period, weighted by the number of patients available for the survival experience.[23] In other words, by using a weighted average of the relative risk, the HR accounts for the fact that some patients (for example, those who already experienced the outcome) were part of the study up to a specific time. Considering this, the interpretation of the HR is similar to that of the relative risk as well.

When authors of a study present their results using relative measures of effect, values closer to 1 (the value at which point the risk or the odds of the event is the same in the exposed group and control group) represent small effects, whereas values further from 1 represent large effects. Once again, how large this magnitude is depends on the outcome of interest.[22]

▸ *How precise was the estimate of the risk?*

The uncertainty in the measure of association, owing to the fact that only a sample of all the population of interest is being observed, usually is described with confidence intervals (CI). A CI is a plausible range of values within which the true value actually will lie given the data observed in a study.[25] The narrower the CI, the more certain the researchers are of the estimate of effect. Similarly to what was described for interpreting the magnitude of the treatment effect, the interpretation of the width of the CI depends on the clinical context.[25]

> **Box 4.4. Your Assessment of the Results of the Observational Study You Identified**
>
> You find that men who have fewer teeth have 1.26 times the odds of having physical complaints (such as pain of upper extremity, tinnitus, and dizziness) than men who have more teeth, and that women who have fewer teeth have 1.18 times the odds of having physical complaints than women who have more teeth. The confidence intervals range from 1.11 to 1.43 for men and 1.06 to 1.32 for women. Your judgment indicates that these numbers represent associations of small magnitude, and that the estimate for men is more precise than that for women (see the Supplemental Table[10] at the end of this chapter for details and explanation). Regarding the outcome mortality, you see that there are no numerical results provided, so you cannot do a critical appraisal of the results.

How Can I Apply the Results to Patient Care?

Ultimately, it is necessary to assess to what extent the results of a study are applicable to a particular context. When evaluating the applicability of articles about harm, you should consider the following factors:

▸ *Were the study patients similar to the patients in my practice?*

To confidently apply the results to your patients, you should ensure that the patients in your practice are similar to those recruited for the study. Clinicians should look to a description of the patients participating in an observational study to determine how similar the study participants are to their own patients. If the characteristics of the included patients are similar to the patients in their practice, clinicians can confidently apply the results. If there is any characteristic that differs, such as age, medical history, or the biology of the exposure on the outcome, clinicians should assess if this difference is reason enough to think that the effect of the intervention would be different in their practice and decide to what extent the results are applicable.[21]

For example, the association between using a hard toothbrush (exposure) and having dental cervical lesions (outcome) may not be the same in a population of patients with a high prevalence of bruxism compared with a population of patients with a low prevalence of this condition. Therefore, the clinician must be careful when applying results from a study that recruited the former patients to the latter.

▸ *Was the follow-up sufficiently long?*

A study must follow up with patients for a period long enough that the exposure could have had an effect on the outcome.[21] For instance, when determining whether chronic rhinosinusitis increases the risk of chronic periodontitis, Keller and colleagues[17] followed up with patients for five years after they had been diagnosed with chronic rhinosinusitis. Clinicians applying the results from this observational study to inform their clinical decisions should assess whether five years is a period long enough to be a contributing factor in the development of chronic periodontitis.

▸ *Is the exposure similar to what might occur in my patient?*

Just like patients' characteristics, the exposure may not be exactly the same in all patients. For example, in the study to determine whether periodontal disease was a risk factor for implant failure,[5] approximately two-thirds of the exposed patients had severe chronic periodontitis. Therefore, clinicians must note if the results presented were for patients with chronic periodontitis, no matter what the severity, when they consider applying the results to patients with moderate chronic periodontitis. When the exposure is an external agent, such as fluoride in water, it is important to consider the dose and duration of the exposure.

▸ *Are there any benefits that offset the risks associated with the exposure?*

Even though risk factors generally are associated with undesirable consequences, they may also be associated with some benefits. For instance, even though having fluoride in water may increase the risk of patients experiencing dental fluorosis, it may decrease the risk of patients experiencing dental caries. It is necessary, therefore, to determine whether it is worthwhile to eliminate potentially harmful exposure. When one of the outcomes is unacceptable and there are no additional benefits from the exposure, this decision is straightforward; however, in many cases, the clinician may need to decide on the balance between the outcome and the potential benefits of the exposure.

> **Box 4.5. Your Assessment of the Applicability of the Observational Study You Identified**
>
> When assessing the applicability of the results, you noted that the patients enrolled in this study belonged to a rural population, which makes them likely to have important differences in aspects such as oral health care and occupation, causing differences between that study population and your clinic population in both exposure and outcome. For the study population, tooth extraction may be one of the few available treatment options, and rehabilitation after the tooth extraction may take different paths when compared with the options available to patients living in an urban area (see the Supplemental Table[10] at the end of this chapter for more details). Because your practice is in a big city, you decide that this evidence is not entirely applicable to your patient.

Conclusion

Observational studies are the best type of study to inform clinical decisions about harm. Critical appraisal skills allow clinicians to optimally use the results of studies to inform their clinical practice. The critical appraisal of observational studies focuses on aspects of risk of bias, the results, and applicability.

Box 4.6. What You Say to Your Patient

Despite the fact that the abstract of the study suggests that the number of teeth is associated with physical complaints, the risk of bias, the moderate magnitude association reported, and the limitations in applicability make you conclude that this evidence is not enough to claim that such an association actually exists and is important enough to worry about. You discuss this with your patient and suggest that he undergo oral rehabilitation because of the other benefits it would have, but you make it clear that this may not be one of the causes of his physical complaints. Even though your patient did not ask, you let him know that there is also not enough evidence to claim that there may be an association between functional tooth number and mortality.

References

1. Brignardello-Petersen R, Carrasco-Labra A, Glick M, Guyatt GH, Azarpazhooh A. "A practical approach to evidence-based dentistry: understanding and applying the principles of EBD." *JADA* 2014;145(11):1105–1107.

2. Chapter 2 of this book was based on Brignardello-Petersen R, Carrasco-Labra A, Booth HA, et al. "A practical approach to evidence-based dentistry: II: how to search for evidence to inform clinical decisions." *JADA* 2014;145(12):1262–1267.

3. Brignardello-Petersen R, Carrasco-Labra A, Glick M, Guyatt GH, Azarpazhooh A. "A practical approach to evidence-based dentistry: III: how to appraise and use an article about therapy." *JADA* 2015;146(1):42–49.

4. Grimes DA, Schulz KF. "An overview of clinical research: the lay of the land." *Lancet* 2002;359(9300):57–61.

5. Levin L, Ofec R, Grossmann Y, Anner R. "Periodontal disease as a risk for dental implant failure over time: a long-term historical cohort study." *J Clin Periodontol* 2011;38(8):732–737.

6. Claus EB, Calvocoressi L, Bondy ML, Schildkraut JM, Wiemels JL, Wrensch M. "Dental x-rays and risk of meningioma." *Cancer* 2012;118(18):4530–4537.

7. Okada T, Ikebe K, Inomata C, et al. "Association of periodontal status with occlusal force and food acceptability in 70-year-old adults: from SONIC Study." *J Oral Rehabil* 2014;41(12):912–919.

8. Grimes DA, Schulz KF. "Cohort studies: marching towards outcomes." *Lancet* 2002;359(9303):341–345.

9. Schulz KF, Grimes DA. "Case-control studies: research in reverse." *Lancet* 2002;359(9304):431–434.

10. Fukai K, Takiguchi T, Ando Y, et al. "Associations between functional tooth number and physical complaints of community-residing adults in a 15-year cohort study." *Geriatr Gerontol Int* 2009;9(4):366–371.

11. Guyatt GH, Straus S, Meade MO, et al. "Therapy." In: Guyatt GH, Rennie D, Meade MO, Cook DJ, editors. *Users' Guide to the Medical Literature: A Manual for Evidence-Based Clinical Practice.* 2nd ed. New York, NY: McGraw-Hill; 2008. p. 67–86.

12. Fletcher R, Fletcher S. "Introduction." In: Fletcher R, Fletcher S, editors. *Clinical Epidemiology: The Essentials.* 4th ed. Baltimore, MD: Lippincott Williams & Wilkins; 2005. p. 1–16.

13. Grimes DA, Schulz KF. "Bias and causal associations in observational research." *Lancet* 2002;359(9302):248–252.

14. Hernan MA, Hernandez-Diaz S, Robins JM. "A structural approach to selection bias." *Epidemiology* 2004;15(5):615–625.

15. Kennedy CC, Jaeschke R, Keitz S, et al. "Tips for teachers of evidence-based medicine: adjusting for prognostic imbalances (confounding variables) in studies on therapy or harm." *J Gen Intern Med* 2008;23(3):337–343.

16. Tripepi G, Jager KJ, Dekker FW, Wanner C, Zoccali C. "Bias in clinical research." *Kidney Int* 2008;73(2):148–153.

17. Keller JJ, Wu CS, Lin HC. "Chronic rhinosinusitis increased the risk of chronic periodontitis: a population-based matched-cohort study." *Laryngoscope* 2013;123(6):1323–1327.

18. Chugal NM, Clive JM, Spangberg LS. "A prognostic model for assessment of the outcome of endodontic treatment: effect of biologic and diagnostic variables." *Oral Surg Oral Med Oral Pathol Oral Radiol Endod* 2001;91(3):342–352.

19. Bernabe E, Vehkalahti MM, Sheiham A, Aromaa A, Suominen AL. "Sugar-sweetened beverages and dental caries in adults: a 4-year prospective study." *J Dent* 2014;42(8):952–958.

20. Chaffee BW, Feldens CA, Vitolo MR. "Association of long-duration breastfeeding and dental caries estimated with marginal structural models." *Ann Epidemiol* 2014;24(6):448–454.

21. Levine M, Ioannidis J, Haines T, Guyatt GH. "Harm (observational studies)." In: Guyatt GH, Rennie D, Meade MO, Cook DJ, editors. *Users' Guide to the Medical Literature: A Manual for Evidence-Based Clinical Practice.* 2nd ed. New York, NY: McGraw-Hill; 2008. p. 363–381.

22. Brignardello-Petersen R, Carrasco-Labra A, Shah P, Azarpazhooh A. "A practitioner's guide to developing critical appraisal skills: what is the difference between clinical and statistical significance?" *JADA* 2013;144(7):780–786.

23. "Glossary." In: Guyatt GH, Rennie D, Meade MO, Cook DJ, editors. *Users' Guide to the Medical Literature: A Manual for Evidence-Based Clinical Practice.* 2nd ed New York, NY: McGraw-Hill; 2008. p. 769–808.

24. Norman G, Streiner D. "Logistic Regression." In: Norman G, Streiner D, editors. *Biostatistics: The Bare Essentials.* 3rd ed. Hamilton, ON, Canada: BC Decker; 2008. p. 159–166.

25. Guyatt GH, Walter S, Cook D, Wyer P, Jaeschke R. "Confidence intervals." In: Guyatt GH, Rennie D, Meade MO, Cook D, editors. *Users' Guides to the Medical Literature: A Manual for Evidence-Based Clinical Practice.* 2nd ed. New York, NY: McGraw Hill; 2008. p. 99–107.

A version of this chapter originally appeared in the February 2015 edition of *JADA* (Volume 146, Issue 2, Pages 94–101. e1). It has been reviewed and updated for accuracy and clarity by the editors of *How to Use Evidence-Based Dental Practices to Improve Your Clinical Decision-Making.*

Supplemental Table. Example of a Critical Appraisal of an Article Regarding Harm*

1. How Serious Is the Risk of Bias?

Were patients similar for prognostic factors that are known to be associated with the outcome (or did statistical adjustment level the playing field)?	Probably yes. Although the tables and text were not completely clear regarding the balance of prognostic factors, the researchers adjusted for the main confounding factors (age, systemic diseases, denture use) when assessing the relationship between functional tooth number and mortality physical complaints. However, there were other prognostic factors, such as socioeconomic level and physical disabilities, for which the researchers did not account.
Were the circumstances and methods for detecting the outcome similar?	Probably yes. It can be inferred from the article that the study authors measured the outcomes (physical complaints and mortality) using the same methods, irrespective of the exposures that a given patient had; however, the authors did not describe this.
Was the follow-up sufficiently complete?	For the outcome mortality, the authors reported having more patients at follow-up (5,684) than at baseline (5,584), which decreased trust in the reporting of the numbers of patients lost to follow-up. There was no information provided regarding the number of patients lost to follow-up, if any, or the reasons for it.

2. What Are the Results?

How strong was the association between exposure and outcome?	The associations between the prognostic factor "number of functional teeth" and the outcome "physical complaints" were reported separately for men (odds ratio [OR] = 1.26) and women (OR = 1.18). These values meant that men who had fewer teeth had 1.26 times the odds of having physical complaints compared with those who had more teeth, and that women who had fewer teeth had 1.18 times the odds of having physical complaints than those who had more teeth. Even though these numbers represented associations of small to moderate magnitude, it is not clear from the article whether they were calculated considering one tooth of difference or more than one tooth. Therefore, it is safer to conclude that the magnitude of the association is small.
	Regarding the outcome mortality, the authors only reported that "Physical complaints were not a significant factor of survival rate of either men or women." However, no numerical data were provided, which made it impossible to appraise these results.
How precise was the estimate of the risk?	The 95% CIs[†] reported by sex were somewhat precise and did not include extreme values. For men, the CI of physical complaints was 1.11 to 1.43, and for women it was 1.06 to 1.32. In both groups, the upper limit of the CI may have reflected an effect that was important in clinical practice; however, in women the lower extreme of the CI represented an association of small magnitude, which made it less precise (in other words, the CI of men represented a moderate association in both extremes, whereas the CI for women represented a small to moderate association. Therefore, the CI for the association in men was more precise).

3. How Can I Apply the Results to My Patient Care?

Were the study patients similar to the patients in my practice?	Probably not. The population in the study seemed to be rural, given that their main economic activity was agriculture. This situation could lead to important differences regarding access to health care services and education if the results were applied to urban populations. On the other hand, a rural population may have had such a different lifestyle compared with urban populations (for example, sedentary or active), modifying completely the health indicators and morbidity and mortality risks.
Was follow-up sufficiently long?	Probably yes. For the outcome of mortality, 15 years seemed to be an appropriately long follow-up so that an association between the number of functional teeth could have had any influence on mortality, at least in older patients. However, depending on the main mechanism of this association considered to be plausible by the clinician, this judgment regarding the length of follow-up could change.
Is the exposure similar to what might occur in my patient?	Probably yes. Tooth loss is a reality in both rural and urban populations. However, it is very likely that rural populations are at higher risk of tooth extraction, with lack of access to restorative or conservative therapies, compared with more urbanized populations. This would cause a limitation in applicability if the population of interest were urban.
Are there any benefits that are known to be associated with exposure?	In this particular type of population (rural), tooth extraction may be the only way to manage extended caries, severe periodontitis, and other conditions. On the other hand, and on the basis of the study results, tooth loss (reduction in the number of functional teeth) would increase the risk of physical complaints, but would not increase the risk of mortality. Therefore, the benefits of the exposure would outweigh the potential harms in patients for whom dental extractions were the only available treatment.

* *Source:* Fukai and colleagues.[10]
† CI = Confidence interval.

Chapter 5. How to Appraise and Use an Article about Diagnosis

Romina Brignardello-Petersen, D.D.S., M.Sc., Ph.D.; Alonso Carrasco-Labra, D.D.S., M.Sc., Ph.D.; Michael Glick, D.M.D.; Gordon H. Guyatt, M.D., M.Sc.; and Amir Azarpazhooh, D.D.S., M.Sc., Ph.D.

Introduction

In the previous chapters in this book, we introduced the process of evidence-based dentistry (EBD)[1] and explained how to search for evidence to inform clinical practice[2] and how to use articles about therapy or prevention[3] and harm.[4] In this chapter, we explain how to use an article to inform clinical decisions regarding questions of diagnosis. We introduce and describe the basic concepts needed to understand diagnostic test studies, and we explain how to use the concepts to appraise such studies critically. In subsequent chapters we will describe how to use other types of study designs.

Box 5.1. Clinical Scenario

During a meeting of the clinicians in your practice, a colleague raises the idea of acquiring a new laser device to help with the diagnosis of caries. This clinician explains that a sales representative described how this device was excellent for detecting noncavitated occlusal carious lesions, and your colleague wants to know your opinion. Because you believe that evidence is necessary to inform this important decision for your practice, you tell your colleague that you need to conduct a literature search and a critical appraisal to inform your opinion.

Clinical Questions of Diagnosis

Dentists face diagnosis questions every day. With most patients, dentists need to use diagnostic tests before they can establish a course of action to follow. In the context of everyday practice, a diagnostic test can refer to any test performed in a laboratory or any information obtained from a medical history or clinical examination that is used to confirm or rule out a specific diagnosis.[5] Dental radiographs are a common diagnostic test used by clinicians in many dental specialties, but other procedures such as performing a vitality test and measuring probing depths can be considered diagnostic tests as well.

When facing diagnosis questions, clinicians need to modify the classic Population, Intervention, Comparison, Outcome (PICO) framework for stating questions. The population is the patients of interest (that is, those to whom we will apply the diagnostic test when there is suspicion of a condition or disease). The intervention is the diagnostic test (that is, the test in which we are interested in learning). The comparison is a test we use as a reference to compare the diagnostic test against—this is called the reference standard (or gold standard).[6] Finally, the outcomes are either the health consequences after using the diagnostic test or the measures that describe the performance of a diagnostic test. Both of these cases are described later in this chapter. Table 5.1 shows examples of diagnostic test questions and their PICO components.

Table 5.1. Examples of Diagnosis Questions and the Population, Intervention, Comparison, Outcome Framework

Clinical Question	Population	Diagnostic Test	Reference Standard	Outcomes
How useful is cone-beam computed tomography at detecting the proximity of third-molar roots with the inferior alveolar nerve?	Patients undergoing third-molar extraction surgery	Cone-beam computed tomography	Direct observation of the inferior alveolar nerve when performing the surgery	True positives, true negatives, false positives, and false negatives
How useful is the oral pathologist's clinical observation for diagnosing an oral mucosal lichen planus?	Patients with oral mucosal lesions compatible with oral mucosal lichen planus	Pathologist's observation	Biopsy plus histologic confirmation	True positives, true negatives, false positives, and false negatives
How useful is the laser fluorescence device for detecting noncavitated occlusal caries lesions extending into the dentin?	Patients who might have a noncavitated occlusal caries lesion extending into the dentin	Laser fluorescence device	Direct observation of the caries lesion after performing an enameloplasty	True positives, true negatives, false positives, and false negatives

What Study Design Best Addresses Questions About Diagnosis?

Clinicians can answer diagnostic questions by conducting studies using one of the following two types of designs: randomized clinical trials and cross-sectional studies. Ideally, a study's investigators would treat a diagnostic test as an intervention. Researchers would randomize patients to receive one of two diagnostic strategies, which for the purposes of this chapter we will call strategy A and strategy B. Clinicians would manage patients according to the results of the test, including providing whatever interventions they think might be appropriate on the basis of test results. Ultimately, they would measure patient-important outcomes in the group whose participants received test strategy A and the group whose participants received test strategy B.

For example, when assessing how useful laser fluorescence is for detecting early interproximal carious lesions, researchers should randomly assign patients to undergo diagnosis with either laser fluorescence or bite-wing radiographs. Then clinicians would treat patients according to the results of the test the patients received, either laser fluorescence or bite-wing radiographs. The investigators would follow up with all patients to determine, for example, how many participants in each group have carious lesions extending into the dentin and what is each participant's need for restorations (outcomes). To date, we have not been able to identify any of these study designs in the dental literature, and therefore, they will not be further covered in this chapter.

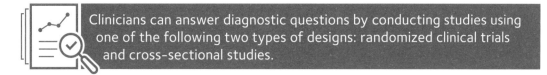

> Clinicians can answer diagnostic questions by conducting studies using one of the following two types of designs: randomized clinical trials and cross-sectional studies.

In studies whose investigators address the accuracy of a diagnostic test, a group of patients undergo both tests (that is, the diagnostic test and the reference standard). The reference standard is considered to be the way to know whether the disease or condition is truly present or absent. The investigators compare the results of the diagnostic test with the reference standard as a way to determine the diagnostic properties of the diagnostic test.

For example, with the aim of assessing the accuracy of thermal and electrical dental pulp tests to diagnose pulp vitality, Villa-Chavez and colleagues[7] conducted the cold, hot, or electrical pulpal tests (three different diagnostic tests) in 110 patients. They used as the reference standard the direct observation of the pulp after opening the pulp chamber, and then they estimated the sensitivity, specificity, predictive values, and accuracy of each of the diagnostic tests by comparing the results with those of the reference standard.

Ideally, clinicians would have available the results of systematic reviews of primary studies addressing test properties. We found that few such systematic reviews have been published in the dental literature. In the absence of reviews, clinicians look to the results of the best single primary diagnostic studies to inform their practice. In this chapter, we address such studies; in subsequent chapters, we will describe how to use systematic reviews.

Critically Appraising a Study Assessing the Properties of a Diagnostic Test to Inform Clinical Decisions

The process of using an article from the dental literature involves three steps: an assessment of the risk of bias, an assessment of the results themselves, and an assessment of the applicability of the results.[9]

How Serious Is the Risk of Bias?

The extent to which a study's results are likely to be correct for the sample of patients enrolled depends on how well the study was designed and conducted.[10] Factors to consider in judging the risk of bias of diagnostic test studies include whether any of the patient's conditions presented a diagnostic dilemma, whether the reference standard was appropriate and independent from the diagnostic test, whether the investigators independently interpreted the results of both tests and did not know the results of the other investigators, and whether all patients underwent both the diagnostic test and the reference standard irrespective of the results of the diagnostic test.[11] Table 5.2[8,12–14] lists questions that address the risk of bias associated with diagnostic tests used in studies and presents examples from the dental literature.

 The process of using an article from the dental literature involves three steps: an assessment of the risk of bias, an assessment of the results themselves, and an assessment of the applicability of the results.[9]

Table 5.2. Examples of the Critical Appraisal of the Validity of the Results of Studies About Diagnosis

Question	Examples	Explanation
Did participating patients present a diagnostic dilemma?	"135 patients (161 impacted teeth) . . . who underwent additional examination by cone-beam CT* because of panoramic features suggesting a close relationship of the tooth root to the mandibular canal were included."[12] "Each surface had to meet one of the three listed criteria to be included in the study: macroscopically intact occlusal fissure that exhibited absolutely no signs of caries; occlusal fissure with a discolored, brown or black area at the clinical examination without cavitation; grey discoloration from the underlying dentin without enamel breakdown."[8]	In both examples, the authors indicated that patients included in the study had characteristics that presented a diagnostic dilemma, such as features suggesting proximity of the third-molar root to the alveolar canal, or occlusal appearances representing a spectrum of patients, ranging from those who seemed healthy to those who seemed diseased. Therefore, in both of these examples, there is a low risk of bias on the basis of this criterion.
Did investigators compare the results of a test with an appropriate, independent reference standard?	"Panoramic and cone-beam CT features were correlated with the intraoperative findings, that is, the presence or absence of the inferior alveolar neurovascular bundle exposure at the time of extraction."[12] "All teeth included in the study underwent endodontic treatment, and the presence or absence of bleeding pulp in the pulp chamber on access was used as a true positive or true negative."[13]	In the first example, the reference standard was the direct observation of the inferior alveolar neurovascular bundle during surgery, which most clinicians would agree is the best method to diagnose proximity of the third-molar roots with the alveolar canal. In the second example, the clinician must judge how appropriate it is that only bleeding was considered as a sign of pulp vitality and whether this may have affected the results of the study. In both cases, the reference standard was independent from the diagnostic test, which was the cone-beam CT scan and thermal tests, respectively.

Question	Examples	Explanation
Were those investigators who interpreted the test and reference standard blinded to the other results?	"LFE[†] scores were analyzed using the manufacturer's cutoff points, taking into account the absence of a histological examination and the in vivo nature of the study. VE[‡] and RE[§] data were analyzed using the ICDAS II[¶] method (Table 5.3), and modified criteria were validated in vivo by the method of . . ."[14]	When the authors described the way in which the tests were interpreted, they did not mention whether this was done by different clinicians or by the same clinician in a blinded fashion. Therefore, clinicians should consider the potential for bias owing to this factor.
Did investigators perform the same reference standard with all patients regardless of the results of the test under investigation?	"The validation method for diagnosis (gold standard) was determined by tissue eradication or enameloplasty using an invasive fissure sealing kit. . . . However, not all fissures could be validated as this is an invasive method. Thus, for ethical reasons, opening of the cavities occurred only in cases when both examiners agreed to the presence of dentin caries."[8]	The authors mentioned not applying the reference standard to some patients, which is not appropriate (that is, it seems likely that the authors assumed that those patients were healthy). There is a risk that the investigators misclassified those patients for whom a substandard reference was used, which could have biased the results. Because this misclassification was done owing to ethical reasons, the clinician should judge how likely it is that bias could have occurred and what the magnitude of this bias could have been.

* CT = computed tomography.
† LFE = laser fluorescence examination.
‡ VE = visual examination.
§ RE = radiographic examination.
¶ ICDAS = International Caries Detection and Assessment System.

Table 5.3. Calculation and Interpretation of Likelihood Ratios*

	Calculation	Interpretation
Likelihood Ratio for Positive Test (LR+)	$\dfrac{\text{Sensitivity}}{1-\text{Specificity}} = \dfrac{0.86}{1-0.89} = 7.81$	When the result of the diagnostic test is positive, the probability of having the disease is high. The exact probability of having the disease depends on the pretest probability and the specific LR+ result.[†]
Likelihood Ratio for Negative Test (LR–)	$\dfrac{1-\text{Sensitivity}}{\text{Specificity}} = \dfrac{1-0.86}{0.89} = 0.16$	When the result of the diagnostic test is negative, the probability of having the disease is low. The exact probability of having the disease depends on the pretest probability and the specific LR– result.[†]

* Described on the basis of numbers from Figure 5.2.
[†] The pretest probability is specific to individual patients and is estimated by the physician on the basis of the patient's medical history and clinical examination results. The shift from pretest to posttest probabilities can be estimated easily using an LR nomogram.[11,17]

▸ *Did participating patients present a diagnostic dilemma?*

Researchers performing diagnostic test studies should select patients who are representative of those to whom the test would be applied in clinical practice. For the results of a diagnostic test to be useful, the results have to discriminate between patients who have and patients who do not have the target condition (for example, in our scenario, the target condition was noncavitated occlusal caries lesion extending to the dentin) when there is a diagnostic dilemma. If patients clearly had the target condition, or clearly did not, there would not be a need to apply the diagnostic test, and in the setting of a study, the accuracy of the test would be overestimated. For example, if a patient had a cavitated mesio-occlusal carious lesion, the clinician would have no need to use a laser fluorescence device to confirm the presence of a carious lesion. In this case where it is so obvious that the carious lesion is present, the device will result in a correct diagnosis most (if not all) of the time. Therefore, for a diagnostic test study to provide a trustworthy assessment of the value of the test, researchers must include patients with early manifestations of the disease, in whom there is doubt regarding the diagnosis, similar to the patients whom clinicians will see in their daily practices.[11]

▸ *Did investigators compare the test with an appropriate, independent reference standard?*

An appropriate reference standard is also a key aspect in assessing the risk of bias of diagnostic test studies. As described previously, clinicians assess the properties of the diagnostic test by comparing the results with the reference standard, which is considered to be the truth.[5,11] Clinicians should consider two aspects when assessing whether the reference standard is appropriate. First, the reference standard should be the test that is accepted most widely as the definitive test to establish a diagnosis.[5] For example, to diagnose oral squamous cell carcinoma, the reference standard is a biopsy and histologic confirmation. Sometimes, however, using the reference standard is only the best available method for diagnosing a target condition instead of the ideal method. For example, to identify a carious lesion extending into the dentin, the reference standard would be to use a combination of clinical signs and radiograph images, as opposed to extracting the tooth and performing a histologic confirmation. Considering this example, the clinician should judge whether the reference standard used in the study is an acceptable way to arrive at a definitive diagnosis.

Second, the reference standard should be independent from the diagnostic test. This means that the diagnostic test should not be part of the reference standard. For example, if the diagnostic test used to diagnose pulpal vital status was a cold test, and the reference standard was a combination of responses from thermal and electrical tests, the diagnostic test would not be independent from the reference standard. Including the test as part of the reference standard leads to overestimation of test accuracy.[11]

▸ *Were the investigators who interpreted the test and reference standard blinded to the other results?*

Another factor to consider when appraising the risk of bias of a diagnostic test study is whether the investigators who interpreted the results of the diagnostic test and the reference standard were blinded to the results of the other test.[11] Many tests, such as radiographs or histologic confirmation, require interpretation by specialists. If the investigators who interpreted the diagnostic test or reference standard were aware of the results of the other test, they may have been influenced subconsciously when they interpreted the results of the diagnostic test or reference standard. Again, the result would be an overestimate of the accuracy of the diagnostic test.

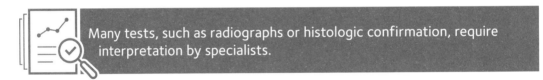

Many tests, such as radiographs or histologic confirmation, require interpretation by specialists.

▸ *Did investigators apply the same reference standard to all patients regardless of the results of the test under investigation?*

Finally, it is important that researchers apply the same reference standard to all patients, irrespective of the results obtained with the diagnostic test.[11] Researchers could overestimate the accuracy of the diagnostic test if only those patients diagnosed as "target positive" by the results of the diagnostic test undergo confirmation with the reference standard, because they would not detect patients wrongly classified as "target negative" by the results of the diagnostic test. For instance, in the example in Table 5.2,[8] some patients who tested negative in the diagnostic test did not undergo the reference standard, and therefore, it is possible that some of these patients had lesions but nevertheless were classified as not having lesions. Again, such misclassification will make the test look more accurate than it really is.

What Are the Results?

After assessing to what extent bias may influence the results of a diagnostic test study, clinicians must review the results to determine how to apply the test in clinical practice. The outcomes of diagnostic test studies reflect the ability of the test to discriminate between target-positive patients and target-negative patients. When thinking about test results, clinicians can consider the probability of being target positive before the test is conducted (pretest probability) and the probability of being target positive after the test is conducted (posttest probability).

The most commonly used measures of accuracy in diagnostic test studies are sensitivity, specificity, probability of having the target condition if the test result is positive (that is, the posttest probability if the test result is positive or—in an unfortunate choice of words—the positive predictive value), probability of having the target condition if the test result is negative (that is, posttest probability if the test result is negative—or, in an even worse choice of terms and meaning—the probability of not having the target condition if the test result is negative [that is, the negative predictive value]), and likelihood ratios. All of these measures are defined and explained below.

Because the diagnostic test is being compared with a reference standard, if the diagnostic test is a yes-no or dichotomous test (either positive or negative, rather than presenting a range of results), patients could be classified correctly as target positive (true positive), correctly classified as target negative (true negative), incorrectly classified as target positive (false positive), and incorrectly classified as target negative (false negative).

Assessments of the accuracy of a diagnostic test are made on the basis of this classification (Figure 5.1). Sensitivity is the capacity of the test to correctly classify target-positive patients, whereas specificity is the ability to correctly classify target-negative patients.[15,16] Posttest probabilities, sometimes referred to as predictive values, reflect the likelihood of patients being target positive in those studies whose investigators used positive and negative tests in the particular sample studied.[16]

Figure 5.1. Outcomes of a Diagnostic Test Study Based on the Relationship between the Results From the Diagnostic Test and the Reference Standard

		Reference Standard	
		Diseased	**Healthy**
Diagnostic Test	**Diseased**	True positive	False positive
	Healthy	False negative	True negative

$$\text{Sensitivity} = \frac{\text{True positive}}{\text{True positive} + \text{False negative}}$$

$$\text{Specificity} = \frac{\text{True negative}}{\text{True negative} + \text{False positive}}$$

$$\text{Posttest probability (if test is positive)} = \frac{\text{True positive}}{\text{True positive} + \text{False positive}}$$

$$\text{Posttest probability (if test is negative)} = 1 - \frac{\text{True negative}}{\text{True negative} + \text{False negative}}$$

Posttest probabilities when test results are positive or negative are what clinicians want to know. Unfortunately, the posttest probabilities reported in a particular study will only be accurate for clinicians' use if their patients have the same pretest probability as the population studied, which likely will be true for only a few patients.

The posttest probability of having the target condition if the test is positive is sometimes referred to as the positive predictive value. Unfortunately, instead of reporting the posttest probability of having the target condition if the test is negative (that is, the intuitive way to think of the situation), the investigators of studies often report the posttest probability of not having the target condition if the test is negative; this is referred to as the negative predictive value.[5,15] Figure 5.2 provides an example of how these outcomes are calculated. Because all of these outcomes are proportions or probabilities, they can range from 0 to 1 (or from 0% to 100%), and thus, values closer to 1 reflect greater accuracy, or a greater posttest probability, of a patient's having the target condition.

The likelihood ratio (LR) is an outcome that helps clinicians moving from a pretest probability to a posttest probability of having the target condition. This number can range from zero to infinity. An LR of 1 indicates that the posttest probability of having the target condition is the same as the pretest probability. In other words, when the LR is 1, the test result has provided no useful information. Large LRs imply large increases in posttest probabilities relative to the pretest probabilities, whereas LRs close to zero imply large decreases in posttest probabilities relative to pretest probabilities.[11,17] As a rule of thumb, LRs higher than 5.0 or lower than 0.2 mean that the diagnostic test is useful for arriving at a diagnosis.[11] Unfortunately, investigators do not commonly report the LR in diagnostic test studies in dentistry; however, it can be

Figure 5.2. Calculation of Diagnostic Test Studies Outcomes

		Reference Standard	
		Diseased	Healthy
Diagnostic Test	Diseased	180	30
	Healthy	20	170

$$\text{Sensitivity} = \frac{180}{180 + 20} = 0.9$$

$$\text{Specificity} = \frac{170}{170 + 30} = 0.85$$

$$\text{Posttest probability (if test is positive)} = \frac{180}{180 + 30} = 0.86$$

$$\text{Posttest probability (if test is negative)} = 1 - \frac{170}{170 + 20} = 0.11$$

calculated easily using the sensitivity and specificity values reported frequently in these studies (Table 5.3[11,17]). After LRs have been calculated, they can be used to move from specific pretest to posttest probabilities by using mathematical formulas, or more easily, graphical tools such as the Fagan nomogram.[17]

In summary, when appraising the results of a diagnostic test study, clinicians should look at sensitivity, specificity, and predictive values, which ideally should be close to 1. Calculating the LR for positive and negative results also can be valuable, although clinicians need to keep in mind the fact that the pretest probabilities differ among patients and individual patients in a clinical practice may not have the same pretest probability as that of the patients in the study.

Box 5.4. Your Assessment of the Results of the Study You Identified

You find that the likelihood ratio (LR) of a positive test is 3.68, which is a somewhat large value and indicates that the test produces moderate shifts from pretest to posttest probabilities. For instance, in a patient with a 40% pretest probability, if the test is positive, the posttest probability is 71%. In addition, the LR negative is 0.09, a small LR that indicates that a negative result with the laser fluorescence test will be helpful for ruling out the presence of caries lesions (see the Supplemental Table[8] at the end of this chapter for more details). For instance, in the same patients with a 40% pretest probability, a negative result of the test would result in a posttest probability of 5.7%. Therefore, you conclude that the laser fluorescence device is accurate for confirming or ruling out the presence of caries lesions.

How Can I Apply the Results to Patient Care?

Finally, it is necessary to assess to what extent the results of a study are applicable to a particular context. The following factors should be considered when evaluating the applicability of results published in articles about diagnosis.

▸ *Will the reproducibility of the test results and its interpretation be satisfactory in my clinical setting?*

First, it is necessary to judge whether the diagnostic test had adequate reproducibility (that is, whether the study yielded the same results when reapplied to the same patient in the study). The investigators of diagnostic test studies often report inter-rater reproducibility, intra-rater reproducibility, or both. These values range from 0 to 1, and values closer to 1 represent better reproducibility. For example, Jablonski-Momeni and colleagues[18] reported that the "intra-class correlation coefficient (ICC) was 0.89" when using a fluorescence-based camera for detecting occlusal carious lesions. This is a high value that makes us confident that, in a study setting, the results of the diagnostic test would be highly reproducible.

Clinicians, however, need to consider whether the test will be equally reproducible in their own clinical setting. Limitations of reproducibility include lack of optimal training or experience in applying the test or interpreting its results, or limitations in the maintenance or calibration of the necessary equipment.

▸ *Are the study results applicable to the patients in my practice?*

If the patients in the study had different characteristics than the patients to whom the results would be applied, the performance of the test could change. A test could have different properties when evaluated in patients with a different mix of disease severity or comorbidities that could confuse the diagnosis.[11] For example, if investigators assessed a diagnostic test for detecting interproximal carious lesions in a population with enamel defects, a clinician can expect that the test would perform differently when used in patients without these defects. Therefore, the clinician should look at the selection criteria and characteristics of the patients included in the study and judge whether they are similar to the patients in their practice.

▸ *Will the test results change my management strategy?*

A third aspect clinicians have to consider when judging the extent to which a test will be useful in their practice is the frequency with which results with LRs far from 1.0 occur. For instance, consider a positive test that has an LR of 1.5 (extremely uninformative) and a negative test that has an LR of 0.1 (leading to large decreases in posttest versus pretest probability). This will be a useful test if the negative result occurs frequently, but not if it is rarely seen.

▸ *Will patients be better off as a result of the test?*

This final point requires clinicians to consider the consequences of applying a diagnostic test.[11] When the consequences of not diagnosing a disease are severe, it is likely that the clinician would want to apply the diagnostic test. The consequences of false-positive and false-negative results should be considered as well. Other considerations include possible adverse effects from having the test if it is invasive as well as taking on the financial cost of the test and addressing issues of convenience and burden. These judgments require clinical expertise.

Conclusion

The investigators of the best studies of diagnostic test accuracy will enroll a population in whom there is genuine uncertainty about the diagnosis, and these investigators will undertake a blinded comparison between the test and a reference standard to patients. The critical appraisal of diagnostic test studies focuses on aspects of risk of bias, results, and applicability. Clinicians should apply these guidelines using their best judgment.

References

1. Brignardello-Petersen R, Carrasco-Labra A, Sash P, Azarpazhooh A. "A practitioner's guide to developing critical appraisal skills: what is the difference between clinical and statistical significance?" *JADA* 2013;144(7):780–786.

2. Chapter 2 of this book was based on Brignardello-Petersen R, Carrasco-Labra A, Booth HA, et al. "A practical approach to evidence-based dentistry: II: how to search for evidence to inform clinical decisions." *JADA* 2014;145(12):1262–1267.

3. Brignardello-Petersen R, Carrasco-Labra A, Glick M, Guyatt GH, Azarpazhooh A. "A practical approach to evidence-based dentistry: III: how to appraise and use an article about therapy." *JADA* 2015;146(1):42–49.e1.

4. Brignardello-Petersen R, Carrasco-Labra A, Glick M, Guyatt GH, Azarpazhooh A. "A practical approach to evidence-based dentistry: IV: how to use an article about harm." *JADA* 2015;146(2):94–101.e1.

5. Fletcher R, Fletcher S. "Diagnosis." In: Fletcher R, Fletcher S, editors. *Clinical Epidemiology: The Essentials.* 4th ed. Baltimore, MD: Lippincott Williams & Wilkins; 2005. p. 35–58.

6. Guyatt GH, Meade MO, Richardson S, Jaeschke R. "What is the question?" In: Guyatt GH, Rennie D, Meade MO, Cook DJ, editors. *Users' Guide to the Medical Literature: A Manual for Evidence-Based Clinical Practice.* 2nd ed. New York, NY: McGraw-Hill; 2008. p. 17–28.

7. Villa-Chavez CE, Patino-Marin N, Loyola-Rodriguez JP, et al. "Predictive values of thermal and electrical dental pulp tests: a clinical study." *J Endod* 2013;39(8):965–969.

8. Costa AM, Paula LM, Bezerra AC. "Use of Diagnodent for diagnosis of non-cavitated occlusal dentin caries." *J Appl Oral Sci* 2008;16(1):18–23.

9. Guyatt GH, Straus S, Meade MO, et al. "Therapy." In: Guyatt GH, Rennie D, Meade MO, Cook DJ, editors. *Users' Guide to the Medical Literature: A Manual for Evidence-Based Clinical Practice.* 2nd ed. New York, NY: McGraw-Hill; 2008. p. 67–86.

10. Fletcher R, Fletcher S. "Introduction." In: Fletcher R, Fletcher S, editors. *Clinical Epidemiology: The Essentials.* 4th ed. Baltimore, MD: Lippincott Williams & Wilkins; 2005. p. 1–16.

11. Furukawa TA, Strauss S, Bucher HC, Guyatt GH. "Diagnostic tests." In: Guyatt GH, Rennie D, Meade MO, Cook D, editors. *Users' Guides to the Medical Literature: A Manual for Evidence-Based Clinical Practice.* 2nd ed. New York, NY: McGraw Hill; 2008. p. 419–438.

12. Tantanapornkul W, Okouchi K, Fujiwara Y, et al. "A comparative study of cone-beam computed tomography and conventional panoramic radiography in assessing the topographic relationship between the mandibular canal and impacted third molars." *Oral Surg Oral Med Oral Pathol Oral Radiol Endod* 2007;103(2):253–259.

13. Jespersen JJ, Hellstein J, Williamson A, Johnson WT, Qian F. "Evaluation of dental pulp sensibility tests in a clinical setting." *J Endod* 2014;40(3):351–354.

14. Sinanoglu A, Ozturk E, Ozel E. "Diagnosis of occlusal caries using laser fluorescence versus conventional methods in permanent posterior teeth: a clinical study." *Photomed Laser Surg* 2014;32(3):130–137.

15. Grimes DA, Schulz KF. "Uses and abuses of screening tests." *Lancet* 2002;359(9309):881–884.

16. Fields MM, Chevlen E. "Screening for disease: making evidence-based choices." *Clin J Oncol Nurs* 2006;10(1):73–76.

17. Fagan TJ. "Letter: nomogram for Bayes theorem." *N Engl J Med* 1975;293(5):257.

18. Jablonski-Momeni A, Heinzel-Gutenbrunner M, Klein SM. "In vivo performance of the VistaProof fluorescence-based camera for detection of occlusal lesions." *Clin Oral Investig* 2014;18(7):1757–1762.

A version of this chapter originally appeared in the March 2015 edition of *JADA* (Volume 146, Issue 3, Pages 184–191. e1). It has been reviewed and updated for accuracy and clarity by the editors of *How to Use Evidence-Based Dental Practices to Improve Your Clinical Decision-Making.*

Supplemental Table. Critical Appraisal of an Article About Diagnosis*

Guide	Explanation
Are the Results Valid?	
Did participating patients present a diagnostic dilemma?	Some of them. Teeth included in the study could be at any stage of the disease, ranging from healthy to decayed appearance. There was a subgroup of healthy teeth that were excluded from the sample after the teeth had been enrolled. In addition, when looking more closely at the proportion of teeth from each category included, the results showed that only teeth with signs of being decayed were included for the assessment of the diagnostic test properties. This indicates that the accuracy of the diagnostic test probably was overestimated.
Did investigators compare the results of the test with an appropriate, independent reference standard?	Yes, the reference standard was fissure eradication or enameloplasty, a method that most clinicians would agree is the best available to diagnose noncavitated carious lesions.
Were the investigators interpreting the test and reference standard blinded to the other results?	Probably not. It is not clear from reading the description of the methods whether the clinicians who applied the different diagnostic tests were the same clinicians who applied all the tests. If the clinicians were the same, then they were not blinded to the results of the other tests, as the clinicians may have recognized the patients they were examining.
Did investigators perform the same reference standard with all patients regardless of the results of the test under investigation?	No, owing to ethical reasons, only patients classified as sick underwent confirmation with the reference standard. This could have resulted in an overestimation of the accuracy of the diagnostic test.
What Are the Results?	
What LRs[†] were associated with the range of possible test results?	The positive LR (that is, LR+) value was 3.68. This means that a positive test result would lead to moderate to low shifts in pretest to posttest probabilities of having noncavitated occlusal carious lesions. The negative LR (that is, LR–) value was not reported by the investigators of this article, but it can be calculated using the sensitivity and specificity values. Because the sensitivity is 0.93 and the specificity is 0.75, the LR– value is 0.09. This means that, when the test is negative, the change from pretest to posttest probability of being healthy would be important, and the disease could be ruled out with more confidence.

Guide	Explanation
How Can I Apply the Results to My Patients' Care?	
Will the reproducibility of the test result and its interpretation be satisfactory in my setting?	Inter-rater and intra-rater reproducibility values ranged from 0.730 to 0.747, which represents substantial agreement according to the criteria followed by the authors. The laser device assessed in this study seems to be easy to use and its results easy to interpret; therefore, it is likely that the study results could be applied to many settings. However, the clinician should assess whether there would be any limitation in his or her practice.
Are the results applicable to the patients in my practice?	The study investigators included permanent molars and premolars with and without apparent carious lesions from 26 patients aged 10 to 13 years. Clinicians should consider whether their patients might have any different features that could alter the performance of the test.
Will the results change my management strategy?	Probably not. The LR shows that the diagnostic test alone would not be enough to confirm or rule out the diagnosis of noncavitated carious lesions.
Will patients be better off as a result of this test?	Probably not. Even though the consequence of not diagnosing a noncavitated carious lesion could be severe, potentially leading to pulp necrosis, the test results were not accurate enough. Conventional methods performed better than the diagnostic test. Therefore, patients are unlikely to benefit from the additional use of this diagnostic test.

* *Source:* Costa and colleagues.[8]
† LR = likelihood ratio.

Chapter 6. How to Use a Systematic Review and Meta-Analysis

Alonso Carrasco-Labra, D.D.S., M.Sc., Ph.D.; Romina Brignardello-Petersen, D.D.S., M.Sc., Ph.D.; Michael Glick, D.M.D.; Gordon H. Guyatt, M.D., M.Sc.; and Amir Azarpazhooh, D.D.S., M.Sc., Ph.D.

In This Chapter:

Knowledge Synthesis and Translation

What Is the Difference Between Narrative and Systematic Reviews?

Why Are Systematic Reviews Considered to Be a Study Design?

Critically Appraising Systematic Reviews to Inform Clinical Decisions

- How Serious Is the Risk of Bias?

- What Are the Results?

Anatomy of a Meta-Analysis

- How Can I Apply the Results to Patient Care?

Conclusion

Introduction

In the previous chapters in this book, we introduced the process of evidence-based dentistry (EBD)[1] and explained how to search for evidence to inform clinical practice[2] and how to use articles about therapy,[3] harm,[4] and diagnosis.[5] In this chapter, we explain how to use a systematic review to answer a clinical question, introduce and describe the basic concepts for understanding the design of a systematic review, and explain how to use these concepts to critically appraise such studies. In addition, readers will learn how to interpret and use the results presented in the systematic review to inform clinical decisions. In a subsequent chapter, we describe how to use evidence-based clinical practice guidelines.

Box 6.1. Clinical Scenario

While working at a clinic in a remote rural location, you meet with a 55-year-old woman who has been referred to you for treatment of open caries on tooth #20, which the referring clinician has diagnosed as having irreversible pulpitis. After conducting a clinical examination, you recommend that the tooth be extracted. The patient asks if she will need to attend many follow-up appointments, because traveling from her home to your clinic is a burden. Among other measures, you decide to minimize your patient's risk of having alveolar osteitis (dry socket) as a postoperative complication. You have been in the habit of prescribing chlorhexidine in cases such as this one; however, you wonder if this medication is actually of any use in decreasing the patient's risk of experiencing dry socket. You consult the Cochrane Library and find a recently published systematic review that addresses this issue.[6]

Knowledge Synthesis and Translation

Keeping updated in knowledge related to any clinical discipline is challenging. According to the Medline (PubMed) Trend Database,[7] more than 30,000 randomized controlled trials (RCTs) were published in 2012. Of these, approximately 1,500 were dental trials. This overwhelming amount of information can be impossible to manage for any health care provider, including dentists. Systematic reviews represent an efficient way to learn about the available evidence for an intervention or exposure.

According to the Cochrane Collaboration,[8] a systematic review is defined as "a review of a clearly formulated question that uses systematic and explicit methods to identify, select, and critically appraise relevant research, and to collect and analyze data from the studies that are included in the review." Like primary observational studies and randomized controlled trials, systematic reviews represent a type of study that requires implementation in a manner that minimizes the risk of bias. If these bias-reducing strategies (that is, the systematic review process) are in place, then readers can trust that the appropriate analysis will provide the best available estimate of the effect of an intervention or exposure.[8]

What Is the Difference Between Narrative and Systematic Reviews?

Authors of many articles published in the dental literature refer to their work as "reviews"; only a small number of these articles, however, are systematic reviews. For this reason, clinicians interested in using review articles must be able to distinguish between narrative and systematic reviews. In narrative reviews, authors discuss one or more aspects related to a particular condition or disease (that is, etiology, diagnosis, prognosis, or therapy and management). Although this type of review may be useful for dental students (and sometimes dentists) who are interested in background information, the failure of authors to systematically collect and process the data makes the conclusions that arise from such articles potentially misleading.[9,10] In contrast, authors of trustworthy reviews use systematic, transparent, and comprehensive methods to retrieve, select, critically appraise, and summarize all the available evidence regarding the effectiveness of an intervention, prognosis, and diagnosis questions. Although it is possible to have systematic reviews that focus on prognosis and diagnosis (and harm) issues, in this chapter, we will focus on therapy (and harm) issues. Table 6.1[11] presents additional details regarding the difference between narrative and systematic reviews.

One of the key limitations of systematic reviews and meta-analyses is that the summary estimates produced are only as trustworthy as the results of the primary studies that inform the review.[12] Thus, the authors of rigorously conducted systematic reviews still may report low-quality evidence that warrants only weak inferences.

Table 6.1. Differences Between Narrative and Systematic Reviews*

Characteristic	Narrative Reviews	Systematic Reviews
Clinical Question of the Review	Seldom reported, or addressed several broad questions	Focused question specifying population, intervention or exposure, and outcome
Search for Primary Studies	Seldom reported; if reported, not comprehensive	Comprehensive search of databases of evidence resources
Selection of Primary Studies	Seldom reported; if reported, often biased sample of studies	Explicit selection criteria for primary studies
Assessment of the Risk of Bias of Primary Studies	Seldom reported; if reported, not usually systematic	Risk of bias of primary studies assessed
Methods to Summarize the Included Studies' Results	Usually qualitative nonsystematic summary	Synthesis is systematic (qualitative or quantitative)

* Reprinted with permission of *JAMA* and The JAMA Network from Guyatt and colleagues.[11]

Why Are Systematic Reviews Considered to Be a Study Design?

Systematic reviews and evidence-based clinical practice guidelines represent the most valuable documents that can inform clinical decision-making.[12] Review authors start by defining a clear and focused research clinical question in a way that is similar to that described in a previous chapter in this book, which addressed the framing of a question using the Population, Intervention, Comparison, Outcomes (PICO) approach (see Chapter 2).[2] The components of this PICO question correspond with the eligibility criteria outlined by the authors of the studies that are included in the review. For example, if the author specifies the population of interest as patients after tooth extraction, eligible studies must enroll such patients, and only such patients. Authors of systematic reviews should present clearly the population or type of patients, clinical intervention or exposure of interest, the comparator for such an intervention, and the selection of patient-important outcomes.

After specifying all these criteria, review authors should describe their methods in a protocol that, ideally, should be published or made available to users. Many reasons support the authors' explicit and transparent declaration of selection criteria and methods in systematic reviews. Investigators have described important discrepancies between the selection of outcomes and methods when comparing them before the review starts with after the final manuscript is published.[13] Ideally, reviewers will describe the comprehensive search for all the available (published and unpublished) evidence they have conducted. As a result of this process, researchers should screen a set of references at the level of title and abstract first, and complete study reports later, to establish whether the articles retrieved meet the selection criteria (Figure 6.1[11]). Having identified all the relevant studies, reviewers abstract data that are related to the studies' characteristics, risk of bias assessment, and results. Finally, they summarize the evidence and assess the quality of the body of evidence[14] (Figure 6.1[11]).

Figure 6.1. Process of Conducting a Systematic Review

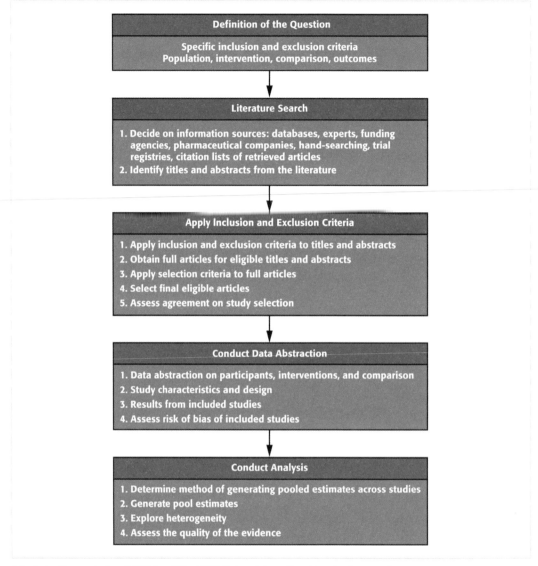

Definition of the Question

Specific inclusion and exclusion criteria
Population, intervention, comparison, outcomes

Literature Search

1. Decide on information sources: databases, experts, funding agencies, pharmaceutical companies, hand-searching, trial registries, citation lists of retrieved articles
2. Identify titles and abstracts from the literature

Apply Inclusion and Exclusion Criteria

1. Apply inclusion and exclusion criteria to titles and abstracts
2. Obtain full articles for eligible titles and abstracts
3. Apply selection criteria to full articles
4. Select final eligible articles
5. Assess agreement on study selection

Conduct Data Abstraction

1. Data abstraction on participants, interventions, and comparison
2. Study characteristics and design
3. Results from included studies
4. Assess risk of bias of included studies

Conduct Analysis

1. Determine method of generating pooled estimates across studies
2. Generate pool estimates
3. Explore heterogeneity
4. Assess the quality of the evidence

Adapted with permission of *JAMA* and The JAMA Network from Guyatt and colleagues.[11]

Box 6.2. The Study You Found

You consult the Cochrane Library and find a recently published systematic review whose authors aimed to assess the effects of local interventions on the prevention and treatment of alveolar osteitis (dry socket) after tooth extraction.[6] Reviewers identified 21 trials, and among these, the authors of 18 trials, which included more than 2,370 participants, reported results related to the prevention of dry socket. Although the authors of the systematic review reported more than 10 intrasocket interventions, they found limited evidence for each of these interventions.

Critically Appraising Systematic Reviews to Inform Clinical Decisions

As described in previous chapters, the process of using an article from the dental literature involves assessing the risk of bias, assessing the results, and assessing the applicability of the results.[14]

How Serious Is the Risk of Bias?

The probability that the results of a systematic review are correct depends on whether reviewers identified, retrieved, selected, critically appraised, and summarized all the relevant studies.[15] Table 6.2[16–21] presents examples of the aspects to consider when assessing the risk of bias of a systematic review.

Table 6.2. Examples Illustrating Critical Appraisal of the Risk of Bias of a Systematic Review

Aspect	Example	Explanation
How Serious Is the Risk of Bias?		
Did the review include explicit and appropriate eligibility criteria?	"Population: orthodontics patients of either gender, any age and any type of malocclusion (Class I, II, or III) and crowding treated with fixed multibrackets on both arches with first molars included over the course of at least 12 months. Intervention: only in vivo studies on human participants involving different oral health motivation strategies, and oral and dental hygiene techniques and procedures. Comparison: no treatment or usual care (the gold standard), or inactive control. Outcome: as a primary outcome, the following data were evaluated: plaque index (PI) and gingival index (GI). The secondary outcomes considered were carious lesions and the presence/absence of white spot."[16]	The reviewers aimed to answer the question "whether it is clinically possible to avoid plaque increase and prevent permanent teeth lesions in orthodontics patients, and in particular, whether prophylactic procedures performed by the dental hygienist are efficacious in reducing the risk of demineralization in orthodontics patients fitted with multibracket appliances."[16] The authors described in detail the different components of the research question. These components represented the selection criteria (inclusion and exclusion criteria). The criteria described here reflect a sensitive and focused question. The outcomes defined in the review were classified as patient-important.

Aspect	Example	Explanation
Was the search for relevant studies detailed and exhaustive?	"Relevant articles were identified in any language by searching MEDLINE (from 1950 to September 2011), the entire Cochrane Library (from 1990 to September 2011), CINAHL Nursing database (from 1980 to September 2011), and the University of Michigan School of Dentistry 'Dentistry and Oral Sciences' database (EBSCO host) (from 1990 to September 2011). The final search update was performed on September 19, 2011. To locate potentially relevant studies in MEDLINE, exploded MeSH terms and key words were used to generate sets for the following themes: 1) periodontitis; 2) preterm birth; and 3) scaling treatment. We then found the intersection of these terms using the Boolean term 'AND.' This basic approach was modified as necessary to search each electronic database (see Supplementary Appendix 3 in the online *Journal of Periodontology*). No limitations in the search were used."[17] "To locate unpublished trials, *ClinicalTrials.gov* and abstracts of scientific conferences were searched (National Academy for State Health Policy's 20th Annual State Health Policy Conference, Denver, Colorado, October 15, 2007; 34th National Conference of Indian Society of Periodontology, Dharwad, India, December 3-5, 2009)."[17]	Study authors described every electronic database consulted during the review searching process along with the time frame searched. They also reported the complete search strategy in an online supplementary appendix. Additionally, they searched for "grey literature" in clinical trials registries and conference abstracts. One potential limitation in this review is that the authors did not include EMBASE among the included databases for searching. Some reports show that systematic reviews including one or a few databases have a higher risk of missing relevant studies compared with reviews including all of the most important databases.[18] The Cochrane Handbook suggests that at least MEDLINE, EMBASE, and CENTRAL should be consulted in every systematic review search.[19] The possibility that this review missed some relevant primary studies cannot be discarded.

Aspect	Example	Explanation
Were the primary studies of high methodological quality?	"We performed the risk-of-bias assessment for the included trials by using the Cochrane Collaboration's risk-of-bias assessment tool, which incorporated six domains: random sequence generation, allocation concealment, masking, completeness of outcome data, risk of selective outcome reporting and risk of other bias."[20] "Using the predetermined six domains for risk-of-bias assessment, we determined three of the five RCTs* to have a high risk of bias, whereas we judged two to have an unclear risk of bias and none to have a low risk of bias."[20]	The authors presented a table with a detailed description of the risk of bias for each of the included studies. This analysis showed that most of the studies were judged as having a high risk of bias. The rest of the studies were classified as unclear risk of bias, which raises concerns about the review results.
Were assessments of studies reproducible?	"Two review authors (Anneli Ahovuo-Saloranta [AAS] and Helenab Forss [HF]) independently carried out the selection of papers on the basis of the title, keywords and abstract, and the decisions about eligibility. The full text of every study considered for inclusion was obtained. If the information relevant to the inclusion criteria was not available in the abstract or if the title was relevant but the abstract was not available, the full text of the report was obtained."[21] "Data were extracted independently and in duplicate by two review authors (AAS, HF) using a previously prepared data extraction form. The extraction form was pilot-tested independently by two review authors in the previous review version (AAS, Anne Hiiri [AH]) with a sample of studies to be included."[21]	Authors provided an exhaustive explanation about all the methodological steps involved to minimize the risk of mistakes and arbitrary judgments during the review process. Critical steps were conducted independently and in duplicate.

* RCT = randomized controlled trial.

▸ *Did the review present explicit and appropriate eligibility criteria?*

Consider a systematic review whose author intended to pool the effects of all antibiotics for treating all types of maxillofacial infections. Now, consider a review whose author intended to pool the results of the effects of fluoride varnishes for reducing the incidence of carious lesions in children and adolescents. Clearly, the first review would be excessively broad in its scope; equally clearly, the second review would be satisfactorily narrow.

What makes a systematic review question too broad? There are pathophysiological and microbiological aspects of maxillofacial infections and of the mechanism of the action of antibiotics that suggest that treatment effects vary across different types of patients (different types of infections) and interventions (different types of antibiotics).[11] A single pooled estimate summarizing all these data would not be applicable to any specific group of patients or any specific antibiotic, and therefore, it would be of no use to the clinician. On the other hand, results from the more focused question are likely to be similar for children and adolescents, for the available fluoride varnishes, and for the available approaches to identifying carious lesions. This similarity of effect across patients, interventions, and outcomes is what legitimizes the single pooled estimate of effect.[22]

▸ *Was the search for relevant studies exhaustive?*

Secure estimates of treatment effect require a comprehensive search for eligible studies. Unfortunately, even a search that includes all the relevant electronic databases may be insufficient. If the authors of a primary study selectively report and publish research results according to the effect (that is, studies favoring the intervention get published; studies that are negative do not), then the results will be a systematic overestimate of effect (that is, publication bias).[23,24] One way to mitigate this issue is to search and include "gray literature," which includes documents such as dissertations, conference abstracts, personal correspondence, records of studies' methods and results found in investigators' file drawers or on their hard drives, and policy documents.[25,26]

When assessing whether the search strategy was comprehensive, users should focus on which databases the authors consulted, and whether the systematic reviewers restricted their search to resources published in one particular language or to only published reports.[19] To learn more about specific databases and their characteristics, please refer to Chapter 2.

▸ *Did the primary studies have a low risk of bias?*

The credibility of the results of a systematic review is as only as great as the credibility of the primary studies included. Assessing credibility requires addressing the risk of bias associated with the primary studies that are included in a systematic review. Studies assessed as having a high risk of bias may overestimate treatment effects by up to 150%.[27] Thus, when the risk of bias across the included studies is low, credibility increases.[11] Different primary study designs are associated with specific sets of potential biases and, consequently, require reviewers to follow specific checklists to assess the risk of bias. For issues of therapy addressed in RCTs, key considerations include concealment of randomization, blinding, and minimizing loss to follow-up.[5,28]

▸ *Were the selection and assessment of primary studies reproducible?*

All of the steps that investigators perform when conducting a systematic review (Figure 6.1[11]) are susceptible to error.[29] For example, including and excluding studies from the review requires making judgments. Likewise, errors may occur during data abstraction: for example, investigators found that 20 of 34 reviews conducted by the Cochrane Cystic Fibrosis and Genetic Disorders Group included errors such as miscalculations and misinterpretation of data from the primary studies.[30] Independent, duplicate eligibility review and data extraction with resolution of discrepancies can minimize such errors and other unintentional or subconscious bias.[31] Hence, users of systematic reviews should check whether reviewers conducted screening and data extraction in duplicate.

Box 6.3. Your Assessment of the Risk of Bias of the Systematic Review You Identified

The authors of the systematic review[6] defined a sufficiently narrow range of patients, interventions, comparisons, and outcomes, and they conducted a comprehensive search that included reviewing several databases and making an effort to retrieve unpublished data. The reporting by authors of the included primary studies was poor, and the result was that risks of bias ratings were often assessed as unclear risk of bias. Finally, the authors of the systematic review reported that they selected the studies in duplicate and independently. Thus, you determine that this systematic review has a low to moderate risk of bias, and you proceed to read and interpret the results.

What Are the Results?

After assessing the magnitude of the risk of bias, clinicians must consider the results—in particular, the magnitude and the precision of the treatment effects—and the implications for patient care. Industry-supported reviews of drugs tend to rank eligible studies at low risk of bias, and although showing similar treatment effects, provide more positive and favorable conclusions when compared with Cochrane systematic reviews on the same clinical question. Ideally, clinicians should look for reviews that are not funded by industry, and if none of these are available, clinicians should exercise skepticism about authors' inferences.[32]

Evaluating the results of a systematic review requires clinicians to consider whether effects are similar across studies, as well as to assess the magnitude and the precision of the effects. Table 6.3[20,21] presents examples of assessments of the results of systematic reviews in dentistry.

Table 6.3. Examples Illustrating Critical Appraisal of the Results of a Systematic Review

Example	How Large Was the Treatment Effect?	How Precise Was the Estimate of Treatment Effect?
"Additionally, we noted no significant difference in the likelihood of clinical success between primary molars treated with MTA* and primary molars treated with FC† (RR‡= 1.01; 95 percent confidence interval [CI], 0.98-1.05) during the observational period, as shown in Figure 6.2."[20]	The RR for having clinical success when treating a primary molar with MTA compared with FC is 1.01. This represents a 1% increase in the probability of experiencing clinical success using MTA compared with FC. The point estimate in this case is suggesting that there may be no difference between using MTA compared with FC to have clinical success when treating primary molars.	The 95% CI§ (0.98-1.05) suggested in the lower limit a 2% reduction on clinical success when using MTA compared with FC. On the other hand, the upper limit shows that there may be a 5% increase in clinical success when using MTA compared with FC. Since it is likely that both extremes of the CI would lead to a similar clinical action (because both an RR reduction of 2% and 5% can be considered clinically irrelevant to prefer MTA over FC), this CI could be considered to be precise or narrow enough.
"Resin-based sealant compared with no sealant: Compared to control without sealant, second or third or fourth generation resin based sealants prevented caries in first permanent molars in children aged 5 to 10 years (at 2 years of follow-up odds ratio (OR) 0.12, 95% confidence interval (CI) 0.07 to 0.19."[21] "If we were to assume that 40% of the control tooth surfaces were decayed during 2 years of follow-up (400 carious teeth per 1,000), then applying a resin-based sealant will reduce the proportion of the carious surfaces to 6.25% (95% CI 3.84% to 9.63%); similarly if we were to assume that 70% of the control tooth surfaces were decayed (700 carious teeth per 1,000), then applying a resin-based sealant will reduce the proportion of the carious surfaces to 18.92% (95% CI 12.28% to 27.18%)."[21]	Authors presented relative and absolute estimates. In relative terms, resin-based sealants compared with no sealant reduce the proportion of carious surfaces by 88%. Although this seems to be a large treatment effect, this should be expressed in absolute terms to appreciate the complete benefit of sealants. When expressing the results in absolute terms using as reference two hypothetical populations, one with 40% (moderate baseline risk) of tooth surfaces decayed and another one with 70% (high baseline risk), use of resin-based sealants reduces this proportion to 6.25% and 18.92%, respectively. In both populations, the effect seems to be large and clinically relevant.	Authors presented CIs for both relative and absolute estimates. In relative terms, using resin-based sealants compared with no sealant shows an impressive 93% reduction in the proportion of carious surfaces in its lower limit. The upper limit still suggests a large treatment effect of 81% reduction in the outcome. Since both extremes are showing clinically relevant and large treatment effects, the CI is precise or narrow enough. In absolute terms, for the moderate risk population, the CI shows a reduction from a baseline risk of 40% to 3.8% in the lower limit and 9.6% in the upper limit. This large reduction in absolute terms in both extremes of the CI suggests that these results are precise. For the high-risk population, the lower limit of the CI shows a reduction from a 70% baseline risk to 12.3% in the lower limit and 27.2% in the upper limit. Both extremes suggest a large treatment effect. This CI also can be considered precise enough.

* MTA = mineral trioxide aggregate.
† FC = formocresol.

‡ RR = relative risk.
§ CI = confidence interval.

▸ *Were the results similar from study to study?*

Systematic reviewers collect data on characteristics of the eligible studies, particularly related to patients, interventions, exposures, comparisons, and outcomes measures. The results of primary studies may differ, and variation in these characteristics may be responsible for the differences. When results differ and remain unexplained, the reader's confidence in the pooled estimates should decrease. The following list offers four ways to assess whether the results of primary studies are sufficiently similar to maintain confidence in the pooled summary estimate[11]:

- The point estimates (that is, the estimates of treatment effect): these estimates should be similar among trials; the more they differ, the greater the concern regarding inconsistency.

- The overlapping of the confidence intervals (CIs): the more overlap across CIs, the less the concern regarding inconsistency.

- The statistical test for heterogeneity (χ^2): this test assesses whether the point estimates of the individual study results are the same (relative risk [RR] study 1 = RR study 2 = RR study 3). The lower the P value, the more the concern regarding inconsistency (increasing concern as the P value decreases below 0.1, 0.05, 0.01, or 0.001).

- The I^2 statistic: this estimate represents the percentage of heterogeneity in effect estimates across trials owing to real variability between them.[33] As a rule of thumb, I^2 values higher than 50% may represent large heterogeneity.

The greater the heterogeneity identified, the more compelling the need for reviewers to explore possible explanations for between-study variability. Ideally, reviewers will, before looking at the data, have generated a priori possible explanations of heterogeneity in the as-yet unknown study results. If heterogeneity remains unexplained, the confidence in the estimates of effect (quality of the evidence) decreases[34] (Figure 6.2[35-38]).

▸ *What are the overall results of the review?*

Sometimes systematic reviewers are not able to conduct a meta-analysis to obtain a single estimate of the effect across all the included studies. Reasons include incomplete outcome reporting, as well as substantial differences across patients, interventions, and outcomes. In situations in which it is not possible or appropriate to conduct a meta-analysis, reviewers present results of individual studies in tables.

Often, however, reviewers are able to conduct a meta-analysis and present a pooled estimate that represents the weighted average effect of the intervention under study. Pooled estimates (that is, the meta-analysis result) are usually expressed in the same way as the results from primary studies. For dichotomous outcomes (such as the presence of any carious lesion or the occurrence of an infection event), clinicians will find RR, RR reduction, risk difference, or odds ratios (OR). For continuous outcomes, like probing depth, quality of life, and the amount of trismus, reviewers may use mean difference or standardized mean difference.[5]

Each trial's results contribute a particular "weight" of data to the final pooled estimate. The results of trials whose investigators described a small number of events have less weight compared with the results of trials whose investigators described a large number of events. If the authors of studies report the same outcome of interest but using different units, the results still can be pooled and presented in standard deviation (SD) units (for example, a standardized mean difference of 0.5 means that the treatment intervention effect in comparison with the control is 0.5 SD).

To learn where to find the primary studies' point estimates and the pooled (summary) estimate in a meta-analysis, readers should refer to Figure 6.2.[35-38]

Figure 6.2. Meta-Analysis on the Effect of Initiating Brushing with Fluoride Toothpaste after Age of Two Years versus before Age of Two Years on the Development of Fluorosis

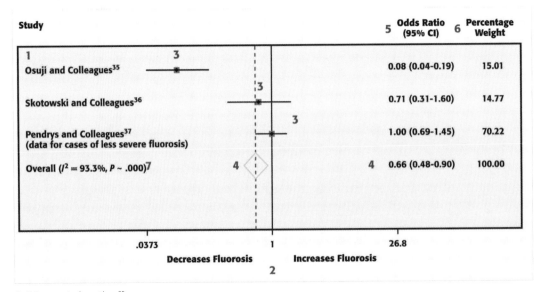

1. Primary study author.[35]
2. Line of no effect.
3. Study point estimate and 95% confidence interval.[35-37]
4. Pooled (summary) estimate.
5. Exact point estimate and confidence intervals (CI).
6. Weight of each included study.
7. Statistical test and estimates to assess heterogeneity.

Adapted with permission of *The Journal of the American Dental Association* from Wright and colleagues.[38]

Anatomy of a Meta-Analysis

In general, a forest plot (that is, the figure reporting a standard meta-analysis) has the following components:

- study identifier, which can be the name of the study author, as well as the year of publication or the name of the study;

- vertical line of no effect (in other words, when there is no difference between the two groups under comparison, the point estimate lies on this line);

- point estimate and 95% CI for each primary study;

- pooled (summary) estimate, which corresponds with the vertical component of the diamond, and its 95% CI, which corresponds to the horizontal component of the diamond;

- measure of association used and exact point estimates and CIs of each primary study, in numbers;

- weight of each included study, expressed as a percentage;

- statistical test and I^2 statistic of heterogeneity.

Figure 6.2[35-38] illustrates these elements in a meta-analysis.

Consider the following clinical question: To avoid fluorosis, should children initiate brushing with fluoride toothpaste before or after two years of age? A recently published systematic review included a meta-analysis of three primary studies that showed a 34% reduction in the development of fluorosis when brushing after age two (OR = 0.66; 95% CI, 0.48-0.90).[38] Figure 6.2[35-38] shows a forest plot presenting the review results.

▸ *How precise were the results?*

Every meta-analysis should provide a point estimate and a CI. A CI can be defined as a plausible range of values within which the true effect actually lies.[39] Thus, the CI expresses the degree of uncertainty around the point estimate. Narrow CIs represent precise results (that is, a large number of participants or events), whereas wide CIs represent imprecise results (that is, a small number of participants or events).

To determine whether the CI is too wide, clinicians should focus on both boundaries of the CI and judge what these boundaries are suggesting, either including or excluding any important benefit or harm.[39] For example, a systematic review that summarized the role of antibiotic prophylaxis for preventing inflammatory complications after tooth extraction showed that the use of this intervention both preoperatively and postoperatively slightly increases the risk of complications by 9% (RR = 1.09; 95% CI, 0.40-2.94).[40] However, the lower boundary of the CI suggests a 60% reduction in complications, whereas the upper limit shows an increase in the risk of having complications of 194%. Because CI boundaries include appreciable benefit and important harm, the evidence leaves clinicians with uncertainty regarding the effect of the intervention: the evidence is consistent with major benefit, has no effect at all, or has appreciable harm. Therefore, this CI is imprecise (that is, too wide).

Consider another example from the same review assessing the effect of preoperative antibiotic prophylaxis on the outcome "local sign of infection." The meta-analysis that included seven studies showed a 71% reduction in this outcome (RR = 0.29; 95% CI, 0.15-0.54). The CI indicates what can be considered an appreciable benefit in both limits. The boundary consistent with the largest plausible treatment effect suggests a reduction of 85% (1.00-0.15) and the upper limit shows a 46% reduction in local signs of infection (1.00-0.54). At either extreme of the CI, the intervention seems to be highly effective. Hence, this CI is sufficiently precise.[40] To learn where to find in the forest plot of a meta-analysis the primary studies' and pooled (summary) estimates' 95% CI, see Figure 6.2.[35–38]

▸ *What is the overall quality of the evidence (also known as confidence in the estimate of effect)?*

The Grading of Recommendations Assessment, Development, and Evaluation (GRADE) Working Group is an international collaboration created in the year 2000 with the purpose of developing a common, sensible, and transparent approach to rating quality of evidence and grading strength of recommendations (*www.gradeworkinggroup.org*). GRADE defines quality of the evidence in the context of a systematic review as "the extent of confidence that an estimate of effect is correct."[41] Clinicians need to learn not only about the best estimates of an intervention's benefits and harmful consequences but also what is the quality or certainty of these estimates. In the GRADE approach, evidence from RCTs starts as high-quality evidence. However, the following five factors can decrease the certainty in the estimates from high to moderate, low, or very low[42]:

- Risk of bias of the included studies[43]

- Inconsistency of the results across studies[34]

- Indirectness of the identified evidence compared with the review's research question components[44]

- Imprecision of the results of the primary studies[45]

- Suspicion of publication bias[46]

Review authors should explore each of these factors and present their findings in the results, discussion, and conclusion sections of the manuscript (Table 6.4). For example, the quality of the evidence can be moderate for the outcome "alveolar osteitis," which means that the investigators are moderately confident that the estimates of effect calculated are close to the truth. On the other hand, for the same intervention, a single investigator or a group of investigators can have low-quality evidence for the outcome "adverse effect," which means that the investigators are extremely uncertain about the estimate for this outcome. Clinicians may proceed differently when the reviewers assess all included patient-important outcomes as high or at least moderate quality evidence, as compared with when the quality is low or very low. Examples of systematic reviews in dentistry that have used the GRADE approach are published by the Cochrane Oral Health Group and others.[47–49]

Table 6.4. Grading of Recommendations Assessment, Development, and Evaluation Approach to Assess the Quality of the Evidence in Systematic Reviews of Randomized Controlled Trials

Issue – Randomized Trials Start High but Move Down Because of Serious Issues Related to:	Criteria
Risk of bias[43]	• Randomization • Allocation concealment • Blinding • Lost to follow-up • Selective outcome reporting
Imprecision[45]	• Confidence intervals are too wide • Small number of participants and events
Indirectness[44]	• Included studies showing differences from the clinical review question regarding the population, intervention, comparison, and outcomes included
Inconsistency[34]	• Presence of heterogeneity among the included studies identified analyzing the similarities between point estimates, overlap of confidence intervals, and statistical methods to detect heterogeneity (χ^2 test and I^2 estimate)
Publication bias[46]	• Asymmetry of the funnel plot • No comprehensive searching methods • Small sample size trials • All trials industry funded • All included studies showing positive and "hard to believe" treatment effects

Box 6.4. Your Assessment of the Results of the Systematic Review You Identified

The authors of the systematic review of interventions for preventing alveolar osteitis (dry socket)[6] reported that moderate quality evidence suggests that the use of chlorhexidine rinse reduces the risk of experiencing alveolar osteitis by 42% (relative risk [RR] = 0.58; 95% confidence interval [CI], 0.43-0.78).[2] The CI suggests an appreciable benefit associated with the use of chlorhexidine at both the lower and upper limit (that is, a 57% reduction and a 22% reduction). Regarding the heterogeneity of the included studies, individual study point estimates are similar and the CIs overlap widely. The P value of the χ^2 test for heterogeneity was .36 and the I^2 estimate was 6%, indicating that heterogeneity was low. In summary, the results of the systematic review suggest a potentially large reduction in the risk of experiencing alveolar osteitis when patients use chlorhexidine rinse, with a precise CI and negligible heterogeneity across studies (Figure 6.3[50-53]).

Figure 6.3. Meta-Analysis on the Effect of Chlorhexidine Rinse versus Placebo for Preventing Dry Socket (Alveolar Osteitis)[50-53]

Study or Subgroup	Chlorhexidine Rinse n/N	Placebo n/N	Risk Ratio M-H, Random, 95% CI	Weight	Risk Ratio M-H, Random, 95% CI
Delilbasi and Colleagues,[50] 2002	13/62	14/59		18.5%	0.88 (0.45-1.72)
Hermesch and Colleagues,[51] 1998	25/136	40/135		40.0%	0.62 (0.40-0.96)
Larsen,[52] 1991	12/144	28/134		20.3%	0.40 (0.21-0.75)
Ragno and Szkutnik,[53] 1991	10/40	20/40		21.2%	0.50 (0.27-0.93)
Total (95% CI)	382	368		100.0%	0.58 (0.43-0.78)

Total events: 60 (chlorhexidine rinse), 102 (placebo)

Heterogeneity: $\tau^2 = 0.01$; $\chi^2 = 3.20$, $df = 3$, $P = .36$; $I^2 = 6\%$

Test for overall effect: $z = 3.66$ ($P = .00026$)

Test for subgroup differences: Not applicable

0.5 0.7 1 1.5 2

Favors Chlorhexidine Rinse   Favors Placebo

CI = confidence interval. M-H = Mantel Haenszel.
Reproduced with permission of John Wiley and Sons from Daly and colleagues.[6]

How Can I Apply the Results to Patient Care?

In these final steps, clinicians should determine to what extent the results of the review are applicable to their particular context. Factors to consider when applying the results are whether the investigators considered all of the patient-important outcomes, what is the overall quality of the evidence (also known as the certainty of the estimates of effect), and whether the benefits are worth the costs and potential risks.

▸ *Were all patient-important outcomes considered?*

A patient-important outcome means that if the patient were informed that only this outcome would change after implementing an intervention, the patient still would consider receiving the intervention even if it is associated with adverse effects, additional burdens, or costs.[54,55] Frequently, authors of systematic reviews do not report the negative aspects (that is, adverse effects) of the intervention under study.[56,57] Users should avoid making clinical decisions without considering all patient-important outcomes. The costs and burdens of the intervention also can be considered patient-important outcomes. Other examples of patient-important outcomes in dentistry are tooth loss, pain, swelling, and tooth discoloration.

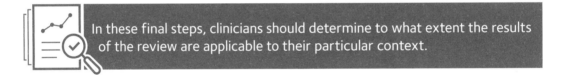

In these final steps, clinicians should determine to what extent the results of the review are applicable to their particular context.

▶ *Are the likely treatment benefits worth the potential harms and costs?*

Finally, when considering whether to administer a treatment to patients, the clinicians should consider the balance in benefits and harms, costs,[11] and treatment burdens.[58] Patients' values and preferences (that is, "the collection of goals, expectations, predispositions, and beliefs that people have for certain decisions and their potential outcomes"[59]) and the context of the health system are required for conducting this balancing exercise.

Box 6.5. Your Assessment of the Applicability of the Systematic Review You Identified

The review of alveolar osteitis[6] presents all the important outcomes. Although the systematic review's authors did not summarize adverse effects by using meta-analysis, they did include a tabulated, per-study report that showed that the most common adverse events were reversible alterations of taste and staining of teeth. The benefit of a 42% reduction in the risk of experiencing alveolar osteitis, which was supported by evidence of moderate quality, seems to outweigh the mild adverse events.

Conclusion

The amount of scientific information available for clinical decision-making is overwhelming. Clinicians interested in informing their decisions with the best available evidence need high-quality and comprehensive summaries. When conducted and reported appropriately, systematic reviews provide crucial information for informing clinical decisions. However, the results of systematic reviews are susceptible to bias. Clinicians need to critically appraise systematic reviews to inform their decisions adequately. The critical appraisal of a systematic review focuses on aspects of risk of bias, results, and applicability. Clinicians should apply these guidelines to achieve the best possible results for their own practices.

Box 6.6. What You Say to Your Patient

After having a discussion with your patient, you prescribe the use of a chlorhexidine rinse and plan to check the patient's progress at the follow-up appointment. A week after you extracted the tooth, you determine that the patient has no signs of developing alveolar osteitis, and that the surgical wound is healing well. The Supplemental Table[6] at the end of this chapter presents a detailed description of the critical appraisal conducted in this review.

References

1. Brignardello-Petersen R, Carrasco-Labra A, Glick M, Guyatt GH, Azarpazhooh A. "A practical approach to evidence-based dentistry: understanding and applying the principles of EBD." *JADA* 2014;145(11):1105–1107.

2. Chapter 2 of this book was based on Brignardello-Petersen R, Carrasco-Labra A, Booth HA, et al. "A practical approach to evidence-based dentistry: II: how to search for evidence to inform clinical decisions." *JADA* 2014;145(12):1262–1267.

3. Brignardello-Petersen R, Carrasco-Labra A, Glick M, Guyatt GH, Azarpazhooh A. "A practical approach to evidence-based dentistry: III: how to appraise and use an article about therapy." *JADA* 2015;146(1):42–49.e1.

4. Brignardello-Petersen R, Carrasco-Labra A, Glick M, Guyatt GH, Azarpazhooh A. "A practical approach to evidence-based dentistry: IV: how to use an article about harm." *JADA* 2015;146(2):94–101.e1.

5. Brignardello-Petersen R, Carrasco-Labra A, Glick M, Guyatt GH, Azarpazhooh A. "A practical approach to evidence-based dentistry: V: how to appraise and use an article about diagnosis." *JADA* 2015;146(3):184–191.e1.

6. Daly B, Sharif MO, Newton T, Jones K, Worthington HV. "Local interventions for the management of alveolar osteitis (dry socket)." *Cochrane Database Syst Rev* 2012;12:CD006968.

7. Corlan AD. "Medline trend: automated yearly statistics of PubMed results for any query; 2004." Available at: http://dan.corlan.net/medline-trend.html. Accessed February 17, 2015.

8. Green S, Higgins J. "Glossary." *Cochrane Handbook for Systematic Reviews of Interventions* 4.2.5. The Cochrane Collaboration; 2005. Available at: *http://community.cochrane.org/glossary*. Accessed March 3, 2015.

9. Oxman AD, Guyatt GH. "The science of reviewing research." *Ann N Y Acad Sci* 1993;703:125–133.

10. Antman EM, Lau J, Kupelnick B, Mosteller F, Chalmers TC. "A comparison of results of meta-analyses of randomized control trials and recommendations of clinical experts: treatments for myocardial infarction." *JAMA* 1992;268(2):240–248.

11. Guyatt GH, Jaeschke R, Prasad K, Cook DJ. "Summarizing the evidence." In: Guyatt GH, Rennie D, Meade MO, Cook DJ, editors. *Users' Guide to the Medical Literature: A Manual for Evidence-Based Clinical Practice.* 2nd ed. New York, NY: McGraw-Hill; 2008. p. 523–542.

12. Murad MH, Montori VM, Ioannidis JP, et al. "How to read a systematic review and meta-analysis and apply the results to patient care: users' guides to the medical literature." *JAMA* 2014;312(2):171–179.

13. Page MJ, McKenzie JE, Kirkham J, et al. "Bias due to selective inclusion and reporting of outcomes and analyses in systematic reviews of randomised trials of healthcare interventions." Cochrane Database Syst Rev 2014;10:MR000035.

14. Guyatt GH, Rennie D, Meade MO, Cook DJ, editors. *Users' Guide to the Medical Literature: A Manual for Evidence-Based Clinical Practice.* 2nd ed. New York, NY: McGraw-Hill; 2008.

15. Fletcher R, Fletcher S. "Introduction." In: Fletcher R, Fletcher S, editors. *Clinical Epidemiology: The Essentials.* 4th ed. Baltimore, MD: Lippincott Williams & Wilkins; 2005.

16. Migliorati M, Isaia L, Cassaro A, et al. "Efficacy of professional hygiene and prophylaxis on preventing plaque increase in orthodontic patients with multibracket appliances: a systematic review." *Eur J Orthod.* 2015;37(3):297-307.

17. Kim AJ, Lo AJ, Pullin DA, Thornton-Johnson DS, Karimbux NY. "Scaling and root planing treatment for periodontitis to reduce preterm birth and low birth weight: a systematic review and meta-analysis of randomized controlled trials." *J Periodontol* 2012;83(12):1508–1519.

18. Song F, Eastwood AJ, Gilbody S, Duley L, Sutton AJ. "Publication and related biases." *Health Technol Assess* 2000;4(10):1–115.

19. Lefebvre C, Manheimer E, Glanville J. "Chapter 6: Searching for studies." In: Higgins JPT, Green S, editors. *Cochrane Handbook for Systematic Reviews of Interventions,* Version 5.1.0 (updated March 2011). The Cochrane Collaboration; 2011. Available at: *www.cochrane-handbook.org.* Accessed February 17, 2015.

20. Marghalani AA, Omar S, Chen JW. "Clinical and radiographic success of mineral trioxide aggregate compared with formocresol as a pulpotomy treatment in primary molars: a systematic review and meta-analysis." *JADA* 2014;145(7):714–721.

21. Ahovuo-Saloranta A, Forss H, Walsh T, et al. "Sealants for preventing dental decay in the permanent teeth." Cochrane Database Syst Rev 2013;3:CD001830.

22. Marinho VC, Worthington HV, Walsh T, Clarkson JE. "Fluoride varnishes for preventing dental caries in children and adolescents." Cochrane Database Syst Rev 2013;7:CD002279.

23. Montori V, Ioannidis J, Guyatt GH. "Advanced topics in systematic reviews: reporting bias." In: Guyatt GH, Rennie D, Meade MO, Cook DJ, editors. *Users' Guide to the Medical Literature: A Manual for Evidence-Based Clinical Practice.* New York, NY: McGraw-Hill; 2008.

24. Hopewell S, McDonald S, Clarke MJ, Egger M. "Grey literature in meta-analyses of randomized trials of health care interventions." Cochrane Database Syst Rev 2007;2:MR000010.

25. Auger CP. *Information Sources in Grey Literature* (Guides to Information Sources). 4th ed. London: Bowker Saur; 1998.

26. McAuley L, Pham B, Tugwell P, Moher D. "Does the inclusion of grey literature influence estimates of intervention effectiveness reported in meta-analyses?" *Lancet* 2000;356(9237):1228–1231.

27. Kunz R, Oxman AD. "The unpredictability paradox: review of empirical comparisons of randomised and non-randomised clinical trials." *BMJ* 1998;317(7167):1185–1190.

28. Higgins JPT, Altman DG, Sterne JAC. "Chapter 8: Assessing risk of bias in included studies." In: Higgins JPT, Green S, editors. *Cochrane Handbook for Systematic Reviews of Interventions,* Version 5.1.0 (updated March 2011). The Cochrane Collaboration; 2011. Available at: *www.cochrane-handbook.org.* Accessed February 17, 2015.

29. Ford AC, Guyatt GH, Talley NJ, Moayyedi P. "Errors in the conduct of systematic reviews of pharmacological interventions for irritable bowel syndrome." *Am J Gastroenterol* 2010;105(2):280–288.

30. Jones AP, Remmington T, Williamson PR, Ashby D, Smyth RL. "High prevalence but low impact of data extraction and reporting errors were found in Cochrane systematic reviews." *J Clin Epidemiol* 2005;58(7):741–742.

31. Buscemi N, Hartling L, Vandermeer B, Tjosvold L, Klassen TP. "Single data extraction generated more errors than double data extraction in systematic reviews." *J Clin Epidemiol* 2006;59(7):697–703.

32. Jorgensen AW, Hilden J, Gotzsche PC. "Cochrane reviews compared with industry supported meta-analyses and other meta-analyses of the same drugs: systematic review." *BMJ* 2006;333(7572):782.

33. Higgins JP, Thompson SG, Deeks JJ, Altman DG. "Measuring inconsistency in meta-analyses." *BMJ* 2003;327(7414):557–560.

34. Guyatt GH, Oxman AD, Kunz R,et al; GRADE Working Group. "GRADE guidelines: 7: Rating the quality of evidence–inconsistency." *J Clin Epidemiol* 2011;64(12):1294–1302.

35. Osuji OO, Leake JL, Chipman ML, Nikiforuk G, Locker D, Levine N. "Risk factors for dental fluorosis in a fluoridated community." *J Dent Res* 1988;67(12):1488–1492.

36. Skotowski MC, Hunt RJ, Levy SM. "Risk factors for dental fluorosis in pediatric dental patients." *J Publ Health Dent* 1995;55(3):154–159.

37. Pendrys DG, Haugejorden O, Bårdsen A, Wang NJ, Gustaven F. "The risk of enamel fluorosis and caries among Norwegian children: implications for Norway and the United States." *JADA* 2010;141(4):401–414.

38. Wright JT, Hanson N, Ristic H, et al. "Fluoride toothpaste efficacy and safety in children younger than 6 years: a systematic review." *JADA* 2014;145(2):182–189.

39. Guyatt GH, Walter S, Cook DJ, Wyer P, Jaeschke R. "Confidence intervals." In: Guyatt GH, Rennie D, Meade MO, Cook DJ, editors. *Users' Guide to the Medical Literature: A Manual for Evidence-Based Clinical Practice.* New York, NY: McGraw-Hill; 2008.

40. Lodi G, Figini L, Sardella A, et al. "Antibiotics to prevent complications following tooth extractions." Cochrane Database Syst Rev 2012;11:CD003811.

41. Guyatt GH, Oxman AD, Kunz R, Vist GE, Falck-Ytter Y, Schunemann HJ; GRADE Working Group. "What is 'quality of evidence' and why is it important to clinicians?" *BMJ* 2008;336(7651):995–998.

42. Balshem H, Helfand M, Schunemann HJ, et al. "GRADE guidelines: 3. Rating the quality of evidence." *J Clin Epidemiol* 2011;64(4):401–406.

43. Guyatt GH, Oxman AD, Vist G, et al. "GRADE guidelines: 4. Rating the quality of evidence–study limitations (risk of bias)." *J Clin Epidemiol* 2011;64(4):407–415.

44. Guyatt GH, Oxman AD, Kunz R, et al; GRADE Working Group. "GRADE guidelines: 8. Rating the quality of evidence–indirectness." *J Clin Epidemiol* 2011;64(12):1303–1310.

45. Guyatt GH, Oxman AD, Kunz R, et al. "GRADE guidelines 6: rating the quality of evidence–imprecision." *J Clin Epidemiol* 2011;64(12):1283–1293.

46. Guyatt GH, Oxman AD, Montori V, et al. "GRADE guidelines: 5. Rating the quality of evidence–publication bias." *J Clin Epidemiol* 2011;64(12):1277–1282.

47. Brignardello-Petersen R, Carrasco-Labra A, Araya I, et al. "Is adjuvant laser therapy effective for preventing pain, swelling, and trismus after surgical removal of impacted mandibular third molars? A systematic review and meta-analysis." *J Oral Maxillofac Surg* 2012;70(8):1789–1801.

48. Carrasco-Labra A, Brignardello-Petersen R, Yanine N, Araya I, Guyatt G. "Secondary versus primary closure techniques for the prevention of postoperative complications following removal of impacted mandibular third molars: a systematic review and meta-analysis of randomized controlled trials." *J Oral Maxillofac Surg* 2012;70(8):e441–e457.

49. Ebrahim S, Montoya L, Busse JW, Carrasco-Labra A, Guyatt GH. "Medically Unexplained Syndromes Research Group. The effectiveness of splint therapy in patients with temporomandibular disorders: a systematic review and meta-analysis." *JADA* 2012;143(8):847–857.

50. Delilbasi C, Saracoglu U, Keskin A. "Effects of 0.2% chlorhexidine gluconate and amoxicillin plus clavulanic acid on the prevention of alveolar osteitis following mandibular third molar extractions." *Oral Surg Oral Med Oral Pathol Oral Radiol Endod* 2002;94(3):301–304.

51. Hermesch CB, Hilton TJ, Biesbrock AR, et al. "Perioperative use of 0.12% chlorhexidine gluconate for the prevention of alveolar osteitis: efficacy and risk factor analysis." *Oral Surg Oral Med Oral Pathol Oral Radiol Endod* 1998;85(4):381–387.

52. Larsen PE. "The effect of a chlorhexidine rinse on the incidence of alveolar osteitis following the surgical removal of impacted mandibular third molars." *J Oral Maxillofac Surg* 1991;49(9):932–937.

53. Ragno JR, Szkutnik AJ. "Evaluation of 0.12% chlorhexidine rinse on the prevention of alveolar osteitis." *Oral Surg Oral Med Oral Pathol* 1991;72(5):524–526.

54. Akl EA, Briel M, You JJ, et al. "LOST to follow-up Information in Trials (LOST-IT): a protocol on the potential impact." *Trials* 2009;10:40.

55. Brignardello-Petersen R, Carrasco-Labra A, Shah P, Azarpazhooh A. "A practitioner's guide to developing critical appraisal skills: what is the difference between clinical and statistical significance?" *JADA* 2013;144(7):780–786.

56. Norris SL, Moher D, Reeves BC, et al. "Issues relating to selective reporting when including non-randomized studies in systematic reviews on the effects of healthcare interventions." *Research Synthesis Methods* 2013;4(1):36–47.

57. Page MJ, McKenzie JE, Forbes A. "Many scenarios exist for selective inclusion and reporting of results in randomized trials and systematic reviews." *J Clin Epidemiol* 2013;66(5):524–537.

58. Andrews JC, Schunemann HJ, Oxman AD, et al. "GRADE guidelines 15: Going from evidence to recommendation-determinants of a recommendation's direction and strength." *J Clin Epidemiol* 2013;66(7):726–735.

59. Guyatt GH, Prasad K, Schünemann HJ, Jaeschke R, Cook DJ. "How to use a patient management recommendation." In: Guyatt GH, Rennie D, Meade MO, Cook DJ, editors. *Users' Guide to the Medical Literature: A Manual for Evidence-Based Clinical Practice.* New York, NY: McGraw-Hill; 2008.

A version of this chapter originally appeared in the April 2015 edition of *JADA* (Volume 146, Issue 4, Pages 255–265. e1). It has been reviewed and updated for accuracy and clarity by the editors of *How to Use Evidence-Based Dental Practices to Improve Your Clinical Decision-Making.*

Supplemental Table. Example of Critically Appraising a Systematic Review.*

1. How Serious Is the Risk of Bias?	
1a. Did the review include explicit and appropriate eligibility criteria?	Yes. The authors described in detail the type of participants, interventions, comparisons, outcome measures, and characteristics of the types of studies to include in the review. (See criteria for considering studies for this review section.)
1b. Was the search for relevant studies detailed and exhaustive?	Yes. Review authors searched MEDLINE, EMBASE, CENTRAL, and the Cochrane Oral Health Group registry. There was no restriction by language of publication, and they also searched for unpublished data by means of contacting investigators, experts, and other organizations. These searches were complemented by screening the reference lists of the identified studies. Finally, a complete description of the search strategy and search terms was provided in the article.
1c. Were the primary studies of high methodological quality?	Probably not. Using the Cochrane risk of bias tool, authors reported that only 30% of the included RCTs[†] appropriately concealed the allocation sequence. In addition, only 25% of the studies implemented appropriate strategies for blinding participants, personnel, and outcome assessors.
1d. Were the selection and assessments of studies reproducible?	Yes. Both screening of title and abstract and full text were conducted independently and in duplicate. The data extraction process was conducted in the same way. A flowchart describing the number of references at every stage of the study also was provided.
2. What Are the Results?	
2a. Were the results similar from study to study?	Regarding the heterogeneity of the included studies, the point estimates seemed to align relatively close to each other, and the confidence intervals showed large overlapping. The P value of the χ^2 test for heterogeneity (yes-no test) was 0.36, which did not allow rejecting the hypothesis that the estimates of the primary studies were the same. The I^2 estimate was only 6%, which was consistent with the previous findings of the analysis of heterogeneity. In summary, heterogeneity seemed negligible across included studies.
2b. What are the overall results of the review?	The meta-analysis including four RCTs showed that the use of chlorhexidine rinse reduced the risk of having alveolar osteitis (dry socket) in 42% of patients (relative risk = 58%). This represents a large treatment effect on reducing the incidence of the outcome.

2c. How precise were the results?	The 95% confidence interval suggests an appreciable benefit at both the lower and upper limit (95% confidence interval, 0.43-0.78) with a 57% reduction in the lower limit and a 22% reduction on the outcome in the upper limit. Because both extremes show that the intervention provides important benefits, the results are precise.
2d. What is the overall quality of the evidence? (Also known as certainty on the estimates of effect)	The quality of the evidence for the outcome presence of alveolar osteitis (dry socket) was moderate owing to serious issues of risk of bias that were described in the section on risk of bias of this critical appraisal. For the outcome adverse events, the quality of the evidence was low owing to serious issues of risk of bias and inconsistency.

3. How Can I Apply the Results to my Patient Care?

3a. Were all patient-important outcomes considered?	Probably yes. For the prevention of alveolar osteitis (dry socket), reviewers considered the proportion of participants presenting with dry socket within one week post-treatment as the main outcome for effectiveness. In addition, authors collected data on any reported adverse event in the included studies.
3b. Are the benefits worth the costs and potential risks?	Yes. The benefit is clinically relevant measured in patient-important outcomes. Although some adverse events were reported—taste disturbance and stained tooth—these are reversible and considered by many patients as tolerable to prevent the occurrence of alveolar osteitis. Chlorhexidine rinse is an inexpensive medication.

Conclusion: The results of the systematic review are likely to be correct, although there is some concern about the risk of bias of the included studies. The magnitude of effect shows a large reduction in the incidence of alveolar osteitis (dry socket) when using chlorhexidine rinse in a preventive way. The applicability assessment shows that this intervention can be implemented with a minimum burden to patients at a reasonable cost and with no severe adverse effects.

* *Source:* Daly and colleagues.[6]
† RCT = randomized controlled trial.

Chapter 7. How to Use Patient Management Recommendations from Clinical Practice Guidelines

Alonso Carrasco-Labra, D.D.S., M.Sc., Ph.D.; Romina Brignardello-Petersen, D.D.S., M.Sc., Ph.D.; Michael Glick, D.M.D.; Gordon H. Guyatt, M.D., M.Sc.; Ignacio Neumann, M.D., M.Sc., Ph.D.; and Amir Azarpazhooh, D.D.S., M.Sc., Ph.D.

In This Chapter:

Evidence-Based Clinical Practice Guidelines

Structured Process of Developing Management Recommendations

Where to Find Clinical Practice Guidelines

Critically Appraising Patient Management Recommendations

Conclusion

Introduction

In previous chapters of this book, we provided an overview of evidence-based clinical practice,[1] explained how to search for[2] and critically appraise articles about therapy,[3] harm,[4] and diagnosis,[5] and described how to use systematic reviews.[6] In this chapter, we define clinical practice guidelines, describe the process of developing guidelines and the basic components of a recommendation, and provide a structure for determining the trustworthiness of recommendations about patient management included in clinical practice guidelines.

Box 7.1. Clinical Scenario

You meet with a 63-year-old edentulous patient who was referred to your practice for full-mouth rehabilitation with dental implants. During the physical examination, the patient mentions that he has a prosthetic hip joint implant, which was placed five years ago. Although you are aware that for many years the standard of care was to provide antibiotic prophylaxis to patients with joint implants before performing invasive dental procedures, you also know that this practice has been questioned in recent years. The patient, who has received antibiotic prophylaxis routinely for dental procedures since having his joint replacement, is skeptical about proceeding without a prophylactic regimen. When planning the patient's dental implant surgery, you decide to consult the available recommendations about the use of antibiotic prophylaxis in patients with prosthetic joints and share with your patient the available evidence on this matter.

Evidence-Based Clinical Practice Guidelines

According to the Institute of Medicine[7] of the National Academies, clinical practice guidelines are "statements that include recommendations intended to optimize patient care that are informed by a systematic review of evidence and an assessment of the benefits and harms of alternative care options." Although the authors of evidence-based guidelines follow a systematic process to identify, select, assess, and summarize evidence, they rely on the consensus of a group of decision makers, also known as a guideline panel. After reviewing the evidence, the panel typically recommends a specific course of action on the basis of the implications for those who may be affected by the recommendation. The panel's mission is to interpret the available evidence and to consider the clinical context in which the recommendations will be applied.

Because of differences in clinical contexts and in clinicians' attitudes toward benefits and harms, members of various guideline panels might evaluate the same body of evidence but not necessarily make the same recommendations. For example, there are major discrepancies between the recommendations formulated by guideline panels from the American Heart Association (AHA)[8] and the National Institute for Health and Care Excellence (NICE)[9] regarding the use of antibiotic prophylaxis for preventing infective endocarditis in patients who are at risk for developing this condition and who are undergoing invasive dental procedures. In 2008, both of these guideline panels[8,9] conducted rigorous systematic reviews that showed similar results. Although the AHA recommended the use of prophylaxis for patients with particular cardiac conditions, NICE recommended against its use in all patients, regardless of the perceived susceptibility of the patient to develop infective endocarditis. In this case, AHA guideline panelists placed a higher value on the potential benefit of the intervention than the adverse events and cost, whereas NICE panelists considered that the risk and cost of antibiotic prophylaxis outweighed the minimal benefits of administering the intervention.

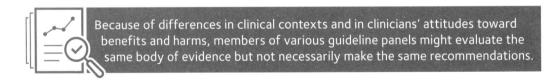

Because of differences in clinical contexts and in clinicians' attitudes toward benefits and harms, members of various guideline panels might evaluate the same body of evidence but not necessarily make the same recommendations.

Structured Process of Developing Management Recommendations

Decision-making is ubiquitous in clinical practice. Consciously or unconsciously, clinicians weigh the potential short- and long-term benefits and harms, burden of the treatment, and costs associated with alternative courses of action to arrive at a decision consistent with the patient's best interest.[10] By consulting guidelines whose authors have documented in a systematic manner both the evidence and the rationale for specific recommendations, clinicians can make sound decisions about clinical options for typical patients.

The process of developing recommendations begins when an institution or an organization defines a health care problem as a priority and initiates a call to develop guidelines to address the health care problem. After defining the scope of the guideline (for example, focusing on primary, secondary, or tertiary care) and the target audience (for example, dentists or other health care professionals who contribute to the management of oral conditions), the institution or organization selects a panel of experts and charges the panel with the task of defining the questions the guideline will answer. These questions include details about patients, clinical options (that is, one or more courses of action), and target outcomes. Using the questions, the panel (which may be expanded to include other collaborators such as information specialists and clinical epidemiologists) undertakes systematic searches of the literature to identify the highest quality available evidence, arrive at the best estimates of benefits and harms, and assess their certainty or confidence in those estimates. On the basis of evidence summaries generated from this process, the panel formulates and grades the strength of the recommendations. After producing and publishing the guideline, the panel can monitor its implementation and update the guideline when new evidence emerges (Figure 1).[10,11]

Figure 7.1. The Process of Developing and Updating Clinical Guidelines

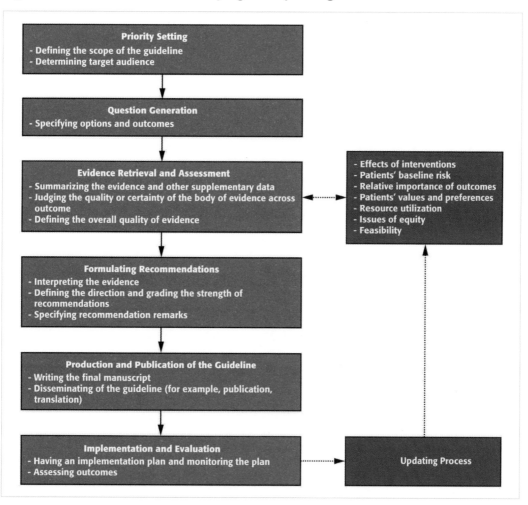

Where to Find Clinical Practice Guidelines

Specific databases presenting full versions or brief summaries of evidence-based clinical practice guidelines are available (see Chapter 2). For example, by using the Trip database (*www.tripdatabase.com*), clinicians can find references to guidelines, which are organized according to the region in which they were developed, and links to full texts of guidelines. Databases that provide summaries of guidelines relevant to dentistry include the National Guideline Clearinghouse (*www.guideline.gov*) and the American Dental Association (ADA) Center for Evidence-Based Dentistry (*http://ebd.ADA.org/en/evidence*).

Box 7.2. The Clinical Practice Guideline You Found

You discover that in 2012, the American Academy of Orthopedic Surgeons (AAOS) and the American Dental Association (ADA) guideline panel[12] conducted a systematic review to inform practitioners about the use of antibiotic prophylaxis in patients with prosthetic joints who required invasive dental procedures, and accordingly, formulated a recommendation. In 2014, the ADA Council on Scientific Affairs formed a new guideline panel with the mission of reformulating and further clarifying the 2012 recommendation.[12,13] This guideline panel[13] updated the systematic review from 2012,[12] focusing on outcomes important to patients and therefore disregarding the evidence about surrogate outcomes (for example, bacteremia). The panel formulated the new recommendation using the ADA's system to assess the level of certainty and strength of the recommendation. Because you want to use the most updated document to select the course of action to take with your patient, you decide to review the ADA recommendation that was published in January 2015[13] on this topic.

Critically Appraising Patient Management Recommendations

Regardless of whether the recommendations address preventive, diagnostic, or therapeutic interventions, clinicians need to determine the extent to which a clinical practice guideline provides trustworthy recommendations.

Are the Recommendations Clear and Comprehensive?

Optimal recommendations use a standardized format that clearly describes the suggested course of action, which alternatives were considered, and to which group of patients and under what specific clinical circumstances the recommendations apply.[14]

Clinicians should only follow guidelines when dealing with "typical" patients because exceptions can arise. For example, a clinician should amend all recommendations regarding antibiotics or anesthetics if a patient is allergic to a particular drug. Also, if a clinician is determining the course of action in the case of a patient who might need antibiotic prophylaxis before undergoing dental procedures, for example, the clinician should consider whether the patient has had a prior joint infection or an immune deficiency.

The extent to which guidelines should address the more common of the atypical or unusual clinical situations is a matter for the guideline panel to consider. For example, the authors of clinical guidelines may face criticism for failing to address the likelihood of multimorbidity, which commonly occurs in patients in a clinical practice.

In whatever way a panel decides to address atypical or unusual clinical situations, it is likely that they will find it impossible to foresee all the idiosyncratic situations that could arise in patient care. This is one reason that following clinical guidelines should not supersede following a clinician's judgment; instead, clinical guidelines should provide the sort of guidance that, it is hoped, will apply to most or even nearly all of the situations that typically confront clinicians. Therefore, clinicians should anticipate that guidelines will address a broad range of patients, including most of the kinds of patients that a clinician is likely to see. Guidelines that do not do this provide only limited assistance for clinical care.

▸ *Is the recommended intervention clear and actionable?*

Sometimes recommendations are too vague to provide a clear course of action to clinicians. For example, consider the following recommendation: In children, teenagers, or young adults undergoing cancer treatment—"if any invasive dental procedure is required, this should be undertaken by either a consultant or specialist pediatric dentist as appropriate."[15] Although this recommendation attempts to inform clinicians about the type of dental professional to whom they should refer a cancer patient who requires an invasive dental procedure, it fails to be specific, referring to this professional as a "consultant" (any dental professional in any specialty can be classified as a consultant). In addition, the recommendation provides two options (consultant or specialist pediatric dentist) without offering clear guidance about when or how to choose either option. An additional limitation is the use of the expression "as appropriate," without providing additional information about how clinicians should determine what is and what is not appropriate. Another issue that may influence clinicians' ability to act on a recommendation is a potential discrepancy between the intended population or type of patients that the panel members defined and the type of patient a clinician has in the dental chair. The credibility of recommendations is lower when the guideline panel's definition of the patients is vague or when the patients are different from the ones the clinician wants to apply the recommendations to.

Another example is provided in the guideline addressing the prevention of orthopedic implant infection in patients undergoing dental procedures, which was developed by the American Academy of Orthopedic Surgeons (AAOS) and the ADA in 2012.[12] The authors declared, "We are unable to recommend for or against the use of topical oral antimicrobials in patients with prosthetic joint implants or other orthopedic implants undergoing dental procedures," and graded the recommendation as "inconclusive."[12,16] Clinicians interested in using topical oral antimicrobials in this type of patient would find no guidance from the AAOS and ADA guideline[12] and, forced to rely on their own resources (in situations in which they perhaps cannot spend the time nor have the skills to make their own assessment of the relevant evidence), could become understandably frustrated. In contrast, a guideline by the ADA Council on Scientific Affairs[13] states the following: "In general, for patients with prosthetic joint implants, prophylactic antibiotics are not recommended prior to dental procedures to prevent prosthetic joint infection."[13] In this case, a clear course of action is defined (although it would be optimal if the recommendation were worded so that it is clearly a recommendation against prophylaxis, such as, "We recommend against the use of prophylaxis," omitting the potentially frustrating qualification "In general" that suggests that there are exceptions that the recommendation has not specified).

▸ *Is the alternative clear?*

Many times, for a particular clinical problem, clinicians may use a range of potentially effective treatments. When formulating recommendations, the guideline panel should state explicitly what options they considered. If the alternative course of action is not stated clearly, the recommendation remains ambiguous. For example, consider the following recommendation: "Advise adults that use of sucrose-free polyol (xylitol only or polyol combinations) chewing gum for 10 to 20 minutes after meals may reduce incidence of coronal caries."[17] Should clinicians advise patients to use chewing gum for 10 to 20 minutes after meals as opposed to not chewing gum at all, or when toothbrushing is not possible, or in addition to toothbrushing? This recommendation is unclear about whether chewing gum can replace toothbrushing or whether it should be considered an adjuvant measure to reduce the risk of coronal caries. Moreover, it is unclear whether clinicians simply should provide patients with information or encourage use of the gum. Recommendation statements should be clear and complete enough to be used and interpreted without the need to read the full text of the guideline.

▸ *Were all the relevant outcomes important to patients explicitly considered?*

For any recommendation, the guideline panel should determine the balance between the benefits and the harms. This balance depends on the outcomes that were identified as being relevant for decision-making. Clinicians assessing the trustworthiness of recommendations should judge whether the panel considered all patient-important outcomes. A patient-important outcome is an outcome for which—even if it were the only outcome improved by treatment—the patient still would consider receiving the intervention, in the face of some adverse effects, costs, and burden.[18,19]

Examples of patient-important outcomes in dentistry include having a prosthetic joint infection after undergoing an invasive dental procedure, oral health–related quality of life, tooth loss, pain, trismus, aesthetic issues, or dental implant failure. Surrogate outcomes may not be considered to be important individual outcomes, but they are associated with patient-important outcomes. Unfortunately, the effects of interventions on surrogates do not guarantee beneficial effects on the associated patient-important outcomes.[20] Surrogate outcomes in dentistry include bacteremia after an invasive dental procedure, levels of pocket probing depth, clinical attachment level, and bleeding on probing.[21] When guideline panels use surrogate outcomes to determine the balance between benefits and harms, the resulting recommendations are less credible than when the guideline panel bases recommendations on patient-important outcomes.

Was the Recommendation Made on the Basis of the Best Current Evidence?

Guideline panelists formulating recommendations should use the best available current evidence. Clinicians using recommendations should focus on the methodology of the systematic review(s) conducted to identify, select, assess, and summarize the relevant evidence. To determine the credibility of this process, users of clinical guidelines should determine whether the literature search was comprehensive, reproducible, and current.[6]

Recommendations made on the basis of the results of systematic reviews whose authors used suboptimal or unclear methods are less credible.[14] For example, the longstanding practice of prescribing antibiotic prophylaxis for all patients with prosthetic joints who need invasive dental procedures,[22] probably "just to be on the safe side," was common before 1997, when no guidelines using a systematic approach to review and summarize the literature on the topic were available. In 1997, the ADA and AAOS conducted an exhaustive review of the literature to determine whether antibiotic prophylaxis was effective in these patients.[23] On the basis of all the evidence, the 1997 guideline panel recommended (for the first time in history) against the use of antibiotic prophylaxis in patients with prosthetic joints who were undergoing invasive dental procedures, a situation that determined a dramatic change in clinical practice.[23] The contrast in clinical practice before and after the 1997 recommendation[23] highlights the value of conducting comprehensive systematic reviews of the literature to inform decision-making.

Are Values and Preferences Associated with the Outcomes Appropriately Specified?

Another important issue is the preference or relative importance that patients attribute to some outcomes over others.[14] Patients' values and preferences are expressions that include "patients' perspectives, beliefs, expectations, and goals for health and life. More precisely, they refer to the processes that people use when considering the potential benefits, harms, costs, limitations, and inconvenience of the management options in relation to one another. For some, the term 'values' has the closest connotation to these processes. For others, the connotation of 'preferences' best captures the notion of choice. Thus, we use both words together to convey the concept."[24]

For example, when looking for recommendations about the management of unerupted and impacted mandibular third molars, we noted that the Scottish Intercollegiate Guidelines Network (SIGN)[25] and NICE[26] recommend avoiding the prophylactic surgical removal of these molars unless the eruption process clearly is associated with pathological events such as infection, caries, and cyst formation, among others. Although the American Association of Oral and Maxillofacial Surgeons (AAOMS)[27] provides a similar recommendation when the third molar is affected pathologically, their recommendation also supports the early removal of third molars, even before an associated pathology is apparent: "Whenever possible, treatment should be provided before the pathology has adversely affected the patient's oral and/or systemic health."[27] The panel members explain their rationale as follows: "Treatment of impacted teeth at an early age is associated with a decreased incidence of morbidity and represents an efficient use of health care resources. Treatment at an older age carries with it an increase in the incidence and severity of perioperative and postoperative problems, a longer and more severe period of postoperative recovery, greater anesthetic risk and greater and more costly interference in daily activities and responsibilities."[27]

Why did three guideline panels, using the same evidence collected in a systematic and rigorous manner, provide clinicians with varying recommendations? The SIGN[25] and NICE[26] guideline panels put a higher value on avoiding adverse events associated with the surgical removal of third molars and the potentially unnecessary costs of treating (that is, extracting) otherwise healthy erupted molars. On the other hand, the AAOMS panel[27] placed a higher value on avoiding future pathological or unfavorable events related to the retention of third molars, including having a higher risk for experiencing postoperative adverse events when this type of surgery is required in older patients. Clinicians should look for clear statements about the role that values and preferences played when formulating any recommendation and adjust their decision to meet the values and preferences of their own patients.

Ideally, the results of a systematic review of the available evidence addressing patients' values and preferences should inform the guideline panel and drive the recommendation. The American College of Dentists' ethics handbook[28] states, "Decision processes based on ethical principles always consider the patient's best interests, as well as the patient's values and preferences. Risk management processes and decisions that do not include the perspective of the patient may be unethical."[28] Unfortunately, studies addressing patients' values and preferences are uncommon in the dental literature.[29-33]

When evidence exploring patients' values and preferences is not available, guideline panelists usually rely on the experiences of clinicians who deal with patients and decision-making on a regular basis. Another option is to include at least one patient representative in the process of formulating recommendations.[34] The limitation of these less systematic approaches is the extent to which those invited to the guideline panel meeting are actually representative of the typical patient targeted for a particular recommendation.

Regardless of the sources that the panel used to learn about patients' values and preferences, clinicians using recommendations should look actively for a transparent and explicit description of this matter, and consider what their own patients' values and preferences regarding benefits and risks might be.

Do the Authors Indicate the Strength of Their Recommendations?

The authors of trustworthy recommendations provide clinicians with an assessment of the strength of the recommendations.[14] In doing so, panels may rely on one of many available systems to grade their recommendations. The available systems to grade recommendations— including the Grading of Recommendations Assessment, Development and Evaluation (GRADE) approach,[35] the ADA system,[36] and those used by the U.S. Preventive Services Task Force (USPSTF)[37] and the AHA[38]—use diverse methods to represent confidence in the estimates of effect and the strength of their recommendations.[39,40]

These four systems share two critical features. First, they provide an assessment of the confidence in the effect estimates. In the context of clinical practice guidelines, this assessment of confidence represents the extent to which the estimates support a decision or a recommendation (Figure 7.2[14]).[41] The GRADE approach, which is by far the most widely used system, considers the following four levels of confidence (sometimes also described as *certainty* in the evidence) in the estimates of effect: high, moderate, low, and very low. Risk of bias, imprecision, indirectness, inconsistency, and publication bias can reduce this confidence in a given recommendation. The ADA system includes three levels: high, moderate, and low. This system uses the same domains described for the GRADE approach to determine the confidence in the effect estimates. Clinicians using guidelines should look for the guideline panel's rating of the degree of confidence and the reasons that influenced their assessment.

Figure 7.2. Assessment of the Direction and Strength of Recommendations Using Different Grading Systems

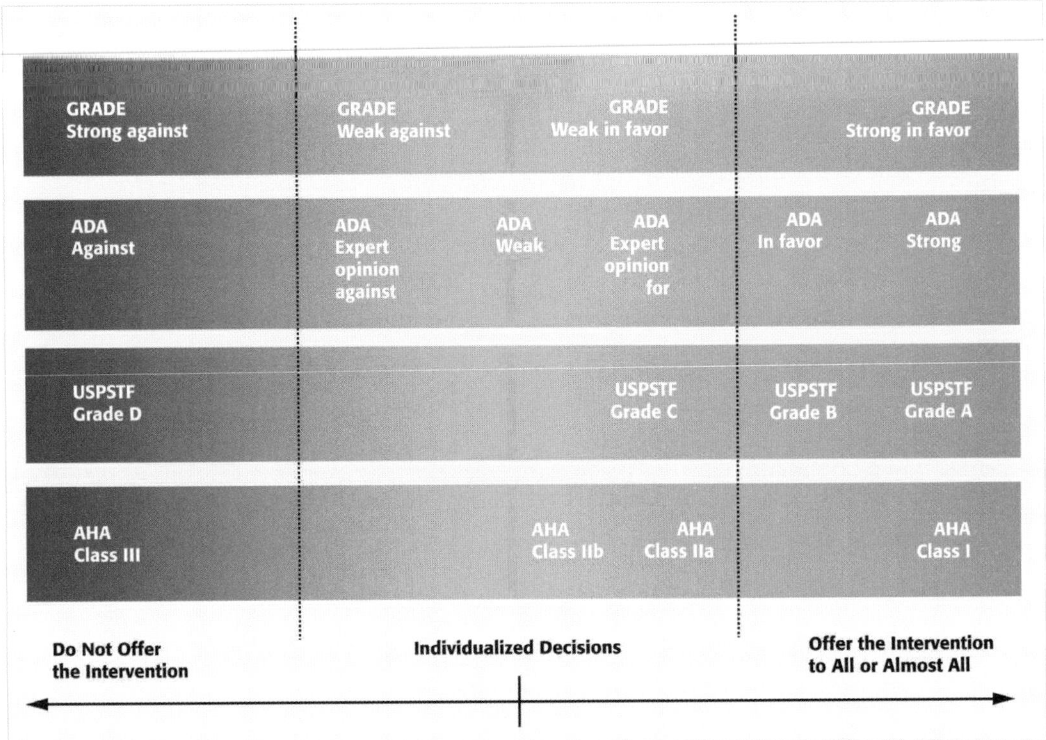

GRADE = Grading of Recommendations Assessment, Development, and Evaluation. ADA = American Dental Association. USPSTF = U.S. Preventive Services Task Force. AHA = American Heart Association.

Adapted with permission of McGraw-Hill Education from Neumann and colleagues.[14]

Second, the systems discriminate between strong and weak recommendations. Whereas the GRADE system uses only two types of recommendations (strong and weak), the ADA system uses the following six grades for recommendations: strong (evidence strongly supports providing this intervention), in favor (evidence favors providing this intervention), weak (evidence suggests implementing this intervention after alternatives have been considered), expert opinion for (evidence is lacking; the level of certainty is low—expert opinion guides this recommendation), expert opinion against (evidence is lacking; the level of certainty is low—expert opinion suggests not implementing this intervention), and against (evidence suggests not implementing this intervention or discontinuing ineffective procedures).[36]

For example, the ADA Council of Scientific Affairs formulated clinical recommendations addressing the use of nonfluoride caries-preventive agents. One of them[17] states the following: "Using 0.12 percent chlorhexidine rinse alone or in combination with fluoride for prevention of coronal caries is not recommended." The guideline panel determined the strength of the recommendation as "against," based on high-quality evidence.[17]

Is the Evidence Supporting the Recommendation Easily Understood?

▸ *For strong recommendations, is the strength appropriate?*

When a strong recommendation is provided, the message for clinicians is clear: "In almost all the cases, just do it."[14] When the right course of action depends on circumstances or is sensitive to patients' values and preferences, such a strong recommendation is likely to have undesirable consequences.

Four domains influence the strength of a recommendation: the magnitude of benefits and harms, certainty in the evidence, patients' values and preferences, and resource utilization.[24] A strong recommendation is more likely when the desirable consequences are many and important and undesirable consequences are few and unimportant; when there is high certainty in the evidence; when most patients place a high value in the desirable consequences; and when net costs are low. On the other hand, a weak or conditional recommendation is more likely when there are few and less important desirable consequences and many and more important undesirable consequences; low certainty in the evidence; low value placed on desirable consequences, or large uncertainty about values and preferences; and high net cost.

In general, clinicians should be cautious when presented with a strong recommendation on the basis of low-quality or very low-quality evidence. In this case, the message from the panel may be contradictory: in most situations clinicians have to implement the intervention (strong recommendation); however, we are uncertain or very uncertain about the evidence supporting this recommendation (low or very low confidence). There are, however, some specific situations that justify formulating a strong recommendation on the basis of low or very low confidence. Some of these exceptional scenarios are life-threatening situations, having equivalence between two options in which one is clearly cheaper or less risky, and when low confidence in the evidence suggests catastrophic harm.[24]

▸ *For weak recommendations, does the information provided facilitate shared decision-making?*

When clinicians are presented with a weak or conditional recommendation, it means that in many cases it is best to follow the suggested course of action; in many other cases, however, the optimal course of action may differ. Guideline panelists should provide clinicians with the information they need when decisions are value- and preference-sensitive, to engage in shared decision-making. Guidelines may provide this information in the remarks attached to each recommendation, in the recommendation rationale section, or in accompanying tables.

Weak recommendations mandate clinicians to engage in a bidirectional exchange of information with their patients—that is, shared decision-making.[42] In this process, clinicians provide patients with the evidence from clinical research, whereas patients share with clinicians their perspectives and values acquired from their own experience, social interaction, and other personal information. At the end of this deliberative process, both actors draw a conclusion and decide on the best course of action.[42,43]

Table 7.1 summarizes the implications of strong and weak recommendations for clinicians, patients, and policy makers.

Table 7.1. Implications for Strong and Weak Recommendations

Recommendation	Implications
Strong Recommendation for a Particular Intervention	*For clinicians:* Most patients should receive the recommended course of action. *For patients:* Most people in this situation would want to follow the recommended course of action, and only a small proportion of people would not want to follow it. *For policy makers:* The recommendation can be adapted as a policy in most situations.
Weak Recommendation for a Particular Intervention	*For clinicians:* Be prepared to help patients make a decision that is consistent with their own values (shared decision-making). *For patients:* Most people in this situation would want the recommended course of action, but many would not. *For policy makers:* There is a need for substantial debate and involvement of stakeholders.

Box 7.5. The Assessment of the Quality of Evidence and Strength of the Recommendation You Identified

You note that the panel who authored the American Dental Association (ADA) guideline published in 2015,[13] using the ADA's grading system for generating clinical recommendations,[36] recommended—on the basis of evidence warranting moderate confidence—against the use of antibiotic prophylaxis in patients with a prosthetic joint undergoing invasive dental procedures. The ADA's grading system explains moderate certainty as follows: "As more information becomes available, the magnitude or direction of the observed effect could change, and this change could be large enough to alter the conclusion. This statement is based on preliminary determination from the current best available evidence, but confidence in the estimate is constrained by one or more factors, such as the number or size of studies; risk of bias of individual studies leading to uncertainty in the validity of the reported results; inconsistency of findings across individual studies; and limited generalizability to the populations of interest."[36] You note that the panel also needs to assess the effect of the intervention; the ADA's language for no effect is "no association." By announcing "moderate" confidence of no association, the direction of the recommendation is "against," and the strength is "strong." With the recommendation "against," the ADA guideline panel means "that evidence suggests not implementing this intervention or discontinuing ineffective procedures."[13]

Given the panel's strong recommendation, you and other clinicians may conclude that in all but exceptional circumstances, the undesirable consequences of antibiotic prophylaxis outweigh the desirable consequences. The panel noted that under exceptional circumstances, the use of antibiotics might be desirable.

Was the Influence of Conflicts of Interest Minimized?

Interpretation of evidence and the process of moving from interpreting evidence to making recommendations are tasks that are susceptible to conflicts of interest. Although investigators have documented the extent of conflicts of interest (particularly financial conflicts of interest) in medical clinical practice guidelines and found them to be considerable,[44-48] clinical guideline panels have not explored the issue in dental guidelines. Intellectual conflicts of interest (for example, attitudes developed as a result of one's own previous research) or professional conflicts of interest (for example, loyalty to one's professional organization) also may influence recommendations.[49] Guidelines should report statements of the authors' conflicts of interest and implement strategies to minimize the impact of these conflicts of interest. Guidelines whose authors fail to report conflicts of interest have weak credibility. For example, a U.S. Preventive Services Task Force guideline addressing the prevention of dental caries in children from birth through age five provided a detailed description of the panel members and their affiliations, potential conflicts of interest, financial disclosure, and the guideline source of funding.[50] Because these disclosures did not suggest any potential conflicts of interest, readers could consider the recommendations to be trustworthy.

On the other hand, in some situations, including the insights of panel members who may have potential intellectual or financial conflicts of interest is necessary to ensure that the panel includes optimal expertise. In such circumstances, clinician users of guidelines should look for documentation of strategies that minimized conflict (for example, ensuring that the chair of the panel does not have any conflicts of interest or having panel members who had conflicts of interest in certain areas recuse themselves during discussion or votes on specific issues).[36,51] Failure to implement such measures in the presence of conflict of interest weakens a guideline's credibility.

Box 7.6. Your Assessment of the Conflict of Interest in the Guideline You Identified

In the section "Preventing bias in an AAOS clinical practice guideline," the American Dental Association guideline panel[12] explained the process of identifying members of the panel who have conflicts of interest, included a detailed description of the potential conflicts of interest of all the members of the American Academy of Orthopedic Surgeons working group, and explained their strategies to deal with such conflicts that included recruiting a methodologist who did not have any conflicts of interest to be a key actor in the guideline development process.[52] When you read this description, you and other clinicians using this guideline can be reassured that the guideline development group made efforts to minimize the effect of conflict of interest, which increases the trustworthiness of the guideline.

Conclusion

Clinicians in need of guidance regarding use of a diagnostic or a therapeutic strategy can benefit from referring to evidence-based recommendations provided by international or local organizations. Because some recommendations are more evidence-based and more credible than others, clinicians should assess each recommendation's credibility. Criteria for a trustworthy guideline include clear and actionable recommendations that were developed on the basis of the best available evidence, patients' values and preferences having been specified appropriately, the provision of a clear indication of the strength of the recommendation, and the use of an effective method to address issues of conflict of interest. Highly credible guidelines can assist clinicians with providing a succinct yet comprehensive summary of the balance between benefits and harms, the certainty of the evidence, patients' values and preferences, and costs of an intervention. However, guidelines cannot cover all types of patients and clinical scenarios, and therefore, oral health care professionals should incorporate their own clinical judgment when determining the most appropriate care.

> **Box 7.7. What You Say to Your Patient**
>
> Because the American Dental Association Council on Scientific Affairs recommendation published in 2015[13] provides a clear and actionable statement that was made on the basis of a comprehensive and rigorous systematic review of the evidence that includes patients' values and preferences associated with the outcomes clearly specified, and that seems to be highly protected against the influence of panel members' conflicts of interest, you decide to discuss the recommendation and supplementary data with your patient. You both decide that the patient will not use antibiotic prophylaxis for this procedure. The Supplemental Table at the end of this chapter provides a summary of this recommendation and the critical appraisal conducted.[12,13]

References

1. Brignardello-Petersen R, Carrasco-Labra A, Glick M, Guyatt GH, Azarpazhooh A. "A practical approach to evidence-based dentistry: understanding and applying the principles of EBD." *JADA* 2014;145(11):1105–1107.

2. Chapter 2 of this book was based on Brignardello-Petersen R, Carrasco-Labra A, Booth HA, et al. "A practical approach to evidence-based dentistry: II: how to search for evidence to inform clinical decisions." *JADA* 2014;145(12):1262–1267.

3. Brignardello-Petersen R, Carrasco-Labra A, Glick M, Guyatt GH, Azarpazhooh A. "A practical approach to evidence-based dentistry: III: how to appraise and use an article about therapy." *JADA* 2015;146(1):42–49.e1.

4. Brignardello-Petersen R, Carrasco-Labra A, Glick M, Guyatt GH, Azarpazhooh A. "A practical approach to evidence-based dentistry: IV: how to use an article about harm." *JADA* 2015;146(2):94–101.e1.

5. Brignardello-Petersen R, Carrasco-Labra A, Glick M, Guyatt GH, Azarpazhooh A. "A practical approach to evidence-based dentistry: V: how to appraise and use an article about diagnosis." *JADA* 2015;146(3):184–191.e1.

6. Carrasco-Labra A, Brignardello-Petersen R, Glick M, Guyatt GH, Azarpazhooh A. "A practical approach to evidence-based dentistry: VI: how to use a systematic review." *JADA* 2015;146(4):255–265.e1.

7. Institute of Medicine of the National Academies. *Clinical Practice Guidelines We Can Trust*. Washington, DC: National Academies Press; 2011.

8. Wilson W, Taubert KA, Gewitz M, et al; American Heart Association. "Prevention of infective endocarditis: guidelines from the American Heart Association: a guideline from the American Heart Association Rheumatic Fever, Endocarditis and Kawasaki Disease Committee, Council on Cardiovascular Disease in the Young, and the Council on Clinical Cardiology, Council on Cardiovascular Surgery and Anesthesia, and the Quality of Care and Outcomes Research Interdisciplinary Working Group" (published correction appears in *JADA*. 2008;139[3]:254). *JADA* 2008;139(suppl):3S–24S.

9. Centre for Clinical Practice, National Institute for Health and Clinical Excellence. "Prophylaxis Against Infective Endocarditis: Antimicrobial Prophylaxis Against Infective Endocarditis in Adults and Children Undergoing Interventional Procedures." NICE clinical guideline 64. London, UK: National Institute for Health and Clinical Excellence; 2008.

10. Guyatt GH, Prasad K, Schünemann H, Jaeschke R, Cook DJ. "How to use a patient management recommendation." In: Guyatt GH, Rennie D, Meade MO, Cook DJ, eds. *Users' Guides to the Medical Literature. A Manual for Evidence-Based Clinical Practice.* 2nd ed. United States: The McGraw-Hill Companies, Inc; 2008. p. 597.

11. *World Health Organization (WHO) Handbook for Guideline Development.* Geneva, Switzerland: World Health Organization; 2012.

12. American Academy of Orthopaedic Surgeons; American Dental Association. "Prevention of Orthopaedic Implant Infection in Patients Undergoing Dental Procedures: Evidence-Based Guideline and Evidence Report." 1st ed. Rosemont, IL: American Academy of Orthopaedic Surgeons; 2012.

13. Sollecito TP, Abt E, Lockhart PB, et al. "The use of prophylactic antibiotics prior to dental procedures in patients with prosthetic joints: evidence-based clinical practice guideline for dental practitioners–a report of the American Dental Association Council on Scientific Affairs." *JADA* 2015;146(1):11–16.e8.

14. Neumann I, Akl EA, Vandvik PO, et al. "How to use a patient management recommendation: clinical practice guidelines and decision analyses." In: Guyatt GH, Rennie D, Meade MO, Cook DJ, eds. *Users' Guides to the Medical Literature: A Manual for Evidence-Based Clinical Practice.* 3rd ed. New York, NY: McGraw-Hill; 2015. p. 531.

15. Glenny AM, Gibson F, Auld E, et al; Children's Cancer and Leukaemia Group (CCLG)/Paediatric Oncology Nurses Forum's (CCLG-PONF) Mouth Care Group. "The development of evidence-based guidelines on mouth care for children, teenagers and young adults treated for cancer." *Eur J Cancer* 2010;46(8):1399–1412.

16. Watters W, Rethman MP, Hanson NB, et al; American Academy of Orthopedic Surgeons; American Dental Association. "Prevention of Orthopaedic Implant Infection in Patients Undergoing Dental Procedures." AAOS-ADA Clinical Practice Guideline Summary. Published December 13, 2012. Available at: *http://www.aaos.org/research/guidelines/PUDP/dentalexecsumm.pdf.* Accessed March 18, 2015.

17. Rethman MP, Beltran-Aguilar ED, Billings RJ, et al; American Dental Association Council on Scientific Affairs Expert Panel on Nonfluoride Caries-Preventive Agents. "Nonfluoride caries-preventive agents: executive summary of evidence-based clinical recommendations." *JADA* 2011;142(9):1065–1071.

18. Akl EA, Briel M, You JJ, et al. "LOST to follow-up Information in Trials (LOST-IT): a protocol on the potential impact." *Trials* 2009;10:40.

19. Brignardello-Petersen R, Carrasco-Labra A, Shah P, Azarpazhooh A. "A practitioner's guide to developing critical appraisal skills: what is the difference between clinical and statistical significance?" *JADA* 2013;144(7):780–786.

20. Aronson JK. "Biomarkers and surrogate endpoints." *Br J Clin Pharmacol* 2005;59(4):491–494.

21. Lee DW. "Validated surrogate endpoints needed for peri-implantitis." *Evid Based Dent* 2011;12(1):7.

22. Lockhart PB. "Antibiotic prophylaxis guidelines for prosthetic joints: much ado about nothing?" *Oral Surg Oral Med Oral Pathol Oral Radiol* 2013;116(1):1–3.

23. "Advisory statement. Antibiotic prophylaxis for dental patients with total joint replacements. American Dental Association; American Academy of Orthopaedic Surgeons." *JADA* 1997;128(7):1004–1008.

24. Andrews JC, Schunemann HJ, Oxman AD, et al. "GRADE guidelines: 15: going from evidence to recommendation–determinants of a recommendation's direction and strength." *J Clin Epidemiol* 2013;66(7):726–735.

25. Scottish Intercollegiate Guidelines Network (SIGN). "Management of Unerupted and Impacted Third Molar Teeth: A National Clinical Guideline." SIGN Publication No. 43. Edinburgh, Scotland: Scottish Intercollegiate Guidelines Network; 1999.

26. *Guidance on the Extraction of Wisdom Teeth.* NICE Technology Appraisal Guidance 1. London, UK: National Institute for Health and Care Excellence; 2000.

27. "The management of impacted third molar teeth." Statement by the American Association of Oral and Maxillofacial Surgeons concerning the management of selected clinical conditions and associated clinical procedures. Clinical paper. Rosemont, IL: American Association of Oral and Maxillofacial Surgeons; 2013.

28. American College of Dentists. *Ethics Handbook for Dentists: An Introduction to Ethics, Professionalism, and Ethical Decision Making.* Gaithersburg, MD: American College of Dentists; 2012.

29. Atchison KA, Gironda MW, Black EE, et al. "Baseline characteristics and treatment preferences of oral surgery patients." *J Oral Maxillofac Surg* 2007;65(12):2430–2437.

30. Liedholm R. "Mandibular third molar removal: patient preferences, assessments of oral surgeons and patient flows." *Swed Dent J Suppl* 2005;175:1–61.

31. Liedholm R, Knutsson K, Lysell L, Rohlin M, Brickley M, Shepherd JP. "The outcomes of mandibular third molar removal and non-removal: a study of patients' preferences using a multi-attribute method." *Acta Odontol Scand* 2000;58(6):293–298.

32. Matthews D, Rocchi A, Gafni A. "Putting your money where your mouth is: willingness to pay for dental gel." *Pharmacoeconomics* 2002;20(4):245–255.

33. Azarpazhooh A, Dao T, Figueiredo R, Krahn M, Friedman S. "A survey of patients' preferences for the treatment of teeth with apical periodontitis." *J Endod* 2013;39(12):1534–1541.

34. Nilsen ES, Myrhaug HT, Johansen M, Oliver S, Oxman AD. "Methods of consumer involvement in developing healthcare policy and research, clinical practice guidelines and patient information material." *Cochrane Database Syst Rev* 2006;3:CD004563.

35. Guyatt GH, Oxman AD, Schunemann HJ, Tugwell P, Knottnerus A. "GRADE guidelines: a new series of articles in the Journal of Clinical Epidemiology." *J Clin Epidemiol* 2011;64(4):380–382.

36. Center for Evidence-Based Dentistry, American Dental Association. *ADA Clinical Practice Guidelines Handbook: 2013 Update.* Chicago, IL: American Dental Association; 2013.

37. U.S. Preventive Services Task Force. "Grade Definitions." 2012. Available at: *http://www uspreventiveservicestaskforce.org/Page/Name/grade-definitions.* Accessed March 18, 2015.

38. American College of Cardiology Foundation; American Heart Association. "Methodology Manual and Policies from the ACCF/AHA Task Force on Practice Guidelines." June 2010. Available at: *http://www.acc.org/guidelines/about-guidelines-and-clinical-documents/methodology.* Accessed March 18, 2015.

39. Atkins D, Eccles M, Flottorp S, et al; GRADE Working Group. "Systems for grading the quality of evidence and the strength of recommendations I: critical appraisal of existing approaches." *BMC Health Serv Res* 2004;4(1):38.

40. Faggion CM Jr. "Grading the quality of evidence and the strength of recommendations in clinical dentistry: a critical review of 2 prominent approaches." *J Evid Based Dent Pract* 2010;10(2):78–85.

41. Balshem H, Helfand M, Schunemann HJ, et al. "GRADE guidelines: 3: rating the quality of evidence." *J Clin Epidemiol* 2011;64(4):401–406.

42. Charles C, Gafni A, Whelan T. "Shared decision-making in the medical encounter: what does it mean? (or it takes at least two to tango)." *Soc Sci Med* 1997;44(5):681–692.

43. Montori V, Elwyn G, Devereaux PJ, Straus SE, Haynes RB, Guyatt G. "Decision making and the patient." In: Guyatt GH, Rennie D, Meade MO, Cook DJ, eds. *Users' Guides to the Medical Literature: A Manual for Evidence Based Clinical Practice.* 3rd ed. New York, NY: McGraw-Hill; 2015.

44. Bhattacharyya N, Lin HW. "Prevalence and reliability of self-reported authorship disclosures in Otolaryngology-Head and Neck Surgery." *Otolaryngol Head Neck Surg* 2009;141(3):311–315.

45. Bindslev JB, Schroll J, Gotzsche PC, Lundh A. "Underreporting of conflicts of interest in clinical practice guidelines: cross sectional study." *BMC Med Ethics* 2013;14:19.

46. Choudhry NK, Stelfox HT, Detsky AS. "Relationships between authors of clinical practice guidelines and the pharmaceutical industry." *JAMA* 2002;287(5):612–617.

47. Neuman J, Korenstein D, Ross JS, Keyhani S. "Prevalence of financial conflicts of interest among panel members producing clinical practice guidelines in Canada and United States: cross sectional study." *BMJ* 2011;343:d5621.

48. Norris SL, Holmer HK, Ogden LA, Selph SS, Fu R. "Conflict of interest disclosures for clinical practice guidelines in the national guideline clearinghouse." *PLoS One* 2012;7(11):e47343.

49. Guyatt G, Akl EA, Hirsh J, et al. "The vexing problem of guidelines and conflict of interest: a potential solution." *Ann Intern Med* 2010;152(11):738–741.

50. Moyer VA; US Preventive Services Task Force. "Prevention of dental caries in children from birth through age 5 years: US Preventive Services Task Force recommendation statement." *Pediatrics* 2014;133(6):1102–1111.

51. Schunemann HJ, Wiercioch W, Etxeandia I, et al. "Guidelines 2.0: systematic development of a comprehensive checklist for a successful guideline enterprise." *CMAJ* 2014;186(3):E123–E142.

52. Hirsh J, Guyatt G. "Clinical experts or methodologists to write clinical guidelines?" *Lancet* 2009;374(9686):273–275.

A version of this chapter originally appeared in the May 2015 edition of *JADA* (Volume 146, Issue 5, Pages 327–336. e1). It has been reviewed and updated for accuracy and clarity by the editors of *How to Use Evidence-Based Dental Practices to Improve Your Clinical Decision-Making.*

Supplemental Table. Example of Critically Appraising Patient Management Recommendations from a Clinical Practice Guideline*

1. Is the Clinical Recommendation Clear and Comprehensive?	
1a. Is the recommended intervention clear and actionable?	Yes. The recommendation is as follows: "In general, for patients with prosthetic joint implants, prophylactic antibiotics are not recommended prior to dental procedures to prevent prosthetic joint infection." Clinicians would easily understand from this statement that, in most cases, prophylactic antibiotics should not be prescribed to patients.
1b. Is the alternative clear?	Yes. The opposite option is prescribing antibiotic prophylaxis. The ADA guideline panel[13] explicitly describes in which exceptional circumstances the alternative approach, providing the antibiotic prophylaxis, could be an option: "For patients with a history of complications associated with their joint replacement surgery who are undergoing dental procedures that include gingival manipulation or mucosal incision, prophylactic antibiotics should only be considered after consultation with the patient and orthopedic surgeon." This information is provided in the remarks of the recommendation and is easily accessible to clinicians.
1c. Were all relevant outcomes important to patients explicitly considered?	Yes. The guideline panel included not only outcomes of effectiveness (for example, prosthetic joint infection) but also outcomes such as antibiotic resistance and adverse events (for example, secondary infections, anaphylaxis, and other allergic reactions, nausea, vomiting, diarrhea).

2. Was the Recommendation Based on the Best Current Evidence?
Yes. The 2012 AAOS-ADA evidence-based guideline and evidence report provides a detailed description of the systematic review conducted to inform the decision-making process. The methods to identify the available evidence are rigorous and described extensively. However, some limitations are the exclusion of studies published in languages other than English and the lack of any description of the methods used to select and assess the evidence. The 2014 ADA guideline panel[13] updated the 2012 search.[12] It is likely that the evidence presented to the guideline panel was the best current available evidence.

3. Are the Patients' Values and Preferences Associated with Outcomes Appropriately Specified?
No. The conducted systematic review did not explicitly look for studies exploring patients' values and preferences for this recommendation. It is uncertain whether such studies actually exist for this scenario. The guideline panel relied on their own perception of patients' values and preferences about the balance between the scarce evidence on the potential benefits and all the adverse events associated with antibiotic prophylaxis. They clearly state that when formulating the recommendation, they placed a higher value on the potential harms over the limited evidence of benefits.

4. Do the Authors Indicate the Strength of Their Recommendations?

The ADA guideline panel[13] provided the following recommendation: "In general, for patients with prosthetic joint implants, prophylactic antibiotics are not recommended prior to dental procedures to prevent prosthetic joint infection." The guideline panel graded the strength of this recommendation as "against," based on a moderate level of certainty.

5. Is the Evidence Supporting the Recommendation Easily Understood?

5a. For strong recommendations, is the strength appropriate?	Yes. The ADA guideline panel[13] assessed the certainty in the evidence as moderate and provided a recommendation against the intervention. The panel also stated that the potential harms outweigh the benefits. The strength seems appropriate.
5b. For weak recommendations, does the information provided facilitate shared decision-making?	The strength of the recommendation was graded as strong against the intervention (see 5a); therefore, this question is not applicable to this recommendation.

6. Was the Influence of Conflicts of Interest Minimized?

In the section "Preventing bias in an AAOS clinical practice guideline," the AAOS panelists[12] explain in detail the process to identify and deal with members of the panel who have conflicts of interest. They also included a methodologist who did not have any conflicts of interest on the panel. The guideline document includes a detailed description of the potential conflicts of interest of all the members of the AAOS working group. The reported conflicts of interests were available and explicitly presented to all members in the panel. All these measures implemented by the guideline development group to minimize the influence of conflict of interest increases the credibility of the recommendation.

Conclusion: The recommendation published in January 2015,[13] provided by the ADA guideline panel addressing the use of antibiotic prophylaxis to prevent prosthetic joint infection in patients undergoing invasive dental procedures, seems to be appropriately developed and trustworthy.

* *Sources:* Watters and colleagues[16] and Sollecito and colleagues.[13]

Chapter 8. How to Appraise an Article Based on a Qualitative Study

Joanna E.M. Sale, Ph.D.; Maryam Amin, D.M.D., M.Sc., Ph.D.; Alonso Carrasco-Labra, D.D.S., M.Sc., Ph.D.; Romina Brignardello-Petersen, D.D.S., M.Sc., Ph.D.; Michael Glick, D.M.D.; Gordon H. Guyatt, M.D., M.Sc.; and Amir Azarpazhooh, D.D.S., M.Sc., Ph.D.

In This Chapter:

When Is Qualitative Research Relevant?

Where to Find Qualitative Studies

Critically Appraising Qualitative Research to Inform Clinical Decisions

Are the Results Credible?

- Was the Choice of Participants or Observations Explicit and Comprehensive?

- Was Research Ethics Approval Obtained?

- Was Data Collection Sufficiently Comprehensive and Detailed?

- Were the Data Analyzed Appropriately, and Were the Findings Corroborated Adequately?

What Are the Results?

How Can I Apply the Results to Patient Care?

- Does the Study Offer Helpful Theory?

- Does the Study Help Me Understand the Context of My Practice?

- Does the Study Help Me Understand Social Interactions in Clinical Care?

Conclusion

Introduction

In previous chapters in this book, we introduced the general steps to pursue evidence-based clinical practice[1] and explained how to search for[2] and critically appraise studies about therapy,[3] harm,[4] diagnosis,[5] systematic reviews,[6] and clinical practice guidelines.[7] In this chapter, we turn to appraising the evidence from a study whose investigators relied on qualitative research.

Qualitative research is an inquiry process that focuses on meaning and interpretation.[8,9] Investigators conducting this type of research aim to explore social or human problems.[8,9] Qualitative researchers often address real-world situations in which complex systems are greater than the sum of their parts.[10] Qualitative researchers not only aim to understand how people think about the world and how they act and behave in it, their study results also can extend beyond patients' personal experiences to explore interactions and processes within organizations or other environments.[11] In the context of evidence-based medicine, the results of qualitative research can be particularly important in helping clinicians to understand patients' values and preferences.[12,13]

Box 8.1. Clinical Scenario

A 48-year-old man who smokes heavily came to your office concerning periodic toothaches. Despite having dental insurance benefits, he had not visited a dentist for the past five years as he had no pain until recently. You noticed widespread caries and moderate periodontal disease. You performed scaling and root planing, restored several teeth, and extracted four nonrestorable teeth. Next, he asks you to replace the extracted teeth with dental implants because his wife recently had a positive experience with a dental implant. You explain that the cost for implants is not covered by his insurance; however, he says that he is willing to make such an investment because "the implants will last a lifetime." You are concerned about making a clinical judgment in this case and are not sure if your patient is a good candidate for dental implants given his smoking and oral hygiene status, as well as his unrealistic expectation for the longevity of the implants. Evidence from the literature may provide insights that would bring further understanding of this patient's expectation and preferences. You therefore seek a relevant study to consult.

When Is Qualitative Research Relevant?

There are numerous reasons for conducting a qualitative study. Qualitative research is relevant when little is known about a topic or to address questions that cannot be answered by quantitative methods. Qualitative research results also can be relevant when a clinician wants to study how potential barriers to care are perceived, to describe a decision-making process, or to examine why interventions work or do not work. Qualitative research results can be influential when examining the kinds of impact (both anticipated and unanticipated) that might be perceived from using different intervention strategies.[14] Qualitative researchers seek in-depth understandings of "what is going on in the world" and also can challenge assumptions about that world and the people who live and interact in it.[15] Investigators of qualitative research studies that are relevant for clinicians address a social phenomenon and seek a theoretical or conceptual understanding of a particular problem.[16] Qualitative researchers in oral health have conducted studies that have addressed issues such as the effect of having natural teeth as a person gets older, dentists' perceptions and experiences of treating people who receive social assistance, experiences of tooth loss and replacement, and oral health preferences in patients with diabetes.[17-20]

 Qualitative research is relevant when little is known about a topic or to address questions that cannot be answered by quantitative methods.

Where to Find Qualitative Studies

It can be difficult to identify qualitative studies because their key words often do not map easily to medical subject headings (MeSH) terms, which are used for indexing articles in MEDLINE, and these types of studies are not always published in journals that are indexed in commonly used databases (see Chapter 2). However, in 2003, the National Library of Medicine introduced "qualitative research" as a MeSH term. To make a search more sensitive, a clinician using PubMed can apply filters such as "qualitative" or "interview" in the title or abstract fields or the term "experience" in the text word field.

> **Box 8.2. The Search for a Qualitative Study**
>
> You are interested in finding a qualitative study that explores patients' values and preferences regarding dental implants. You start with PubMed and enter the search terms "dental implants" and "qualitative research." The search identifies over 100 articles. As you look through the titles and abstracts, you identify and retrieve an article that appears to be particularly relevant.

> **Box 8.3. The Study You Find**
>
> The study you find was written by Grey and colleagues,[21] and the title is "A Qualitative Study of Patients' Motivations and Expectations for Dental Implants." You read the abstract of this research study, which indicates that patients believe that dental implants are just like natural teeth; such a belief, you note, could be problematic. You decide that reading the article may provide further insight into your patient's perspective and his initial decision to request implants.

Critically Appraising Qualitative Research to Inform Clinical Decisions

There are many approaches (also referred to as methodologies or traditions) to conducting qualitative research, including grounded theory, phenomenology, and ethnography. These approaches, in addition to numerous theoretical perspectives, often shape the research question, data collection, data analysis, and choices for promoting rigor in the study. Unlike quantitative research, there is no hierarchy among the approaches in qualitative research; no approach is more likely to get to the "truth" than another.

Over 100 checklists are available to critically appraise a qualitative study.[22] Many of these checklists are procedural in nature, focusing on the methods alone and diverting attention away from the analytic content of the work and the substantive findings.[23] In addition, many checklists consider all qualitative research to be the same, as they fail to acknowledge differences between approaches or variants within each of the approaches.[24] For the purposes of this chapter, we relied on Giacomini and Cook's[16] criteria because these authors specifically developed criteria for use in evidence-based practice. According to these criteria, the process of using the results of a qualitative research study to inform clinical decisions involves assessing the credibility, the results, and the applicability of those results. Below, we describe each of these three steps.

Are the Results Credible?

Investigators have defined credibility as the degree of confidence that a clinician could have that a study's findings represent the "truth."[25,26] Discussions about and techniques for establishing credibility have evolved over the past 30 years since the term was conceptualized. According to our criteria,[16] answering the following questions can provide key insights into the credibility of the findings of a qualitative study.

Was the Choice of Participants or Observations Explicit and Comprehensive?

One of the hallmarks of qualitative research is purposeful (or purposive) sampling.[10,27–29] Purposeful sampling refers to the process of recruiting information-rich cases (for example, people or documents) that promise to provide a full and sophisticated understanding of the phenomenon.[10,30,31] By selecting information-rich cases, qualitative researchers gain efficiency in learning about the issues of central importance to the research.[10]

There are many types of purposeful sampling strategies. These include, but are not limited to, selecting cases that are diverse or heterogeneous as related to dimensions, such as age, that are deemed important to the researchers (maximum variation sampling); selecting a homogeneous sample to describe a particular subgroup in depth (homogenous sampling); using key sources and initial participants to inform the selection of subsequent participants (snowball sampling); and using the categories and theories that are developed during data analysis to inform future sampling (that is, theoretical sampling).[10,29] The researcher's decision to use any one, or a combination, of these sampling strategies often depends on a variety of elements, including what occurs as data are being collected and analyzed, the type of approach within which the researcher is operating (for example, using the data collected to develop theoretical ideas, concepts, models, and formal theories, which is an approach traditionally referred to as grounded theory[32]), and the data collection techniques used (for example, individual interviews, focus groups, or documents). For example, in a qualitative study that explores the perceptions of people who have undergone a particular experience (phenomenological research), the researcher would be sure to choose participants who have undergone the experience of interest (criterion sampling). When qualitative researchers are planning to conduct focus groups, they may prefer homogenous sampling because they want to minimize variation in the sample, such as a power differential among group members.[33] For example, in a study in which the objective was to understand how dentists perceived and experienced treating people who received social assistance,[19] the authors used maximum variation sampling to recruit dentists who had potentially diverse experiences with people living with poverty.

In summary, when assessing whether the researchers' choice of participants or observations was explicit and comprehensive, clinicians should look for some description of purposeful sampling, even if the researchers did not specifically use the term "purposeful."

Was Research Ethics Approval Obtained?

Similar to other types of research studies, qualitative research studies typically require research ethics approval. Several ethical issues are considered to be unique to qualitative research. For example, it is important to realize that participants can shape the data and create ethical dilemmas; the communities being researched are not passive components of the research study.[34] One ethical issue that occurs during analysis is whether participants should have a say in how the researchers interpret their statements.[35] This issue can be especially important to acknowledge if researchers solicit feedback from participants about the study findings (known as "member checking," "member validation," or "respondent validation").[32] Strategies for member checking include sending participants their interview transcripts or summaries of the findings. Some researchers view member checking as a criterion of critical appraisal; however, it might instead be viewed as another way of gathering data that has ethical consequences.[32,36]

Another ethical consideration of qualitative researchers arises when the openness and intimacy of the research leads participants to disclose information that they may later regret having shared.[35,37] To minimize this risk, qualitative researchers are careful to maintain a professional distance from their participants so that they do not lead participants to believe they have entered into a therapeutic relationship.[35] Because of the small sample sizes used in qualitative research, it is important that researchers do not reveal too much information about their study sample (for example, the hospital from which patients were recruited), as there is always the possibility that readers may be able to identify participants.[38] Ethical issues such as those described previously are not always captured by standard applications for research ethics board approval, yet qualitative researchers may need to discuss these issues as they carry out their research.

Was Data Collection Sufficiently Comprehensive and Detailed?

Among the numerous techniques for collecting data for a qualitative study, the most common are one-on-one interviews, focus groups, observations, and documents. An interview is an active process in which interviewer and interviewee, through their relationship, produce knowledge or data.[31,35] Focus groups are distinguished from one-on-one interviews because of the researcher's ability in focus group sessions to explore the interactions among research participants.[39] Researchers can use observations to study behavior in a natural environment, such as publicly accessible spaces,[11] and they can also analyze documents and records. Documents might include public records (for example, government documents, television scripts, minutes of meetings), private documents (for example, letters, medical histories, school records), and photographs.[32]

It is appropriate to use a single technique or a combination of techniques for collecting data in qualitative research. For example, in grounded theory studies, researchers may combine focus groups with interviews.[40,41] In an ethnographic study, researchers may combine observations with interviews.[42] Although using a combination of techniques is not necessary, doing so can allow the researcher to provide an enhanced description of the phenomenon's structure.[40]

It is helpful when qualitative researchers outline the topic areas they covered in the interview.[35] Some journal reviewers like to see the actual interview questions presented in a table. However, individual interview questions or prompts can be revised to adapt to the ongoing data analysis or circumstances in the field.[11] In some instances, a researcher conducts a single interview with each participant; in other studies, researchers conduct multiple interviews.

There are no hard-and-fast rules to determine sample size in qualitative research. The aim of data collection is to obtain a rich description of the phenomenon of study rather than to generalize to a population of interest.[43] Creswell[8] proposed sample sizes for different qualitative approaches; however, many researchers use a standard strategy in which they stop collecting data when they believe that further data collection will add little or no important new information relevant to the analysis (a state of affairs referred to as saturation).

In a similar manner to quantitative researchers, qualitative researchers collect some demographic data (for example, age, sex, race, education status) to describe the sample as well as the context or setting from which the sample was drawn. For example, the setting can be a dental practice, a screening program, a school, or the community.

In summary, in assessing whether data collection was comprehensive and detailed, clinicians should look for descriptions of how the qualitative researchers collected the data (for example, interviews or focus groups), what types of data were collected (for example, the topic areas covered, interview guide questions, contextual information such as the setting from which participants were selected), and how the decision to stop collecting data was made by the study team (for example, they concluded that they had reached saturation).

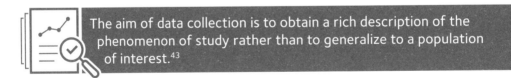

The aim of data collection is to obtain a rich description of the phenomenon of study rather than to generalize to a population of interest.[43]

Were the Data Analyzed Appropriately, and Were the Findings Corroborated Adequately?

In quantitative research, researchers generally conduct analysis separate from, and after, data collection to minimize the risk of bias. This is antithetical to what happens in qualitative research. One key feature of qualitative data analysis is that it is iterative, occurring simultaneously with data collection. The design and process of data collection and analysis is circular in nature; analysis unfolds as a researcher generates data and considers theoretical assumptions, a process referred to as emergent analysis.[32] As a result, researchers can elaborate on and revise the perspective of the phenomenon being studied as data are collected.[32]

Generally, all qualitative analysis involves breaking down data into smaller pieces (that is, coding) and reassembling the pieces to develop an interpretation, a process sometimes referred to as thematic analysis. Themes do not emerge as if they are waiting to be discovered; rather, researchers develop themes on the basis of their interaction with participants and the data collected from participants.[44,45] In other words, after accounting for the data, qualitative researchers determine the different paths they can pursue, each of which might be a separate analysis.[44] Research team members' input can be especially important at this stage of the research, as are the details related to the qualitative approach or tradition, which may provide further guidance as to how analysis should proceed. For example, a description of classic grounded theory outlines prescriptive steps for analysis.[46,47]

The investigators of many qualitative studies stop short of offering an in-depth analysis by providing a list of themes or categories without integrating those themes into a more advanced interpretation.[44] It is important for qualitative researchers to demonstrate that their analysis extends beyond the initial coding of data. When qualitative researchers report their results, they often provide direct quotations from their interviews to support their claims.[22] They also may account for data that do not fit with the themes or concepts or theory developed.[48] Throughout data collection and analysis, qualitative researchers can enhance credibility for their research by critically self-reflecting on their preferences and theoretical predispositions toward the work (for example, by commenting in field notes and memos), a process referred to as reflexivity.[32]

In summary, when assessing whether researchers appropriately analyzed data and corroborated findings, clinicians should determine if the researchers used an iterative process of analysis. In addition, clinicians should look for researchers' explanations of how they developed and then interpreted concepts, themes, or both.

> **Box 8.4. Your Assessment of the Qualitative Research You Identified**
> While reading Grey and colleagues'[21] qualitative research study, your judgment leads you to be concerned about how the authors of the study selected study participants and whether the authors collected sufficient data from their participants. You notice that the authors did not discuss purposeful sampling, nor did they discuss why they stopped recruitment and data collection. You note that although the study appears to have had no concerning ethical issues, the process of data analysis is not entirely clear. You decide to keep reading this study with caution (see Table 8.1 for a more detailed critical appraisal of the article).

Table 8.1 Example of Critically Appraising an Article about Qualitative Research*

Guide	Comments
1. Is qualitative research relevant?	
1a. Is my question about social, rather than biomedical, phenomena?	Yes. The authors sought to understand patients' motivations for seeking implants and their expectations of treatment. The authors did not seek to measure outcomes (for example, patient satisfaction with implants) or determine the efficacy of the implant procedure.
1b. Do I seek theoretical or conceptual understanding of the problem?	Yes. The authors were interested in under-standing a phenomenon rather than making causal or correlational inferences to populations.
2. Are the results credible?	
2a. Was the choice of participants or observations explicit and comprehensive?	Grey and colleagues'[21] study involved interviews with participants. The authors did not report that they conducted purposeful sampling for selecting their participants. They acknowledged that their "small opportunity sample" was a limitation; however, they could have provided more details about how they collected observations from this sample. Eligible patients were adults who were fluent in English and had consulted a restorative dental specialist with an interest in implantology at a private dental practice in Wiltshire, United Kingdom. Although the authors mentioned "a private dental practice," it was not clear whether patients were drawn from more than one restorative dental specialist's practice in Wiltshire. Fifty patients were eligible to participate in the study, and the authors mailed information about the study to these patients. Of the 50 patients, the investigators interviewed only nine patients. The authors gave no explanation of how these nine patients were selected to participate in the study. For example, the authors did not state whether other patients had agreed to participate but then dropped out, whether only nine patients mailed back a response form, or whether more than nine patients mailed back response forms but the authors further selected the sample from these patients.
2b. Was research ethics approval obtained?	Yes, the authors stated that they obtained approval to conduct the study. As stated on page 2, "Approval was gained from the research ethics committees at the University of Bath and the University of the West of England." The authors did not describe any other ethical issues.

Guide	Comments
2c. Was data collection sufficiently comprehensive and detailed?	The authors collected demographic data but did not include some important factors about the participants that might be relevant to describe a clinical scenario, such as participants' highest level of education, socioeconomic status, and race. Also, the investigators collected data through telephone interviews. Although the authors justified this strategy by citing a reference, which indicated that telephone interviews were comparable to face-to-face interviews, face-to-face interviews can create a better rapport between the participant and researcher. Face-to-face interviews also allow the researcher to gauge a participant's nonverbal behavior, such as facial expressions, during the interview.
	The first author conducted all the interviews. The interviews were semistructured, and the first two authors developed the interview schedule (or guide) on the basis of previous literature and with input from the other authors. The authors mentioned that they piloted the interview questions but did not describe with whom they piloted the interview questions. Although it is appropriate to modify the interview questions on the basis of the analysis, the authors did not describe the topic areas of the interview guide. Also, it is not clear whether the authors modified the interview questions on the basis of the piloted questions or whether they modified the questions on the basis of data collection (that is, the interviews conducted with the nine participants). The interviewer also summarized participants' comments at the end of the interview.
	Interviews lasted from 26 to 53 minutes. With a small sample of nine participants (note that this sample size could be considered small, even for a qualitative study), it is important to collect sufficient data to achieve saturation. The authors did not mention how they made the decision to stop collecting data and whether the decision was made because they believed they had reached saturation. If most of the interviews lasted only approximately 30 minutes, a reader might conclude that the authors' data collection strategy was not sufficiently comprehensive.

Guide	Comments
2d. Were the data analyzed appropriately, and were the findings corroborated adequately?	Grey and colleagues[21] did not report that a particular approach, such as grounded theory, had guided their data analysis; however, they did report that they used thematic analysis as described by Braun and Clarke.[45] They reported that they used six steps to analyze the data, but they did not actually describe the analytic process. In a review of Braun and Clarke's analytic process, it is clear that the six steps were as follows: familiarizing yourself with your data, generating initial codes, searching for themes, reviewing themes, defining and naming themes, and producing the report. This process seems reasonable, with the exception that "searching for themes" assumes that the themes were in the data waiting to be discovered. The authors did not discuss the iterative nature of data collection and analysis, so it was not clear whether they analyzed the data simultaneously as they conducted the interviews or whether the investigators conducted the analysis after they had conducted all the interviews. To the benefit of the study, the authors reported that all of the authors had discussed the interpretation of the data, which suggests that several team members with individual expertise contributed to data analysis. On the basis of the affiliations of the authors, the authors' content expertise included psychology, appearance research, oral and dental sciences, and workplace health. It would have been helpful for the authors to have indicated whether anyone on the research team had expertise in qualitative research.

Direct quotations from participants supported the study's findings. However, the authors did not provide accounts from three of the nine participants in the results section. This omission could be related to space limitations in this particular journal; however, it also could have been because the data from these three participants did not "fit" with the overall findings being presented. That stated, with only nine participants, it would be important for the authors to make sure that responses from all of the participants were represented in the results, or it would have been helpful for the authors to have described how data collected from the three participants did not "fit" with the overall findings presented. |

3. What are the results?

	Grey and colleagues[21] reported that their participants described an overarching theme of "normality" in their motivations for requesting, and expectations of having, dental implants. The concept of "normality" encompassed both appearance and function. Regarding appearance, participants described normality in terms of how they felt about themselves and how they behaved in social situations. Participants expected the implants to restore their "normal" appearance so that they could not only regain their internal self-image but also behave naturally in social situations (for example, not having to restrain their smiles or shield their mouths while talking). Regarding

Guide	Comments
	function, participants described their expectations of "normality" in terms of being able to eat and speak as they had before they lost their natural teeth. The authors also discussed how participants' desire to return to "normality" did not mean that participants desired to have perfect teeth or a "Hollywood smile."

4. How can I apply the results to my patient care?

Guide	Comments
4a. Does the study offer helpful theory?	On the basis of Giacomini and Cook's[16] definition of theory, readers could conclude that the results of Grey and colleagues'[21] study do offer helpful theory. Grey and colleagues[21] developed theoretical concepts from their analysis and proposed a visual depiction of these concepts and how they were related (Figure 1 in the article). They identified a central concept of "normality" that was linked to two subthemes of appearance and function. The authors highlighted that this theme of normality was distinct from the expectation of "perfect teeth" and was related to participants restoring their appearance and function rather than improving their function or enhancing their appearance.
4b. Does the study help me understand the context of my practice?	Although the characteristics of the study sample may not be similar to a clinician's own practice population, the findings described by Grey and colleagues[21] may be transferable in that they account for patients' motivations for requesting and expectations regarding having dental implants. If you regularly see patients who are making a decision about implants, reading the study results may help you understand the context of your own practice.
4c. Does the study help me understand social interactions in clinical care?	Assuming that a clinician's patients share similarities with the patients included in this study's sample, we believe that the study can help a clinician understand social interactions in clinical care. The authors proposed that good clinician-patient communication should account for patients' expectations of dental implants. If a patient desires to regain "normality" by receiving a dental implant, the clinician will need to assess whether this is a realistic expectation. The research results also suggest that patients who have this expectation of normality may treat their implants as they treated their previously natural teeth, which, for many, may not entail the thorough cleaning procedures that are necessary for implant longevity. If a patient lost his or her natural teeth owing to poor oral hygiene and periodontal disease, the clinician needs to communicate that the patient may need to improve his or her oral hygiene behaviors, and possibly, address any pre-existing disease, before deciding to get implants.

* *Source:* Grey and colleagues.[21]

What Are the Results?

Investigators usually present the main results of qualitative studies in clinical research as single or multiple concepts (often referred to as themes) that are integrated or linked in some way. The message from the results should be clear in the text. Research reports might include thematic statements as headers in the results section to enhance the accessibility of findings.[49] The results section of a research report may include tables and figures, but this section usually includes quotations or examples of observations to illustrate the concepts or themes presented. The investigators should integrate these quotations or examples of observations into the text along with the claims the quotes or examples support.

Box 8.5. What Are the Results?

Grey and colleagues[21] reported that their participants described an overarching theme of "normality" in their motivations for obtaining and their expectations of having dental implants. The concept of normality encompassed both appearance and function. Regarding appearance, participants described normality in terms of how they felt about themselves and how they behaved in social situations. Participants expected the implants to restore their normal appearance so that they could not only regain their internal self-image but also behave naturally in social situations (for example, they would not have to restrain their smiles or shield their mouths while talking). Regarding function, participants described their expectations of normality in terms of being able to eat and speak as they had before they lost their natural teeth. The authors also discussed how participants' desire to return to normality did not mean that participants desired to have perfect teeth or a "Hollywood smile."

How Can I Apply the Results to Patient Care?

Does the Study Offer Helpful Theory?

Theories provide "lenses" through which clinicians can look at complicated problems.[50] A theory can be central or peripheral to a particular investigation.[51] Theories influence research design, underpin methodology, have implications for how researchers and clinicians analyze and interpret data, and can be developed from the results of a qualitative study.[51,52] Nevertheless, having a resulting formal theory is not required of qualitative studies. Sometimes researchers use diagrams to depict the theories that are developed from a qualitative study, but a visual representation of theories is not a requirement. Clinicians might consider the results of qualitative research to be concepts and relationships.[16] The concepts are the building blocks of theory and they relate to each other in many ways. If a clinician finds that the study results offer concepts or theories that help him or her to understand a clinical scenario, then this newly acquired viewpoint will aid the clinician in providing patient care.

Does the Study Help Me Understand the Context of My Practice?

Rather than describe the generalizability of their research results, qualitative researchers often discuss how their findings may transfer to or fit into contexts outside their particular study.[25] If researchers provide sufficient detail about the circumstances of the situation or case that they studied, clinicians can speculate whether the findings from such a study are applicable to other cases with similar circumstances.[25] Clinicians also can determine whether they can transfer theoretical explanations about the phenomenon to their own clinical scenarios (that is, theoretical generalization).[32]

Does the Study Help Me Understand Social Interactions in Clinical Care?

Qualitative research results offer clinicians insights about understanding social roles, interactions, relationships, and experiences; although the results may not provide a definitive answer to a question, they do provide an understanding into what might be going on.[16] In general, insights from qualitative research results may highlight contextual variables that contribute to patient care, enhance communication between patients and clinicians, offer examples of the contrasting experiences of patients and caregivers, or address assumptions related to medical language that people often take for granted. The results of the study you find can become even more applicable to patient care if they help you understand how to communicate with patients and how patients' and clinicians' social contexts might affect decision-making or the receipt of care.

> **Box 8.6. Your Assessment of the Applicability of the Qualitative Research You Identified**
>
> After assessing the applicability of the results, you conclude that this study offers useful theory and helps you better understand the context of your practice in terms of possible motivations and expectations that your patients may have when seeking implants. The study results also help you understand the interactions that routinely occur between patients and providers when it comes to making clinical decisions (see Table 8.1 for a more detailed critical appraisal of the article[16,21,45]). Thus, you decide that this evidence is applicable to the decision that you and your patient have to make.

 Qualitative research results offer clinicians insights about understanding social roles, interactions, relationships, and experiences.

Conclusion

Because of qualitative researchers' abilities to explore social problems and to understand the perspective of patients, the results of qualitative research studies can provide unique information about patients' fears, worries, goals, and expectations related to dental care. Clinicians should, however, know how to appraise or evaluate the results of these studies to adequately inform their decisions. The critical appraisal criteria we outlined focus on aspects of credibility, the results, and the applicability of those results. By applying these guidelines, clinicians can consider qualitative studies when trying to achieve the best possible results for their own practice.

Box 8.7. What You Say to Your Patient

By reviewing this qualitative study, you learned that patients' pretreatment expectations can strongly influence the treatment outcome and the level of patient satisfaction after treatment. Therefore, it is important to identify your patient's motivation for his treatment choice and to determine his commitment to quit smoking, improve his oral hygiene, and regularly attend appointments for recall and maintenance as needed, because these were the factors that may have contributed to his dental issues. You also need to discuss with the patient the inherent limitations of implants to restore "normality" and the risks associated with implants. By doing so, you will take the necessary steps to correct any misunderstandings or unrealistic expectations that your patient may have developed.

References

1. Brignardello-Petersen R, Carrasco-Labra A, Glick M, Guyatt GH, Azarpazhooh A. "A practical approach to evidence-based dentistry: understanding and applying the principles of EBD." *JADA* 2014;145(11):1105–1107.

2. Chapter 2 of this book was based on Brignardello-Petersen R, Carrasco-Labra A, Booth HA, et al. "A practical approach to evidence-based dentistry: II: how to search for evidence to inform clinical decisions." *JADA* 2014;145(12):1262–1267.

3. Brignardello-Petersen R, Carrasco-Labra A, Glick M, Guyatt GH, Azarpazhooh A. "A practical approach to evidence-based dentistry: III: how to appraise and use an article about therapy." *JADA* 2015;146(1):42–49.e1.

4. Brignardello-Petersen R, Carrasco-Labra A, Glick M, Guyatt GH, Azarpazhooh A. "A practical approach to evidence-based dentistry: IV: how to use an article about harm." *JADA* 2015;146(2):94–101.e1.

5. Brignardello-Petersen R, Carrasco-Labra A, Glick M, Guyatt GH, Azarpazhooh A. "A practical approach to evidence-based dentistry: V: how to appraise and use an article about diagnosis." *JADA* 2015;146(3):184–191.e1.

6. Carrasco-Labra A, Brignardello-Petersen R, Glick M, Guyatt GH, Azarpazhooh A. "A practical approach to evidence-based dentistry: VI: how to use a systematic review." *JADA* 2015;146(4):255–265.e1.

7. Carrasco-Labra A, Brignardello-Petersen R, Glick M, Guyatt GH, Neumann I, Azarpazhooh A. "A practical approach to evidence-based dentistry: VII: how to use patient management recommendations from clinical practice guidelines." *JADA* 2015;146(5):327–336.e1.

8. Creswell JW. *Qualitative Inquiry and Research Design: Choosing Among Five Approaches*. 2nd ed. Thousand Oaks, CA: Sage Publications; 2007.

9. Rice PL, Ezzy D. *Qualitative Research Methods: A Health Focus*. South Melbourne, Victoria, Australia: Oxford University Press; 1999.

10. Patton MQ. *Qualitative Research and Evaluation Methods*. Thousand Oaks, CA: Sage Publications; 2002.

11. Canadian Institutes of Health Research, Natural Sciences and Engineering Research Council of Canada, Social Sciences and Humanitites Research Council of Canada. "Qualitative research." In: *Tri-Council Policy Statement: Ethical Conduct for Research Involving Humans*. 2010:135-145. Available at: *http://www.pre.ethics.gc.ca/eng/archives/tcps2-eptc2-2010/chapter10-chapitre10/#toc10-1*. Accessed June 15, 2015.

12. McCormack JP, Loewen P. "Adding 'value' to clinical practice guidelines." *Can Fam Physician* 2007;53(8):1326–1327.

13. Sackett DL, Rosenberg WM, Gray JA, Haynes RB, Richardson WS. "Evidence based medicine: what is is and what it isn't." *BMJ* 1996;312(7023):71–72.

14. Rist RC. "Influencing the policy process with qualitative research." In: Denzin NK, Lincoln YS, editors. *Handbook of Qualitative Research*. Thousand Oaks, CA: Sage Publications; 1994. p. 545–557.

15. Cheek J, Onslow M, Cream A. "Beyond the divide: comparing and contrasting aspects of qualitative and quantitative research approaches." Advances in Speech-Language Pathology 2004;6(3):147–152.

16. Giacomini M, Cook DJ. "Advanced topics in applying the results of therapy trials: qualitative research." In: Guyatt GH, Rennie D, Meade MO, Cook DJ, editors. *Users' Guides to the Medical Literature: A Manual for Evidence-Based Clinical Practice*. McGraw-Hill; 2008. p. 341–360.

17. Lindenmeyer A, Bowyer V, Roscoe J, Dale J, Sutcliffe P. "Oral health awareness and care preferences in patients with diabetes: a qualitative study." *Fam Pract* 2013;30(1):113–118.

18. Niesten D, van Mourik K, van der Sanden W. "The impact of having natural teeth on the QoL of frail dentulous older people: a qualitative study." *BMC Public Health* 2012;12:839.

19. Bedos C, Loignon C, Landry A, Allison PJ, Richard L. "How health professionals perceive and experience treating people on social assistance: a qualitative study among dentists in Montreal, Canada." *BMC Health Serv Res* 2013;13:464.

20. Rousseau N, Steele J, May C, Exley C. "'Your whole life is lived through your teeth': biographical disruption and experiences of tooth loss and replacement." *Sociol Health Illn* 2014;36(3):462–476.

21. Grey EB, Harcourt D, O'Sullivan D, Buchanan H, Kilpatrick NM. "A qualitative study of patients' motivations and expectations for dental implants." *Br Dent J* 2013;214(1):E1–E5.

22. Dixon-Woods M, Shaw RL, Agarwal S, Smith JA. "The problem of appraising qualitative research." *Qual Saf Health Care* 2004;13(3):223–225.

23. Eakin JM, Mykhalovskiy E. "Reframing the evaluation of qualitative health research: reflections on a review of appraisal guidelines in the health sciences." *J Eval Clin Pract* 2003;9(2):187–194.

24. Sale JE. "How to assess rigour... or not in qualitative papers." *J Eval Clin Pract* 2008;14(5):912–913.

25. Lincoln YS, Guba EG. *Naturalistic Inquiry*. Newbury Park, CA: Sage Publications; 1985.

26. Lincoln YS, Guba EG. "But is it rigorous? Trustworthiness and authenticity in naturalistic evaluation." In: Williams DD, editor. *Naturalistic Evaluation. New Directions for Program Evaluation. No. 90*. San Francisco, CA: Jossey-Boss; 1986. p. 78–84.

27. Patton MQ. *Qualitative Evaluation and Research Methods*. Newbury Park, CA: Sage Publications; 1990.

28. Sandelowski M. "Sample size in qualitative research." *Res Nurs Health* 1995;18(2):179–183.

29. Coyne IT. "Sampling in qualitative research: purposeful and theoretical sampling; merging or clear boundaries?" *J Adv Nurs* 1997;26(3):623–630.

30. Polkinghorne DE. "Phenomenological research methods." In: Valle RS, Halling S, editors. *Existential-Phenomenological Perspectives in Psychology: Exploring the Breadth of Human Experience, With a Special Section on Transpersonal Psychology*. New York, NY: Plenum Press; 1989. p. 41–60.

31. Polkinghorne DE. "Language and meaning: data collection in qualitative research." *J Counseling Psychol* 2005;52(2):137–145.

32. Schwandt TA. *Dictionary of Qualitative Inquiry*. Thousand Oaks, CA: Sage Publications; 2001.

33. Krueger RA. "The future of focus groups." *Qual Health Res* 1995;5(4):524–530.

34. Goodwin D, Pope C, Mort M, Smith A. "Ethics and ethnography: an experiential account." *Qual Health Res* 2003;13(4):567–577.

35. Kvale S, Brinkmann S. *Interviews: Learning the Craft of Qualitative Research Interviewing*. Thousand Oaks, CA: Sage Publications; 2009.

36. Sandelowski M. "Rigor or rigor mortis: the problem of rigor in qualitative research revisited." *ANS Adv Nurs Sci* 1993;16(2):1–8.

37. Smith MW. "Ethics in focus groups: a few concerns." *Qual Health Res* 1995;5(4):478–486.

38. Kaiser K. "Protecting respondent confidentiality in qualitative research." *Qual Health Res* 2009;19(11):1632–1641.

39. Kitzinger J. "The methodology of focus groups: the importance of interaction between research participants." *Sociology of Health & Illness* 1994;16(1):103–121.

40. Lambert SD, Loiselle CG. "Combining individual interviews and focus groups to enhance data richness." *J Adv Nurs* 2008;62(2):228–237.

41. MacKay C, Jaglal S, Sale J, Badley EM, Davis AM. "A qualitative study of the consequences of knee symptoms: 'it's like you're an athlete and you go to a couch potato.'" *BMJ Open* 2014;4(10):e006006.

42. Webster F, Rice K, Dainty K, Zwarenstein M, Durant S, Kuper A. "Failure to cope: the hidden curriculum of emergency department wait times and the implications for clinical training." *Acad Med* 2015;90(1):56–62.

43. Popay J, Rogers A, Williams G. "Rationale and standards for the systematic review of qualitative literature in health services research." *Qual Health Res* 1998;8(3):341–351.

44. Sandelowski M. "Qualitative analysis: what it is and how to begin." *Res Nurs Health* 1995;18(4):371–375.

45. Braun V, Clarke V. "Using thematic analysis in psychology." *Qualitative Research in Psychology* 2006;3(2):77–101.

46. Strauss A, Corbin J. *Basics of Qualitative Research: Grounded Theory Procedures and Techniques.* Newbury Park, CA: Sage Publications; 1990.

47. Strauss A, Corbin J. *Basics of Qualitative Research: Techniques and Procedures for Developing Grounded Theory.* Thousand Oaks, CA: Sage Publications; 1998.

48. Giorgi A. "Concerning a serious misunderstanding of the essence of the phenomenological method in psychology." *J Phenomenological Psychol* 2008;39(1):33–58.

49. Sandelowski M, Leeman J. "Writing usable qualitative health research findings." *Qual Health Res* 2012;22(10):1404–1413.

50. Reeves S, Albert M, Kuper A, Hodges BD. "Why use theories in qualitative research?" *BMJ* 2008;337:a949.

51. Sandelowski M. "Theory unmasked: the uses and guises of theory in qualitative research." *Res Nurs Health* 1993;16(3):213–218.

52. Kelly M. "The role of theory in qualitative health research." *Fam Pract* 2010;27(3):285–290.

A version of this chapter originally appeared in the August 2015 edition of *JADA* (Volume 146, Issue 8, Pages 623–630). It has been reviewed and updated for accuracy and clarity by the editors of *How to Use Evidence-Based Dental Practices to Improve Your Clinical Decision-Making*.

Chapter 9. How to Appraise and Use an Article about Economic Analysis

Lusine Abrahamyan, M.D., M.P.H., Ph.D.; Petros Pechlivanoglou, Ph.D.; Murray Krahn, M.D., M.Sc.;
Alonso Carrasco-Labra, D.D.S., M.Sc., Ph.D.; Romina Brignardello-Petersen, D.D.S., M.Sc., Ph.D.;
Michael Glick, D.M.D.; Gordon H. Guyatt, M.D., M.Sc.; and Amir Azarpazhooh, D.D.S., M.Sc., Ph.D.

Introduction

In the previous eight chapters in this book, we introduced the process of evidence-based dentistry[1] and explained how to search for evidence to inform clinical practice[2] and how to use a research report to inform clinical decisions regarding questions of therapy,[3] harm,[4] diagnosis,[5] systematic reviews,[6] clinical practice guidelines,[7] and qualitative research.[8] In this chapter, we explain how to use an economic analysis to inform clinical and policy decision-making in dentistry. We introduce and describe the basic concepts needed to understand economic analysis, and we explain how to critically appraise such studies.

> **Box 9.1. Clinical Scenario**
> One of your patients, a first-year college student, came to ask for your opinion regarding his third molars, which have not erupted yet. He explained that a friend of his just had two of his mandibular third molars extracted and is planning to extract the remaining two because he was told that the early, prophylactic removal of third molars is less traumatic than the "inevitable late extraction of infected third molars," and that it prevents future teeth crowding. Your patient does not have dental benefits, and he is concerned about his out-of-pocket expenses for extracting these teeth and whether such expenses would be worth the potential benefits and risks of the procedure. You realize that, to answer your patient's question, you need to find an economic analysis whose authors considered both short-term and long-term risks, benefits, and costs for third-molar extraction. You decide to conduct a literature search and a critical appraisal to inform the decision.

Why Economic Analysis in Dentistry?

The economic burden of oral health care is significant, with a reported $111 billion spent on dental care in the United States and $11.7 billion in Canada in 2012.[9,10] Public health agencies invest significant resources in oral health care programs that amounted to $9 billion in 2012 in the United States.[9] Although most of the programs offered are assessed with respect to their effectiveness, whether they represent a good "value for the money" rarely is investigated.

Clinicians daily make treatment decisions not only on the basis of information about the benefits or harms but also on the basis of costs. With a patient's best interest in mind, a clinician needs to assess whether the expected treatment benefits justify the resources used. For example, imagine that you want to buy more advanced three-dimensional (3-D) dental imaging equipment for your practice; does this possible purchase represent a good value for money spent? Or imagine yourself as a policy maker who must decide if the $2 million set aside for a public dental program should be directed toward an oral health prevention program for children or toward a program for adults who have low incomes and who are edentulous. Patients also need to invest their resources (for example, personal income, time off work) in interventions that will provide them with the best value for the money. Over time, such decisions are likely to get more, rather than less, difficult: the projected demographic changes in countries with high and low levels of income, our ever-increasing demand for better care, and increasingly costly health care innovations will continue to strain our already scarce health care resources. All these aspects illustrate the importance of investigating an intervention's effectiveness and safety in conjunction with its efficiency, the balance of costs, and (positive and negative) health consequences.

There are different types of economic analysis that can evaluate the efficiency of a dental intervention. If the dentist is only interested in the overall cost of treating a particular condition, he or she can use a cost analysis, taking into account all resource utilization during and after treatment. This is, however, not a full economic analysis as it does not compare alternative treatments. If the dentist is interested in both the benefits and the costs of two or more treatments, a full economic analysis in the form of cost-effectiveness, cost-utility, or cost-benefit analyses would be a more appropriate source of evidence (Table 9.1[11–14]). In all these types of economic analyses, treatment costs are measured in monetary units.

Cost-Effectiveness Analysis

In a cost-effectiveness analysis (CEA), treatment consequences (that is, benefits and harms) are measured in natural units, such as number of teeth extracted, gingival bleeding rates, or tooth survival. The main outcome of a CEA is the incremental cost-effectiveness ratio (ICER) (that is, the additional cost per additional unit of effect of a candidate intervention compared with an alternative). The results of a CEA can assist clinicians only in making decisions between treatments that share the same clinical effect.

Cost-Utility Analysis

In a cost-utility analysis (CUA), treatment consequences are measured in quality-adjusted life-years (QALYs), which is a combined measure of the duration and quality of life.[15] The advantage of this type of analysis is its transferability, as it offers the means to make comparisons across

Table 9.1. Types of Economic Analyses

Type of Economic Analysis	Measurement of Costs	Measurement of Effectiveness	Example Research Questions
Cost Analysis	Monetary units	None	What is the cost of periodontitis management at a public sector specialist periodontal clinic settings in Malaysia for the first year of periodontal therapy, from the societal perspective?*
Cost-Effectiveness Analysis	Monetary units	Natural units (for example, teeth extracted, gingival bleeding rates, or tooth survival)	What is the cost-effectiveness of implant-supported overdentures, implant-retained overdentures, and complete dentures in patients who are edentulous at three years of follow-up, from the patients' perspective?†
Cost-Utility Analysis	Monetary units	Quality-adjusted life-years	What is the cost-utility of three preventive strategies (that is, no prophylaxis, oral penicillin, and oral cephalexin) in patients with prosthetic joints who are undergoing dental treatment to prevent late prosthetic joint infections at one year follow-up from the patients' perspective?‡
Cost-Benefit Analysis	Monetary units	Single or multiple health outcomes valued in monetary terms (for example, willingness to pay)	What is the value of a four-year caries preventive program among 19-year-olds from a societal and a dental health care perspective?§

* *Source:* Mohd-Dom and colleagues.[11]   ‡ *Source:* Jacobson and colleagues.[13]
† *Source:* Zitzmann and colleagues.[12]   § *Source:* Oscarson and colleagues.[14]

different interventions and different diseases using a common measure (for example, cost per QALY for oral health prevention versus cost per QALY for hypertension prevention). Because of this advantage, CUA is the most common form of economic analysis.

CUA also has limitations: the QALY can be insensitive to improvements in health-related quality of life achieved with dental interventions owing to the fact that few dental interventions are lifesaving or extend life. Furthermore, given that in most settings dental care is paid out of pocket or through private insurance, the need for prioritizing the allocation of resources across dental strategies (for example, investing in a caries prevention program for children or in an oral cancer awareness campaign) is limited. For these reasons, CUAs are rarely used in dentistry.

Cost-Benefit Analysis

In a cost-benefit analysis (CBA), the treatment consequences are evaluated in monetary terms, providing a direct estimate of whether consequences exceed costs.[15] CBA is the least used form of economic analyses, with only few examples in dental literature.

Trial–Based versus Decision Model–Based Economic Analyses

Economic analyses can be conducted alongside clinical studies (trial-based) in which investigators collect patient-level data on health care resource use and costs, along with effectiveness outcomes.[16] These clinical studies include randomized controlled trials (RCTs), observational studies, patient registries, and administrative databases.[17] Constraints of a trial-based economic analysis include the facts that the duration for which costs and outcomes are assessed is limited to the actual study duration, information originating from other similar studies on the treatments of interest is ignored, and collecting data for economic analysis alongside a trial is often resource-intensive.[15,17]

Alternatively, decision models can be used to estimate the long-term (or lifetime) costs and consequences of health care interventions (see Figure 9.1[15,18] for a simplified example of a decision tree). A decision model is a statistical tool that allows clinicians to compare the costs and benefits of two or more alternative clinical decisions while considering the probability of events occurring over a selected period (that is, the time horizon).

Figure 9.1. Example of a Simplified Decision Model Comparing Surgical Removal or Retention of Third Molars

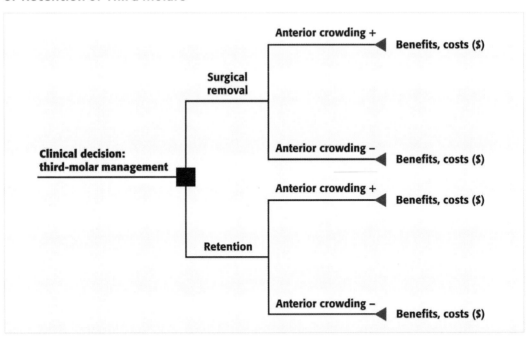

Decision models combine information from multiple sources (for example, randomized controlled trials, literature searches, administrative databases, and expert opinions) to reconstruct the clinical pathways for each alternative intervention under conditions of uncertainty over the time horizon.[15] These models are more suited to evaluate long-term costs and consequences of treatments. This example decision tree considers only one adverse consequence (that is, anterior crowding). A decision tree in which adverse consequences are considered more extensively can be found in the study by Edwards and colleagues.[18]

During your search, you found that the prophylactic extraction of disease-free, impacted third molars remains controversial. The American Association of Oral and Maxillofacial Surgeons, for example, supports the removal of "erupted and impacted third molar teeth even if the teeth are asymptomatic, if there is presence or reasonable potential that pathology may occur caused by or related to the third-molar teeth."[19] In contrast, the investigators of several systematic reviews did not find sufficient evidence to support removal over retention.[20-22] You read that annually in the United States, approximately 10 million third molars are extracted from approximately five million people, with total costs exceeding $3 billion.[23] You found an economic evaluation that compared removal versus retention of asymptomatic, disease-free mandibular third molars, using a decision model.[18] In the abstract of the study, the investigators reported that the probability estimates for different clinical outcomes were obtained from a comprehensive literature review, and the treatment costs were obtained from the National Health Service hospitals in Wales, United Kingdom. The effect of each clinical outcome was assessed among 100 patients attending a single dental hospital. The authors concluded that mandibular third-molar retention was more cost-effective than removal.[18] You obtain the article and conduct a critical review of the methods and results.

Critically Appraising an Economic Analysis to Inform Clinical Decisions

Economic analyses can be critically appraised using three steps: assessing the risk of bias, assessing the results, and assessing their applicability to your patients' care.[24] Below, we describe each of these steps.

How Serious Is the Risk of Bias?

The main research question of an economic analysis should define the patient population, the treatment alternatives, the perspective of evaluation, the type of analysis, and the time horizon for which costs and consequences are to be evaluated. Ideally, economic analyses should compare the new intervention with all standard treatment alternatives.[15] For logistical reasons, however, this is not always feasible. Whatever treatments authors have chosen to compare, we suggest assessing three risk-of-bias criteria: consideration of subgroups, accurate measurement of consequences and costs, and consideration of timing. Table 9.2[12,25-28] presents examples of assessments of the risk of bias in economic analyses. In a critical appraisal process, it is important to evaluate if the new intervention has been compared with a relevant alternative, and if the time horizon of the study was sufficiently long to see the expected costs and consequences of treatments. Components of assessments of the risk of bias in economic analyses that could create a risk of bias are discussed in more details below.

Table 9.2. Critically Appraising the Risk of Bias in Studies of Economic Analysis

Questions	Examples	Explanations
Are results reported separately for relevant patient subgroups?	"The objectives of this study are to examine the utilization of dental sealants and its determinants, evaluate the incremental effectiveness and expenditure associated with sealant placement after correcting the potential selection issue, and explore the differences in sealant's cost-effectiveness among subpopulations Children at relatively high caries risk, as well as children who visited dentists for preventive care more than once a year, had greater odds of receiving sealants."*	In this study, the authors specified subgroup analysis at the study planning phase and included it as part of the study aim. The authors further supported the subgroup analysis by conducting a literature review and by comparing the characteristics of children who visited dentists for preventive care and who either received or did not receive sealants. The cost-effectiveness was evaluated for the full sample and for the selected subgroups. The risk of bias is low on the basis of this criterion.
Were consequences and costs measured accurately?[†]	"For each patient, the costs of delivering treatment were recorded by a research nurse. . . . Laboratory costs were recorded as part of normal hospital policy. . . . All of the dental materials used were recorded and given a unit price . . . [and] the amount of time spent in the dental surgery for each appointment was measured using a stop watch. . . . The total number of clinical appointments was recorded, including unscheduled postoperative care, and the total clinical time calculated for each patient. The cost of professional time per patient was estimated using the highest point of the salary scale for the community dental service in Ireland (€85 185). Based on this salary, the hourly rate for a clinician providing care was €44.37 per hour for 240 8-hour working days per year."[‡]	In this cost-effectiveness analysis, the authors compared the partial removable dental prosthesis and the shortened dental arch for older patients who were partially dentate in a randomized controlled trial that had 12 months of follow-up. The analysis was conducted from the "perspective of a publicly funded body."[‡] The authors described the cost components that were accounted for (that is, laboratory costs, dental materials, clinic visits, and time and cost of professional care) and only some of the sources for unit costs. For example, it is unclear how dental material costs were obtained. Moreover, the reporting of results was not transparent, as authors presented only the total costs per patient without information on frequency of use and unit costs.[†] These limitations entail high risk of bias for this criterion.

Questions	Examples	Explanations
Did investigators consider the timing of costs and consequences?	"Costs were calculated in Euros and future costs discounted at 3% per annum. . . . No such discounting was performed for future effectiveness, since it remains unclear whether and how to discount years of tooth retention."[§]	In this study, the authors used a decision model approach to evaluate the cost-effectiveness of one- and two-step incomplete and complete excavations for caries. They assessed the benefits (that is, tooth retention and vitality) and costs over the patient's lifetime. The authors applied a 3% discounting rate to account for differential timing of costs. Effectiveness measures were discounted neither in their main analysis nor in sensitivity analyses. This limitation may indicate a high risk of bias for this criterion.

* *Source:* Ouyang.[25]
† *Authors' note:* The accuracy of measuring consequences has been covered in previous chapters in this book; here we discuss only costs.
‡ *Source:* McKenna and colleagues.[26]
§ *Source:* Schwendicke and colleagues.[27]

▸ *Are results reported separately for relevant patient subgroups?*

Similar to clinical effectiveness studies, results of economic analyses can vary widely between different patient subgroups. Such variations can be explained by differences in treatment consequences or costs in these subgroups.[29] For example, implant-supported dentures may be more cost-effective than conventional dentures in patients who are edentulous and younger than 60 years but not cost-effective for patients who are 85 years and older, and ignoring this difference can result in misleading interpretation of the results. The subgroups for economic analysis should be defined at the study planning stage and should be reported with the rationale for their selection (for example, to explore heterogeneity in results, to determine policy relevance, or on the basis of a literature review). Once defined, all results should be analyzed for selected subgroups separately.

▸ *Were consequences and costs measured accurately?*

In an economic analysis, the evidence on consequences (that is, clinical effectiveness, safety) may come from a single RCT or an observational study, or, more appropriately, from evidence synthesis (that is, systematic review). The quality of outcomes of an economic analysis depends on the quality of the effectiveness evidence on which it relies. For that reason, systematic collection of the best, unbiased evidence on consequences is important. In previous chapters of this book, we have covered all major issues related to the risk of bias to establish treatment effectiveness,[3] harm,[4] and diagnostic accuracy.[5] Here, we discuss issues pertaining to costs.

The cost components (that is, resources utilized) included in an economic analysis should reflect the perspective assumed. Hence, once you identify the perspective of the economic analysis in the reviewed article, you need to critically appraise whether all relevant cost components have been considered. For example, investigators of a study evaluating from a societal perspective the cost of establishing a community-based oral health promotion program by health educators who do not have an oral health background should consider not only the costs of training the educators (for example, hourly salary, space rental fees, costs of education materials)[30] but also the productivity losses of the participants who attend the sessions. After identifying the cost components and the frequency of their use, unit costs are applied to obtain an estimate of the total costs associated with each patient.

▶ *Did investigators consider the timing of costs and consequences?*

The consequences and costs of health care interventions can occur at different times. For example, although most of the costs for establishing an oral health education program in schools occur at the time of the program launch, the benefit of caries prevention may occur several years later. Investigators of a CEA comparing two alternative approaches for such a program should consider this differential timing of costs and benefits.

As a society and as individual people, we prefer to have resources available to us now, and not later, either because we can invest these resources and receive benefits over time or simply because we prefer good things now to good things later. Time preferences, therefore, play a significant role both in making individual decisions and in influencing public policy.[31]

To adjust for these differential time preferences, especially when the study's time horizon is long, we devalue benefits and costs that accrue later, relative to those that occur earlier. This process of devaluing is called "discounting," and economic analysts apply a discounting rate to costs and outcomes. Most economic evaluation guidelines recommend using either a 3% or a 5% per year discounting of future costs and outcomes to present values.[15] It is, however, debatable if the costs and consequences should be discounted in the same way.[31]

Box 9.3. Your Assessment of the Risk of Bias of the Economic Analysis You Identified

The authors of the study you identified[18] did not specify any subgroups, although they could have considered age and smoking status on the basis of the literature. Effectiveness was estimated by asking patients to rate different scenarios after tooth removal or retention, using a visual analog scale, which is the least preferred method to evaluate health preferences. Furthermore, the variability around the average effectiveness scores was not presented. Only aggregate costs by scenario and by health care resource use were presented, which limited your ability to see, for example, medication costs (see the Supplemental Table[18] at the end of this chapter). The overall time horizon for costs and benefits was not specified, and discounting was not considered. Bearing in mind the identified limitations, you proceed to read the results.

What Are the Results?

To evaluate the results from an economic analysis, you should examine the mean differences in effectiveness and cost between the treatments and the variation around these differences. Conclusions about the cost-effectiveness of the interventions can be made after considering willingness to pay for an incremental cost per unit of benefit. Table 9.3[12,25,32] and indirectly, Figure 9.2[12] (as cited in Table 9.4) present examples and charted information that describes how to critically appraise results of economic analyses.

Table 9.3. Critically Appraising the Results of Economic Analyses

Questions	Examples	Explanations
What were the incremental costs and effects of each strategy?	"For the total follow-up period, the mean cost per child in the experimental group was €496.45 and in the control group was €426.95. The mean incremental cost was €69.50 (95% CI*: 28.25, 110.75). The mean number of DMF[†] increment surfaces was 2.56 in the experimental group and 4.60 in the control group. The mean incremental effectiveness was 2.04 averted DMF surfaces (95% CI: 1.26, 2.82). The ICER[‡] was €34.07 per averted DMF surface."[§]	The authors conducted a cost-effectiveness analysis alongside an RCT[¶] that compared an individually designed, patient-centered preventive program for caries with basic prevention as standard of care in dental clinics in Pori, Finland.[§] The authors presented incremental costs and benefits for each treatment arm and the ICER, with accompanying CIs. The full presentation of incremental costs and effectiveness allows the reader to plot the results on a cost-effectiveness plane.
Do incremental costs and effects differ between subgroups?	"The results from a subgroup analysis show that sealing children at high risk for caries appears to be highly cost effective. In contrast, sealing children at low risk for caries would be much less cost effective. . . . There is no significant difference in ICERs between sealing younger children and sealing older children."[#]	In this study, the authors found that the cost-effectiveness of sealant applications was different by caries risk and by frequency of use of preventive care, but not by age. They concluded that sealant application should not be uniform because it is not always cost-effective.
How much does allowance for uncertainty change the results?	"The cost-effectiveness plane, based on probabilistic sensitivity analysis, showed that for almost all bootstrapped resamples (99.9%) the experimental caries-control regimen was more effective, but more costly. There was very little uncertainty because the bootstrap replications did not straddle other quadrants in the cost-effectiveness plane . . . The curve for acceptability of cost-effectiveness reveals that if the willingness of society to pay for an averted DMF surface is, for example, €40, the probability of an experimental caries-control regimen being considered cost-effective is about 65%."[§]	The authors of this study evaluated the robustness of the ICER by using 5,000 bootstrapping** resamples and found that in almost all resamples the ICER was in the same quadrant (quadrant 1 as per Figure 2). Next, the authors plotted a CEAC[††] in which the probability of being cost-effective was calculated for different values of willingness to pay for an averted DMF surface. Clinicians can use CEAC to see what would be the probability of the described intervention being cost-effective for the threshold values they consider reasonable for their practice.

* CI = confidence interval.
[†] DMF = decayed, missing, and filled.
[‡] ICER = incremental cost-effectiveness ratio.
[§] *Source:* Hietasalo and colleagues.[32]
[¶] RCT = randomized controlled trial.
[#] *Source:* Ouyang.[25]
** Bootstrapping is a technique used to quantify the uncertainty around a random variable based on computer simulations.
[††] CEAC = cost-effectiveness acceptability curve.

Figure 9.2. Cost-Effectiveness Plane for "Complete Denture versus Implant-Retained Overdentures" Comparison[12]

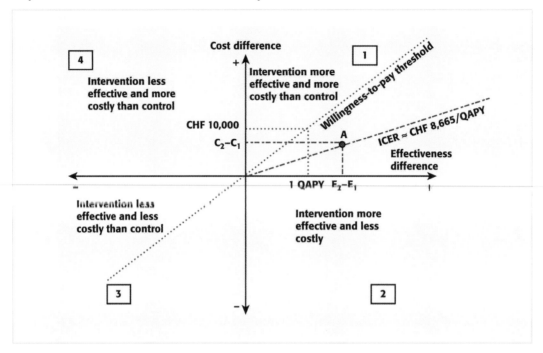

There are four quadrants on a cost-effectiveness plane in which the horizontal line represents the differences in effectiveness and the vertical line represents the differences in costs. Any intervention that is more effective and more costly than the control will have an incremental cost-effectiveness ratio (ICER) located in quadrant 1 and will need a threshold estimate (that is, willingness to pay) to decide if it is cost-effective. An intervention that is more effective and less costly than the control (quadrant 2) always will be a dominant strategy. In contrast, an intervention that is less effective and more costly (quadrant 4) always will be dominated by the control treatment. To decide whether an intervention that is less costly and less effective than the control (quadrant 3) is cost-effective, you need to decide how much loss in effectiveness is acceptable, in comparison with benefiting from cost savings. In this example, E_1 and E_2 are the effectiveness estimates for complete denture. C_1 and C_2 are the cost estimates for implant-retained overdentures. The slope of the line connecting the cost-effectiveness plane origin to point A represents the ICER or the incremental unit cost per incremental unit of effectiveness (that is, 8,665 Swiss francs [CHF] per quality-adjusted prosthesis-year [QAPY]) for the comparison of "implant-retained overdentures versus conventional dentures."[12] If, for example, the maximum willingness to pay for treating edentulism is CHF 10,000 per 1 QAPY, then using implant-retained overdentures would be cost-effective.

Table 9.4. Incremental Costs, Incremental Effectiveness, and Incremental Cost-Effectiveness Ratio*

Strategies	Average 3-Year Cost Per Patient, In CHF,[†] $C^{‡}$	Average 3-Year QAPY[§] Per Patient, $E^{¶}$	Incremental Costs, ΔCHF	Incremental Effects, ΔE (QAPY Gained)	ICER,[#] $\Delta C / \Delta E$ (CHF/QAPY)
Complete Denture	$C_1 = 3{,}675$	$E_1 = 0.86$	NA**	NA	NA
Implant-Retained Overdentures	$C_2 = 8{,}874$	$E_2 = 1.46$	$C_2 - C_1 = 5{,}199$	$E_2 - E_1 = 0.60$	$C_2 - C_1 / E_2 - E_1 = 8{,}665$
Implant-Supported Overdentures	$C_3 = 17{,}837$	$E_3 = 1.57$	$C_3 - C_2 = 8{,}963$	$E_3 - E_2 = 0.11$	$C_3 - C_2 / E_3 - E_2 = 81{,}482$

* *Source:* Zitzmann and colleagues[12] (base-case analysis with 3-year follow-up and 0% discount rate).
  Costs were estimated in 2000 Swiss francs (CHF) (CHF 100 = US $61).
[†] CHF = Swiss franc.
[‡] C = incremental costs.
[§] QAPY = quality-adjusted prosthesis-year.
[¶] E = incremental effectiveness.
[#] ICER = incremental cost-effectiveness ratio.
** NA = not applicable.

▶ *What were the incremental costs and effects of each strategy?*

We will facilitate discussion in this section using the example of CEA by Zitzmann and colleagues,[12] who compared implant-supported overdenture prostheses (four implants), implant-retained overdentures (two implants), and complete dentures (20 patients in each of the three groups) from the patient's perspective in Switzerland, to assess whether implant treatment in the mandible represents value for money spent.[12] The effectiveness was measured in quality-adjusted prosthesis-years (QAPY), a composite estimate of duration of prosthesis use and perceived chewing ability (as measured by a visual analog scale between 0 [the worst possible state] and 1 [the best possible state]). If a patient, for example, reported best possible chewing ability for all three years, the QAPY equaled 3. On the basis of the results of the study, at three years, the average QAPYs per patient were 0.86, 1.46, and 1.57, and the average costs were 2,525 Swiss francs (CHF), CHF 6,935, and CHF 15,805 (CHF 100 = US $61 in 2000) for conventional dentures, implant-retained overdentures, and implant-supported overdentures, respectively.[12]

Table 9.4[12] displays the ICER of implant-retained overdentures versus complete dentures, and implant-supported overdentures versus complete dentures. However, you should not simply look at the ICER value, as it may be deceiving. The ICER is an estimate. Therefore, an intervention that is more effective and more costly than the control treatment can have the same ICER as an intervention that is less effective and less costly than the control. Instead, you first need to evaluate whether the differences in costs and in effectiveness are large enough to have clinical and policy-relevant impact. Next, the differences in costs and effectiveness should be interpreted using a cost-effectiveness plane as shown in Figure 9.2.[12]

▸ *Do incremental costs and effects differ between subgroups?*

In reviewing an economic analysis, you need to consider if the observed benefits, harms, and costs may be different between some patient subgroups. For example, the cost-effectiveness of dental recall examinations may depend on a patient's risk factors. A decision model that evaluated the cost-effectiveness of different recall frequencies of routine dental checks in children found that moving from a six-month to a three-month recall frequency provided only a small benefit in terms of tooth decay and was associated with significantly higher costs.[33] In contrast, moving from a six-month recall schedule to less frequent visits (for example, annual visits or visits every 18 months) increased the risk of dental decay with some cost savings. The cost-effectiveness results, however, were different across the four risk-subgroups that included combinations of patients with differing socioeconomic status (that is, manual or nonmanual workers) and patients living in an area with water fluoridation.[33]

▸ *How much does allowing for uncertainty change the results?*

Economic analyses often combine evidence from different sources to reach an estimate of incremental cost–effectiveness. Because these parameters are sample estimates, they are characterized by uncertainty, known as parameter uncertainty. In addition, the decisions regarding the assumptions of the analysis and the selection of the source of input evidence contribute to the overall uncertainty related to the results of an economic analysis. One advantage of incorporating uncertainty in economic analysis is understanding the consequences of decision-making in the presence of uncertainty.[34]

The effect of uncertainty on the outcomes of the economic analysis usually is studied by making varying assumptions about benefits and costs and examining the impact of these different assumptions on the results (that is, sensitivity analyses). In one-way sensitivity analyses, authors vary only a single variable at a time; in multiway sensitivity analyses, they vary more than one variable simultaneously. For example, Kim and colleagues[35] investigated the cost-effectiveness of endodontic molar retreatment compared with fixed partial dentures and single-tooth implant alternatives for a failed endodontically treated tooth. They investigated the sensitivity of the analyses results on the probability of functional retention (that is, the survival probability) and on the cost input parameters. They concluded that if the survival probability was lower than 77%, the nonsurgical retreatment would become a less cost-effective option compared with the extraction of the failed endodontically treated tooth with the replacement of the same tooth with a fixed partial denture or single implant-supported restoration.

Parameter uncertainty usually is incorporated in economic studies using a probabilistic sensitivity analysis. For example, in a CEA of one- and two-step incomplete and complete excavations for the treatment of deep caries lesions, the authors conducted a probabilistic sensitivity analysis to obtain a distribution of economic analysis outcomes.[27] To achieve this, they first assigned a distribution around each parameter in the model, which represented the uncertainty around the true value of the parameter. Subsequently, they randomly sampled a large number of values from these distributions and calculated the economic outcomes for each set of sampled values. The distribution of the calculated costs and effects captured the underlying uncertainty. The results of probabilistic sensitivity analysis usually are represented using a cost-effectiveness acceptability curve (Figure 9.3[12]).

Figure 9.3. Cost-Effectiveness Acceptability Curve (CEAC) Comparing Implant-Retained Overdentures versus Conventional Dentures

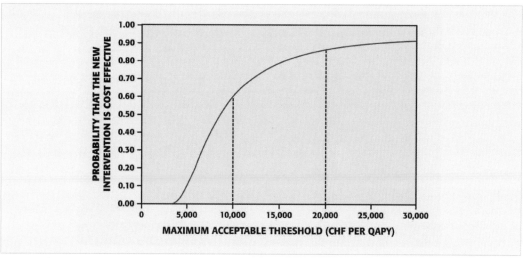

CEAC graphically represents the probability of the intervention (implant-retained overdentures) being cost-effective compared with the control (conventional dentures). This probability is plotted against the range of maximum willingness-to-pay thresholds for 1 unit of effectiveness (that is, quality-adjusted prosthesis-year [QAPY]). For example, the probability that implant-retained overdentures are more cost-effective than conventional dentures is 60% if the threshold is 10,000 Swiss francs (CHF) per QAPY and 86% if the threshold is CHF 20,000 per QAPY.

Source: Zitzmann and colleagues.[12]

Box 9.4. Your Assessment of the Results of the Economic Analysis You Identified

By reviewing the results of the study you identified,[18] you found that the incremental cost of a mandibular third-molar extraction versus retention was £56 (£1 = US $1.64 in 1997), and the incremental effectiveness was −6.2 units (see the Supplemental Table[18] at the end of this chapter for more details). Subsequently, the extraction was more costly and less effective than the retention; hence, it was not cost-effective. For costs, effectiveness, and the incremental cost-effectiveness ratio, the authors presented only their point estimates without variability around the estimates, limiting your ability to judge how uncertain these estimates were. The sources of probability values for events in the model or their ranges were not reported. The authors conducted some sensitivity analyses, but you could not find the list of variables and their values for these analyses. Although the authors reported that the model was sensitive to the probability of pericoronitis being 40%, periodontal disease being 17%, and nonrestorable caries in the second molar being 22%, they did not discuss under which conditions these values could be expected, except for in smokers.[18]

How Can I Apply the Results to My Patient Care?

After you have completed the evaluation of the risk of bias and results of the economic analysis, you will need to assess whether the observed treatment benefits are worth the risks and costs (that is, resource consumption), and whether you can expect similar results in your practice setting.

▸ *Are the viewpoints and setting used in the study relevant to my context?*

Economic analyses can be conducted from different viewpoints or perspectives depending on the type of decision that needs to be made. For example, the costs and consequences can be evaluated from the perspective of a patient, a health care institution (for example, hospital, dental practice), a health care provider (for example, dentist), a third-party payer (for example, private or state insurance), or society in general. The viewpoint of analysis defines which health consequences (that is, benefits and harms) and costs need to be collected for the study. For an economic analysis to be valid, the perspective of the analysis has to match the study's research question. For example, an economic analysis conducted from the patient's perspective should consider patient-important outcomes (for example, health-related quality of life, chewing ability) and costs (for example, insurance premiums, out-of-pocket costs), whereas an economic analysis from the provider's perspective should consider provider-important outcomes (for example, implant success rate, improvements in work environment). Oftentimes, the same economic analysis is conducted from multiple perspectives.

The perspective also defines the cost components that need to be considered in the economic analysis. Dental care-related costs largely can be grouped as direct dental costs (for example, cost of professional time, medications), direct nondental costs (for example, transportation costs for dental visits), and indirect costs (for example, time off work, travel time to seek care, reduced productivity because of the disease, caregiver costs).[15] An economic analysis from the patient's perspective, for example, may consider all relevant dental and nondental costs incurred by the patient in the form of out-of-pocket payments as well as the indirect costs because of lost productivity. In comparison, an economic analysis from the dentist's perspective may consider costs associated with establishing the practice and material costs. Therefore, an economic analysis performed using a patient's perspective may not be applicable to policy makers, because it may be missing important components to consider. Conversely, the results of an economic analysis that adopted a health policy perspective may not be transferrable when considering the cost-effectiveness of an intervention at a patient's level.

Likewise, it is necessary that the setting used in the study is similar enough to the setting in which the results are going to be applied. For example, unit costs for health care resources can be obtained from national formularies, administrative databases, or literature reviews, or through expert opinion. There could be significant variations in the unit costs and charges across different settings. Take the case of the fee for a unit of time for a dental hygiene visit, which can vary significantly depending on the clinic location. You should evaluate whether the authors explicitly stated how they itemized costs, which unit costs were applied and why, and which currency exchange rate was applied. This information also will help you to transfer the results from the setting of the published analysis to your setting. Although the results of treatment effectiveness or harm are relatively transferrable between settings and countries, this is not true for costs.

As a result, the same treatment that could be considered to be a resource-saving treatment in one setting could be considered to be a resource-consuming treatment in another setting.

▸ *Are the treatment benefits worth the risks and costs?*

We already know that after plotting the incremental costs and benefits on the cost-effectiveness plane, any ICER that falls in quadrant 2 (indicating that the intervention is more effective and less costly than control) means that the new intervention should be adopted into practice, and any ICER that falls in quadrant 4 (indicating that the intervention is less effective and more costly than a control) indicates the opposite (Figure 9.2[12]). Most of the innovations, however, cost more than the treatment alternatives in the practice and result in ICERs falling into quadrant 1. For these interventions, clinicians need to critically appraise if the extra benefits are worth the extra costs when the new treatment is adopted into the practice. In a CEA, clinicians can compare the incremental cost per unit of incremental effectiveness with other similar alternatives in practice. Another option would be to compare the ICER against a threshold value (that is, willingness to pay) that society is willing to pay for one unit of outcome. The relevance of these threshold values, however, is still widely debatable.[36] Establishing a monetary threshold for a unit of effectiveness (for example, willingness to pay for one year of best possible chewing ability or 1 QAPY) is not an easy task; the threshold values differ by outcomes, they are not always transferrable between countries, they may change over time, and they can vary depending on who decides on the value (for example, patients with the condition, representatives from general population, health care providers). To increase the applicability of findings, authors use CEACs in situations for which the probability of an intervention being cost-effective is plotted against a range of thresholds, as shown in Figure 9.3.[12]

To fully appreciate the results of an economic analysis, clinicians need to first have an understanding of the notion of opportunity costs. Let us go back to our example in the introduction of this chapter. If you decide to buy a new piece of 3-D dental imaging equipment for your practice, and assuming that you have a fixed budget, you will have to reduce spending by the same amount in a different sector (for example, reducing staff). The benefits are foregone because the expenditure reduction associated with your decision is known as the opportunity cost. Therefore, clinicians always should think about what the opportunity cost of adopting a new treatment into practice would be and how they or society could have otherwise spent this money.

▸ *Can I expect similar costs in my setting?*

Assuming a similar patient population, similar interventions, and a similar expected effectiveness with the economic analysis under review, you need to carefully consider if you can expect similar costs in your practice. To reiterate, total costs in any economic analysis are calculated by multiplying the frequency of utilized cost components by their unit cost. Differences in health care resource utilization frequency between settings and countries can arise because of variable, nonstandardized practice patterns, patient and clinician preferences, health systems' funding sources, and the availability of services.[24] If you expect similar health care resource use rates from your patients, then you should review whether the unit costs in your setting are similar to what were applied in the economic analysis. If the unit costs are different and the authors were transparent in terms of reporting, you can recalculate the total costs by applying the unit costs that are more typical for your setting.

Box 9.5. Your Assessment of the Applicability of Economic Analysis You Identified

After assessing the applicability of the economic analysis,[18] you conclude that although retention appears to be dominant over surgical removal by being more effective and less costly, there are some limitations in the study that may reduce the level of direct applicability of the results to your patient setting (for example, a single health care payer perspective versus a fee-for-service perspective). The authors' viewpoint in the study was that of National Health Service hospitals rather than an individual patient perspective or a societal perspective.[18] This perspective does not match very well the perspective of your first-year college student.

Conclusion

As technologies continue to develop, the need for and the number of economic analyses will increase. Clinicians need to be equipped with adequate knowledge to critically appraise these studies and make decisions that will benefit both patients and society in general.

Box 9.6. What You Say to Your Patient

You explain to your patient that in the absence of disease, retaining the impacted third molars versus removing them prophylactically are two strategies aiming at different outcomes, and hence, comparing these choices is a difficult task. You tell your patient that on the basis of your review of the literature, which focused on assessing an economic analysis conducted by authors in the United Kingdom whose study had methodological limitations,[18] third-molar retention may be more cost-effective than prophylactic removal. You recommend that the patient carefully consider his preferences before making a final decision.

References

1. Brignardello-Petersen R, Carrasco-Labra A, Glick M, Guyatt GH, Azarpazhooh A. "A practical approach to evidence-based dentistry: understanding and applying the principles of EBD." *JADA* 2014;145(11):1105–1107.

2. Chapter 2 of this book was based on Brignardello-Petersen R, Carrasco-Labra A, Booth HA, et al. "A practical approach to evidence-based dentistry: II: how to search for evidence to inform clinical decisions." *JADA* 2014;145(12):1262–1267.

3. Brignardello-Petersen R, Carrasco-Labra A, Glick M, Guyatt GH, Azarpazhooh A. "A practical approach to evidence-based dentistry: III: how to appraise and use an article about therapy." *JADA* 2015;146(1):42–49.e1.

4. Brignardello-Petersen R, Carrasco-Labra A, Glick M, Guyatt GH, Azarpazhooh A. "A practical approach to evidence-based dentistry: IV: how to use an article about harm." *JADA* 2015;146(2):94–101.e1.

5. Brignardello-Petersen R, Carrasco-Labra A, Glick M, Guyatt GH, Azarpazhooh A. "A practical approach to evidence-based dentistry: V: how to appraise and use an article about diagnosis." *JADA* 2015;146(3):184–191.e1.

6. Carrasco-Labra A, Brignardello-Petersen R, Glick M, Guyatt GH, Azarpazhooh A. "A practical approach to evidence-based dentistry: VI: how to use a systematic review." *JADA* 2015;146(4):255–265.e1.

7. Carrasco-Labra A, Brignardello-Petersen R, Glick M, Guyatt GH, Neumann I, Azarpazhooh A. "A practical approach to evidence-based dentistry: VII: how to use patient management recommendations from clinical practice guidelines." *JADA* 2015;146(5):327–336.e1.

8. Sale JEM, Amin M, Carrasco-Labra A, et al. "A practical approach to evidence-based dentistry: VIII: how to appraise an article based on a qualitative study." *JADA* 2015;146(8):623–630.

9. Wall T, Nasseh K, Vujicic M. U.S. Dental Spending Remains Flat Through 2012. Health Policy Institute Research Brief. American Dental Association. January 2014. Available at: *http://www.ADA.org/~/media/ADA/Science%20and%20 Research/HPI/Files/HPIBrief_0114_1.ashx*. Accessed June 30, 2015.

10. Canadian Institute for Health Information (CIHI). National Health Expenditure Trends, 1975 to 2014. Ottawa, Ontario, Canada: CIHI; 2014. Available for download at: *https://secure.cihi.ca/estore/productSeries.htm?pc=PCC52*. Accessed June 30, 2015.

11. Mohd-Dom T, Ayob R, Mohd-Nur A, et al. "Cost analysis of periodontitis management in public sector specialist dental clinics." *BMC Oral Health* 2014;14:56.

12. Zitzmann NU, Marinello CP, Sendi P. "A cost-effectiveness analysis of implant overdentures." *J Dent Res* 2006;85(8):717–721.

13. Jacobson JJ, Schweitzer SO, Kowalski CJ. "Chemoprophylaxis of prosthetic joint patients during dental treatment: a decision-utility analysis." *Oral Surg Oral Med Oral Pathol* 1991;72(2):167–177.

14. Oscarson N, Lindholm L, Kallestal C. "The value of caries preventive care among 19-year olds using the contingent valuation method within a cost-benefit approach." *Community Dent Oral Epidemiol* 2007;35(2):109–117.

15. Drummond MF, Sculpher MJ, Torrance GW, O'Brien BJ, Stoddart GL. *Methods for the Economic Evaluation of Health Care Programmes.* 3rd ed. New York: Oxford University Press; 2005.

16. O'Sullivan AK, Thompson D, Drummond MF. "Collection of health-economic data alongside clinical trials: is there a future for piggyback evaluations?" *Value Health* 2005;8(1):67–79.

17. Drummond MF. "Experimental versus observational data in the economic evaluation of pharmaceuticals." *Med Decis Making* 1998;18(2 suppl):S12–S18.

18. Edwards MJ, Brickley MR, Goodey RD, Shepherd JP. "The cost, effectiveness and cost effectiveness of removal and retention of asymptomatic, disease free third molars." *Br Dent J* 1999;187(7):380–384.

19. American Association of Oral and Maxillofacial Surgeons. "Evidence Based Third Molar Surgery." White Paper. Rosemont, IL: American Association of Oral and Maxillofacial Surgeons; 2013. Available at: *http://www.aaoms.org/ images/uploads/pdfs/evidence_based_third_molar_surgery.pdf*. Accessed July 20, 2015.

20. Mettes TD, Ghaeminia H, Nienhuijs ME, Perry J, van der Sanden WJ, Plasschaert A. "Surgical removal versus retention for the management of asymptomatic impacted wisdom teeth." *Cochrane Database Syst Rev* 2012;6:CD003879.

21. Costa MG, Pazzini CA, Pantuzo MC, Jorge ML, Marques LS. "Is there justification for prophylactic extraction of third molars? A systematic review." *Braz Oral Res* 2013;27(2):183–188.

22. Dodson TB, Susarla SM. "Impacted wisdom teeth. Systematic review 1302." *BMJ Clin Evid* 2014 August. Available at: *http://clinicalevidence.bmj.com/x/systematic-review/1302/overview.html*. Accessed June 30, 2015.

23. Friedman JW. "The prophylactic extraction of third molars: a public health hazard." *Am J Public Health* 2007;97(9):1554–1559.

24. Drummond M, Goeree R, Moayyedi P, Levine M. "Economic analysis." In: Guyatt GH, Rennie D, Meade MO, Cook DJ, editors. *Users' Guides to the Medical Literature: A Manual for Evidence-Based Clinical Practice.* 2nd ed New York, NY: McGraw-Hill; 2008. p. 619–641.

25. Ouyang W. "Cost-effectiveness analysis of dental sealant using econometric modeling 2009." Available at: *http://purl.umn.edu/52377.* Accessed June 30, 2015.

26. ctiveness of tooth replacement strategies for partially dentate elderly: a randomized controlled clinical trial." *Community Dent Oral Epidemiol* 2014;42(4):366–374.

27. Schwendicke F, Stolpe M, Meyer-Lueckel H, Paris S, Dorfer CE. "Cost-effectiveness of one- and two-step incomplete and complete excavations." *J Dent Res* 2013;92(10):880–887.

28. Oscarson N, Kallestal C, Fjelddahl A, Lindholm L. "Cost-effectiveness of different caries preventive measures in a high-risk population of Swedish adolescents." *Community Dent Oral Epidemiol* 2003;31(3):169–178.

29. Sculpher M. "Subgroups and heterogeneity in cost-effectiveness analysis." *Pharmacoeconomics* 2008;26(9):799–806.

30. Marino R, Fajardo J, Calache H, Morgan M. "Cost minimization analysis of a tailored oral health intervention designed for immigrant older adults." *Geriatr Gerontol Int* 2014;14(2):336–340.

31. Severens JL, Milne RJ. "Discounting health outcomes in economic evaluation: the ongoing debate." *Value Health* 2004;7(4):397–401.

32. Hietasalo P, Seppa L, et al. "Cost-effectiveness of an experimental caries-control regimen in a 3.4-yr randomized clinical trial among 11-12-yr-old Finnish schoolchildren." *Eur J Oral Sci* 2009;117(6):728–733.

33. Davenport C, Elley K, Salas C, et al. "The clinical effectiveness and cost-effectiveness of routine dental checks: a systematic review and economic evaluation." *Health Technol Assess* 2003;7(7):iii–v, 1-127.

34. Claxton K. "Exploring uncertainty in cost-effectiveness analysis." *Pharmacoeconomics* 2008;26(9):781–798.

35. Kim SG, Solomon C. "Cost-effectiveness of endodontic molar retreatment compared with fixed partial dentures and single-tooth implant alternatives." *J Endod* 2011;37(3):321–325.

36. Neumann PJ, Cohen JT, Weinstein MC. "Updating cost-effectiveness: the curious resilience of the $50,000-per-QALY threshold." *N Engl J Med* 2014;371(9):796–797.

A version of this chapter originally appeared in the September 2015 edition of *JADA* (Volume 146, Issue 9, Pages 679–689.e1). It has been reviewed and updated for accuracy and clarity by the editors of *How to Use Evidence-Based Dental Practices to Improve Your Clinical Decision-Making.*

Supplemental Table. Example of the Critical Appraisal of an Economic Analysis Study*

Guide	Comments
1. How serious is the risk of bias?	
1a. Are results reported separately for relevant patient subgroups?	No subgroups were specified by the authors. They specified that evidence is scarce regarding the impact of age on surgical morbidity and cited an article that, in fact, reported that the incidence of surgical complications after removal of impacted mandibular third molars was significantly higher in those patients who were older than 24 years compared with patients younger than 24 years.
1b. Were consequences and costs measured accurately?	Unclear. To evaluate consequences, the authors constructed scenarios for each clinical pathway in the decision tree (22 in total). Then they surveyed 100 consecutive patients from a single oral surgery clinic, asking them to rate each scenario on a 100-millimeter VAS,[†] in which 0 mm represented "Things could not be worse" and 100 mm represented "I would not be bothered at all." Mean effectiveness scores then were calculated for each scenario. A VAS is a unidimensional measure and is limited in estimating health preferences.
	For each possible clinical outcome after extraction, retention, or both, the authors estimated direct costs to NHS[‡] hospitals, including costs of diagnostic and surgical equipment, pharmaceutical and surgical supplies, staff costs, and overhead and other equivalent annual costs. Only aggregate costs were presented by cost category (for example, it was unclear what was considered "consumables" or "staff costs"). The sources of unit costs and the year of costs (1997) also were presented.
1c. Did investigators consider the timing of costs and consequences?	No. The costs of third-molar extraction mostly occur immediately and benefits occur later, whereas the opposite may be true for retention. This was not considered by the authors, and no discounting of costs or benefits was applied. Moreover, the model time horizon was not specified at all.
2. What are the results?	
2a. What were the incremental costs and effects of each strategy?	The incremental cost was £56, calculated by subtracting the cost of third-molar retention (£170) from the cost of third-molar extraction (£226). The effectiveness, which was measured by patients' ratings of clinical scenarios on a VAS from 0 to 100 mm, was equal to 63.3 in the removal alternative and 69.5 in the retention alternative. This resulted in an incremental effectiveness of −6.2. Because the third-molar extraction was less effective and more costly than the retention, it was the dominated alternative. Thus, the mandibular third-molar retention was more cost-effective than removal.

2b. Do incremental costs and effects differ between subgroups?	There were no defined subgroups or subgroup analysis.
2c. How much does allowance for uncertainty change the results?	The variability related to the estimates of costs, effectiveness, and ICER§ were not presented, making it impossible to evaluate their precision. The authors specified that the probability of each outcome was calculated as the mean of all incidences from all relevant literature, without referencing literature and providing actual values. It was unclear which type of sensitivity analyses were conducted and using which values, but the authors stated that the ICER was sensitive to specific probability values for pericoronitis, periodontal disease, and unrestorable caries in the second molar.

3. How can I apply the results to patient care?

3a. Are the viewpoints and setting used in the study relevant to my context?	No. Although the authors aimed to establish the cost-effectiveness from "both the health care provider and patient perspective," they considered only the direct costs to NHS hospitals. Furthermore, the authors never specified the patient population to whom this economic analysis could apply, and they presented only aggregate costs (for example, total cost of consumables for pain management), which limited the transferability of costing to other settings.
3b. Are the treatment benefits worth the risks and costs?	This topic was not discussed because the removal of the third molar appeared to be less effective and more costly than its retention. (Authors' note: Figure 9.2 shows that this is the dominated strategy in quadrant 4 on the cost-effectiveness plane). The authors did not discuss what would be an acceptable threshold for a unit of effectiveness if the extraction appeared to be more effective and more costly.
3c. Can I expect similar costs in my setting?	Unclear. The costs were estimated from the perspective of NHS hospitals. It is highly possible that the health care resource utilization and unit costs would be different in other countries in which prophylactic third-molar extraction is not covered by state insurance, and in which most of the extractions are conducted in community-based dental clinics that are run by individual dentists.

* *Source:* Edwards and colleagues.[18]
† VAS = visual analog scale.
‡ NHS = National Health Service.
§ ICER = incremental cost-effectiveness ratio.

Chapter 10. How to Avoid Being Misled by Clinical Studies' Results in Dentistry

Alonso Carrasco-Labra, D.D.S., M.Sc., Ph.D.; Romina Brignardello-Petersen, D.D.S., M.Sc., Ph.D.; Amir Azarpazhooh, D.D.S., M.Sc., Ph.D.; Michael Glick, D.M.D.; and Gordon H. Guyatt, M.D., M.Sc.

In This Chapter:

Guidance on How to Avoid Being Misled by the Results of Clinical Studies

1. Read only the methods and results sections; disregard the inferences.

2. Read synoptic abstracts published in secondary publications (preappraised resources) for evidence-based dentistry.

3. Beware of large treatment effects presented in trials with few events.

4. Beware of statements of statistical significance that claim clinical significance.

5. Beware of differences that are not statistically significant being interpreted as equivalence.

6. Beware of uneven emphasis on benefits and harms.

7. Beware of misleading subgroup analyses.

Conclusion

Introduction

In previous chapters in this book, we presented the process and main principles of evidence-based dentistry (EBD);[1] how to search for evidence;[2] and how to use articles about therapy,[3] harm,[4] diagnosis,[5] systematic reviews,[6] clinical practice guidelines,[7] qualitative studies,[8] and economic evaluations.[9] In this chapter of the book, we offer clinicians guidance on how to avoid being misled by biased interpretations of study results.

Academic competition and conflict of interest have fueled misleading presentations of research findings published in peer-reviewed journals. Regardless of whether a researcher works in academia or in the pharmaceutical industry, there is always a personal interest and a rising pressure to succeed and to provide novel and exciting findings; this pressure often results in interpretations of findings that are far more enthusiastic than the data warrant.[10]

In the area of psychopharmacology, for example, the investigators of 90% to 98% of industry-funded primary studies comparing two drugs reported results that favored the drug produced by their company, particularly when the active comparator drug was a rival product.[11] This situation is not exclusive to primary studies. The investigators of industry-sponsored systematic reviews are less transparent regarding their methods, are less rigorous in their risk of bias assessment, and provide more favorable conclusions toward the study sponsor's drug than are the investigators of reviews that have not been funded by the investigators' industry.[12] When companies employ ghostwriters to produce manuscripts under the names of credible and often well-known researchers, the reported results are likely to be overly favorable.[13]

The involvement of members of a specific industry is not necessary for overenthusiastic interpretations of results. Academic investigators also are subject to the global industry of producing research evidence. The reward system in science involves receiving grants and having research results published, and scientists may believe that overplaying the significance of their work is a requirement for success.[14]

Although guidance and tools to help clinicians recognize study results that have a high risk of bias are widely available,[15,16] researchers have made limited efforts to facilitate the identification of distorted interpretations and misleading presentations of the results of clinical studies. We present the following examples not to criticize investigators, but to illustrate the need to increase awareness among clinicians and encourage them to avoid putting excessive trust in investigators' interpretations of their findings.

Guidance on How to Avoid Being Misled by the Results of Clinical Studies

We present seven criteria that dental professionals can follow to avoid being misled by the results of clinical studies.[17] We illustrate each criterion with a real example from the dental literature, shown in the boxes after each section.

1. Read only the methods and results sections; disregard the inferences.

In not only the discussion but also in the conclusion and the introduction sections of research articles, investigators may provide inferences that differ from those that a less conflicted or involved reader would offer. A number of investigators have addressed the association between funding and the conclusions derived from randomized controlled trials.[18-22] Results have been consistent: researchers are more enthusiastic about new interventions when funding comes from for-profit sources than from not-for-profit sources. In dentistry, investigators have documented that randomized controlled trials in which the authors reported conflicts of interest are more likely to report results supporting the intervention under study than those trials whose authors did not report conflicts of interest (odds ratio [OR] = 2.40; 95% confidence interval [CI], 1.16-5.13).[21]

This situation also affects systematic reviews and meta-analyses of drug interventions. Although industry-sponsored and nonindustry-sponsored reviews (for example, Cochrane systematic reviews) answering the same clinical question report similar treatment effect estimates, the former type of reviews provide more favorable conclusions.[12] In summary, our advice is to read only the methods and the results sections of these articles, skipping the discussion section. However, to apply this guideline, clinicians must be able to assess the rigor of the methods and interpret the results.

2. Read synoptic abstracts published in secondary publications (preappraised resources) for evidence-based dentistry.

Busy clinicians interested in using evidence to inform their clinical practice may not have time to skip the discussion sections of articles and instead critically appraise the evidence, and thus make sense of the results, by themselves. Secondary journals and sources, such as *Evidence-Based Dentistry, Journal of Evidence-Based Dental Practice,* and the American Dental Association's *Evidence Database,* publish synoptic summaries in an abstract format that are accompanied by a brief summary of the original article and a critical appraisal conducted by a team of clinicians and methodologists. These abstracts, developed by independent third parties who have no conflicts of interest, reduce the distortion that the authors of a primary or secondary study may have introduced in the original article. Another objective of this type of synopsis is to educate clinicians about the methodological aspects of different study designs, thereby increasing clinicians' critical appraisal skills.

and other systemic conditions." A synopsis published in the *Journal of Evidence-Based Dental Practice* provided a two-page summary of the original study, including a commentary and analysis.[25] The author of the commentary stated, "It is very unusual for me to have very strong doubts about how a paper that makes such important claims yet has so many shortcomings gets published in a good refereed journal. This is such a paper."[25] After this, the author of the commentary provided a detailed explanation of the study's limitations and the implications of the results in a way that clinicians could understand. The author of the commentary concluded that "the suggested implications for disease management based on the results they report are highly contentious and unjustified."[25]

3. Beware of large treatment effects presented in trials with few events.

Clinicians often are appropriately skeptical of using evidence from the results of only one study and applying it in clinical practice. One argument is that the first studies that investigators conduct to determine the effects of an intervention usually have a small sample size (for example, fewer than 200 participants) and too few events. A meta-epidemiologic study published in the oral medicine and maxillofacial surgery literature showed that the investigators of small randomized trials (that is, those involving fewer than 200 patients) were more likely to report larger and more beneficial effects compared with the investigators of large randomized trials (that is, those involving at least 200 patients) (OR = 0.92; 95% CI, 0.87-0.98; P = .009).[26] Most of the time, our therapeutic interventions target one or two of the many pathologic mechanisms involved in the genesis of a disease.[27] This is why, not only in dentistry but also in medicine in general, few interventions are able to demonstrate a large and real treatment effect.

The results of a systematic survey whose investigators analyzed 85,000 meta-analysis results extracted from 3,082 systematic reviews showed that, in 10% of the cases, the results of the first trial showed statistical significance and a large treatment effect, which afterward proved to be much smaller in comparison with the results that the investigators initially reported.[28] It is important to notice that, when few events are available, even systematic reviews, including meta-analyses, could have this problem. Readers applying this guideline should beware of treatment effects that look "too large to be real," because they are likely to be misleading.

Box 10.3. Example: Does chlorhexidine oral rinse reduce mortality in patients in intensive care units?

The investigators of the first randomized controlled trial that addressed the effectiveness of oropharyngeal decontamination with 0.12% chlorhexidine gluconate oral rinse in patients in intensive care units suggested that this intervention reduces mortality by an astounding 80% (odds ratio [OR] = 0.20; 95% confidence interval [CI], 0.04-0.92).[29] The investigators of this trial enrolled 353 patients and reported 12 deaths. The authors of a subsequent systematic review including 14 trials, 2,111 patients, and 511 deaths demonstrated no benefit; indeed, the best estimate was a 10% increase in mortality (OR = 1.10; 95% CI, 0.87-1.38).[30]

4. Beware of statements of statistical significance that claim clinical significance.

For decades, researchers have been using P values (that is, hypothesis testing methods) to determine whether there is an association between a risk factor and an outcome or to determine whether an experimental intervention applied to one group produces better health outcomes than a control intervention. This P value, although it tells us whether chance may explain differences between interventions, provides no information about the magnitude of the effect or the importance of the findings.[31] Thus, readers who interpret small P values as large treatment effects usually are making a mistake.[32]

To avoid this error, we suggest that clinicians and researchers should focus on CIs and minimal important difference estimates rather than P values in their interpretation of results.[33] CIs provide a range of values, within which the true treatment effect is likely to lie, given the data observed in that particular study. Therefore, using CIs can help clinicians move away from considering trial results to be merely positive, neutral, or negative.[34]

> ### Box 10.4. Example: Is laser therapy effective for reducing facial swelling after sinus lift surgery?
>
> Investigators conducted a randomized controlled trial to determine the effect of neodymium-doped yttrium aluminum garnet (Nd:YAG) laser used for low-level laser therapy (LLLT) on pain, oral health–related quality of life (OHRQoL), and swelling after sinus lift surgery.[35] The authors of the study concluded that "the application of Nd:YAG laser for LLLT was significantly effective in reducing postoperative swelling." In the abstract of the study, they also mentioned, "We observed that the swelling and the OHRQoL in the Nd:YAG group were significantly improved when compared with the control group on the third day after surgery ($P < .05$)." A clinician not familiar with the concept of patient importance may conclude that the laser therapy resulted in an important reduction in facial swelling. A clinician who knows to focus on the magnitude of effect would note a graph showing the results for facial swelling on the third day (expressed in millimeters) in which improvement in facial swelling was only a difference of 2 mm. This difference, although statistically significant, represents a negligible benefit from the patient's point of view. This observation contrasts with the study authors' claim that the Nd:YAG laser for LLLT was significantly effective in reducing swelling.

5. Beware of differences that are not statistically significant being interpreted as equivalence.

A common piece of advice that clinicians hear when using evidence to inform clinical decisions is that the "absence of evidence is not evidence of absence."[36] By convention, *P* values less than 0.05 are considered statistically significant, whereas values greater than 0.05 are called "not significant." A misguided interpretation of results that are not statistically significant ($P > 0.05$) is that the results of a study have demonstrated that there is no important difference between the interventions being tested. Failure to demonstrate a difference does not, however, mean that an important difference does not exist.[36] The sample sizes used in randomized controlled trials often are inadequate, resulting in a lack of power to detect a real and important difference that may exist. The investigators of underpowered trials (that is, trials with a small sample size and a small number of events) often are destined to fail to find statistically significant differences when comparing two interventions. Even when differences fail to reach the conventional *P* value threshold of 0.05, clinicians should not necessarily conclude that interventions are equally effective. The conclusion that no important difference exists usually requires a large sample size. The CI is the best test of whether a sample size is adequate; a CI with a wide range indicates that a reader cannot conclude that no important difference exists. If the upper and lower values of the CI are close together—and neither, if representing the true effect, would constitute an important difference—only then is the conclusion of no important difference warranted.[37]

> **Box 10.5. Example: Is the preoperative injection of methylprednisolone into the masseter muscle more effective than the injection into the gluteal muscle for reducing complications after mandibular third-molar extraction?**
>
> Investigators conducted a randomized controlled trial to determine the effect of the use of preoperative injection of methylprednisolone into the masseter muscle versus into the gluteal muscle to reduce the incidence of postoperative swelling, pain, and trismus after surgical extraction of mandibular third molars.[38] With a total sample of 10 participants, the authors described that, for any of the outcomes, there were differences that were not statistically significant between the two groups. The authors concluded that "[t]he study evidently proves that there is no statistically significant difference between the intrabuccal approach of masseteric injection and gluteal injection of methylprednisolone in terms of pain, swelling and trismus following surgical removal of impacted lower third molars. However, the intrabuccal approach of masseteric injection was found to be more convenient when compared to gluteal injection, for the surgeon as well as the patient. It also has an additional advantage of being a painless steroidal injection on an anesthetized injection site."[38] This conclusion is misleading because the authors interpreted the results that were not statistically significant as having the equivalence of the effectiveness of both techniques, and they provided additional advice to make a clinical decision in favor of the intrabuccal approach. With only 10 participants, the probability of finding any difference, if it exists, is low.

6. Beware of uneven emphasis on benefits and harms.

Clinical decision-making requires the simultaneous consideration of many elements: certainty in the evidence, patient values and preferences, resource utilization, and the balance between benefits and harms.[7,39] The results of randomized controlled trials sometimes inform the effectiveness and safety outcomes in a way that patients and clinicians can see both desirable and undesirable consequences of an intervention. Unfortunately, the investigators of many clinical trials do not report or do not measure adverse effects.[40,41] In other cases, investigators present data about adverse events poorly; for example, the investigators may not provide any event rates for the treatment and the control arm, or they may fail to report the specific definition of the adverse event outcomes. Clinicians using this guideline should actively look for adverse event outcomes that are relevant for decision-making. When these outcomes are not available, clinicians should acknowledge this as a major limitation of the results of a study.

> **Box 10.6. Example: Does the primary closure technique result in fewer postoperative bleeding events than the secondary closure technique after mandibular third-molar extraction?**
>
> The investigators of a systematic review of randomized controlled trials addressed the impact of secondary versus primary closure techniques on the occurrence of the postoperative outcomes of pain, swelling, trismus, infectious complications, and postoperative bleeding.[42] Of the more than 14 studies that met the eligibility requirements, the investigators of only four studies had provided partial information regarding the incidence of postoperative bleeding. This example illustrates the fact that researchers in this area have overemphasized the importance of the beneficial outcomes compared with adverse events such as bleeding. The published results of the identified trials did not allow the authors of the systematic review to provide high-quality estimates for postoperative bleeding that would have facilitated clinical decision-making.

7. Beware of misleading subgroup analyses.

The investigators of clinical studies usually report the average estimates for the specific group of participants under study. Clinicians, on the other hand, try to personalize their prescriptions and indications as much as possible. One way that the investigators of clinical studies may provide the closest evidence possible to the patient is by using subgroup analysis. This type of analysis, conducted in primary studies and systematic reviews, aims to identify a specific subgroup of patients from the population who may respond differently to the treatment than other groups.[43] Although subgroup analyses can be helpful, this type of analysis also can seriously mislead clinicians.

One example of how misleading subgroup analysis can be is the results of the Second International Study of Infarct Survival.[44] The investigators presented an apparent subgroup effect in which patients who had a myocardial infarction and who were born under the zodiac signs of Gemini or Libra experienced an increase in cardiovascular mortality from aspirin use, whereas patients born under other zodiac signs experienced a benefit from aspirin use. No clinician would credit such a subgroup effect; the authors used this example to illustrate the dangers of subgroup analysis.

For clinicians trying to determine to what extent he or she can trust the results of a subgroup analysis in primary studies, researchers have proposed that clinicians ask themselves the following four questions.[43]

- Is it possible that chance can explain the subgroup difference?
- Is the identified subgroup difference consistent across studies?
- Was the subgroup hypotheses among the few tested and specified a priori?
- Is there a solid pre-existent biological rationale to justify the subgroup difference?

In addition to these questions, clinicians also should consider the following question to determine the credibility of subgroup analysis in meta-analyses:[43] was the comparison between subgroups conducted within or between studies? For detailed explanations of these criteria, we suggest referring to guidance published elsewhere.[43] For clinicians applying this guideline, the message is simple: when presented with a subgroup analysis difference, remain skeptical until the results of additional studies confirm the hypothesis

---

Box 10.7. Example: Is scaling and root planing more effective for reducing preterm birth in high- versus moderate-risk group patients?

The authors of a systematic review summarizing the evidence on the effect of scaling and root planing (SRP) in reducing preterm birth and risk of low birth weight conducted a subgroup analysis to explore potential reasons to explain the identified heterogeneity.[45] The review authors conducted a post hoc subgroup analysis and set an arbitrary threshold of 22% risk of prematurity of the populations to divide the studies into two groups: a high-risk group (relative risk [RR] = 0.66; 95% confidence interval [CI], 0.54-0.80; $P < 0.0001$) and a moderate-risk group (RR = 0.97; 95% CI, 0.75-1.24; $P = 0.79$). The authors concluded that there was a "statistically significant effect in reducing risk of preterm birth for SRP in pregnant women with periodontitis for groups with high risks of preterm birth only."[35] Although the test for interaction showed statistically significant results ($P = 0.02$), the authors conducted the subgroup analysis in a post hoc manner (that is, the cutoff point chosen to create the subgroups was not justified, and the difference was established at the level of "between" studies instead of "within" study). The authors of the review appropriately mention in their conclusions that "future research should attempt to confirm these findings and further define groups in which risk reduction may be effective."[5] Clinicians using this guideline should remain skeptical regarding this potential subgroup effect shown in the review and wait for more compelling evidence of such a subgroup difference.

Conclusion

Although clinicians have available a number of guides to critically appraise the risk of bias associated with clinical studies, little guidance exists addressing how to protect patients and clinicians from being misled by the interpretations offered by the authors of clinical studies. In this chapter of the book, we present seven criteria that clinicians can apply to avoid perpetuating misguided interpretations of study results. Clinicians should use these criteria to complement the guides provided in the previous chapters of this book.

References

1. Brignardello-Petersen R, Carrasco-Labra A, Glick M, Guyatt GH, Azarpazhooh A. "A practical approach to evidence-based dentistry: understanding and applying the principles of EBD." *JADA* 2014;145(11):1105–1107.

2. Chapter 2 of this book was based on Brignardello-Petersen R, Carrasco-Labra A, Booth HA, et al. "A practical approach to evidence-based dentistry: II: how to search for evidence to inform clinical decisions." *JADA* 2014;145(12):1262–1267.

3. Brignardello-Petersen R, Carrasco-Labra A, Glick M, Guyatt GH, Azarpazhooh A. "A practical approach to evidence-based dentistry: III: how to appraise and use an article about therapy." *JADA* 2015;146(1):42–49.e41.

4. Brignardello-Petersen R, Carrasco-Labra A, Glick M, Guyatt GH, Azarpazhooh A. "A practical approach to evidence-based dentistry: IV: how to use an article about harm." *JADA* 2015;146(2):94–101.e1.

5. Brignardello-Petersen R, Carrasco-Labra A, Glick M, Guyatt GH, Azarpazhooh A. "A practical approach to evidence-based dentistry: V: how to appraise and use an article about diagnosis." *JADA* 2015;146(3):184–191.e1.

6. Carrasco-Labra A, Brignardello-Petersen R, Glick M, Guyatt GH, Azarpazhooh A. "A practical approach to evidence-based dentistry: VI: how to use a systematic review." *JADA* 2015;146(4):255–265.e1.

7. Carrasco-Labra A, Brignardello-Petersen R, Glick M, Guyatt GH, Neumann I, Azarpazhooh A. "A practical approach to evidence-based dentistry: VII: how to use patient management recommendations from clinical practice guidelines." *JADA* 2015;146(5):327–336.e1.

8. Sale JEM, Amin M, Carrasco-Labra A, et al. "A practical approach to evidence-based dentistry: VIII: how to appraise an article based on a qualitative study." *JADA* 2015;146(8):623–630.

9. Abrahamyan L, Pechlivanoglou P, Krahn M, et al. "A practical approach to evidence-based dentistry: IX: how to appraise and use an article about economic analysis." *JADA* 2015;146(9):679–689.e1.

10. Ioannidis JP. "Why most published research findings are false." *PLoS Med* 2005;2(8):e124.

11. Mandelkern M. "Manufacturer support and outcome." *J Clin Psychiatry* 1999;60(2):122–123.

12. Jorgensen AW, Hilden J, Gotzsche PC. "Cochrane reviews compared with industry supported meta-analyses and other meta-analyses of the same drugs: systematic review." *BMJ* 2006;333(7572):782.

13. Stretton S. "Systematic review on the primary and secondary reporting of the prevalence of ghostwriting in the medical literature." *BMJ Open* 2014;4(7):e004777.

14. Ioannidis JP. "How to make more published research true." *PLoS Med* 2014;11(10):e1001747.

15. Guyatt G, Rennie D, Meade MO, Cook DJ, eds. *Users' Guides to the Medical Literature: A Manual for Evidence-Based Clinical Practice.* 3rd ed. New York, NY: McGraw-Hill; 2015.

16. Higgins JPT, Altman DG, Sterne JAC. "Assessing risk of bias in included studies (Chapter 8)." In: Higgins JPT, Green S, editors. *Cochrane Handbook for Systematic Reviews of Interventions.* Version 5.1.0 (updated March 2011). London, United Kingdom: The Cochrane Collaboration; 2011. Available at: *www.cochrane-handbook.org.* Accessed August 27, 2015.

17. Carrasco-Labra A, Montori VM, Ioannidis JPA, et al. "Advanced topics in applying the results of therapy trials: misleading presentation of clinical trial results (Chapter 13.3)." In: Guyatt G, Rennie D, Meade MO, Cook DJ, eds. *Users' Guides to the Medical Literature: A Manual for Evidence-Based Clinical Practice.* 3rd ed. New York, NY: McGraw-Hill; 2015.

18. Als-Nielsen B, Chen W, Gluud C, Kjaergard LL. "Association of funding and conclusions in randomized drug trials: a reflection of treatment effect or adverse events?" *JAMA* 2003;290(7):921–928.

19. Bekelman JE, Li Y, Gross CP. "Scope and impact of financial conflicts of interest in biomedical research: a systematic review." *JAMA* 2003;289(4):454–465.

20. Bhandari M, Busse JW, Jackowski D, et al. "Association between industry funding and statistically significant pro-industry findings in medical and surgical randomized trials." *CMAJ* 2004;170(4):477–480.

21. Brignardello-Petersen R, Carrasco-Labra A, Yanine N, et al. "Positive association between conflicts of interest and reporting of positive results in randomized clinical trials in dentistry." *JADA* 2013;144(10):1165–1170.

22. Lexchin J, Bero LA, Djulbegovic B, Clark O. "Pharmaceutical industry sponsorship and research outcome and quality: systematic review." *BMJ* 2003;326(7400):1167–1170.

23. Pedrazzi V, Leite MF, Tavares RC, Sato S, do Nascimento GC, Issa JP. "Herbal mouthwash containing extracts of *Baccharis dracunculifolia* as agent for the control of biofilm: clinical evaluation in humans." *ScientificWorldJournal* 2015;2015:712683.

24. Jeffcoat MK, Jeffcoat RL, Gladowski PA, Bramson JB, Blum JJ. "Impact of periodontal therapy on general health: evidence from insurance data for five systemic conditions." *Am J Prev Med* 2014;47(2):166–174.

25. Sheiham A. "Claims that periodontal treatment reduces costs of treating five systemic conditions are questionable." *J Evid Based Dent Pract* 2015;15(1):35–36.

26. Papageorgiou SN, Antonoglou GN, Tsiranidou E, Jepsen S, Jager A. "Bias and small-study effects influence treatment effect estimates: a meta-epidemiological study in oral medicine." *J Clin Epidemiol* 2014;67(9):984–992.

27. Devereaux PJ, Yusuf S. "The evolution of the randomized controlled trial and its role in evidence-based decision making." *J Intern Med* 2003;254(2):105–113.

28. Pereira TV, Horwitz RI, Ioannidis JP. "Empirical evaluation of very large treatment effects of medical interventions." *JAMA* 2012;308(16):1676–1684.

29. DeRiso 2nd AJ, Ladowski JS, Dillon TA, Justice JW, Peterson AC. "Chlorhexidine gluconate 0.12% oral rinse reduces the incidence of total nosocomial respiratory infection and nonprophylactic systemic antibiotic use in patients undergoing heart surgery." *Chest* 1996;109(6):1556–1561.

30. Shi Z, Xie H, Wang P, et al. "Oral hygiene care for critically ill patients to prevent ventilator-associated pneumonia." *Cochrane Database Syst Rev* 2013;8:CD008367.

31. Brignardello-Petersen R, Carrasco-Labra A, Shah P, Azarpazhooh A. "A practitioner's guide to developing critical appraisal skills: what is the difference between clinical and statistical significance?" *JADA* 2013;144(7):780–786.

32. Cleophas TJ. "Clinical trials: renewed attention to the interpretation of the *P* values—review." *Am J Ther* 2004;11(4):317–322.

33. Braitman LE. "Confidence intervals assess both clinical significance and statistical significance." *Ann Intern Med* 1991;114(6):515–517.

34. Guyatt GH, Walter SD, Cook DJ, Jaeschke R. "Confidence intervals: was the single study or meta-analysis large enough? (Chapter 10)." In: Guyatt G, Rennie D, Meade MO, Cook DJ, eds. *Users' Guides to the Medical Literature: A Manual for Evidence-Based Clinical Practice.* 3rd ed. New York, NY: McGraw-Hill; 2015.

35. Ozturan S, Sirali A, Sur H. "Effects of Nd:YAG laser irradiation for minimizing edema and pain after sinus lift surgery: randomized controlled clinical trial." *Photomed Laser Surg* 2015;33(4):193–199.

36. Altman DG, Bland JM. "Absence of evidence is not evidence of absence." *BMJ* 1995;311(7003):485.

37. Mulla SM, Scott IA, Jackevicius CA, You JJ, Guyatt GH. "How to use a noninferiority trial: users' guides to the medical literature." *JAMA* 2012;308(24):2605–2611.

38. Selvaraj L, Hanumantha Rao S, Lankupalli AS. "Comparison of efficacy of methylprednisolone injection into masseter muscle versus gluteal muscle for surgical removal of impacted lower third molar." *J Maxillofac Oral Surg* 2014;13(4):495–498.

39. Andrews JC, Schunemann HJ, Oxman AD, et al. "GRADE guidelines: 15—going from evidence to recommendation: determinants of a recommendation's direction and strength." *J Clin Epidemiol* 2013;66(7):726–735.

40. Ioannidis JP, Evans SJ, Gotzsche PC, et al; CONSORT Group. "Better reporting of harms in randomized trials: an extension of the CONSORT statement." *Ann Intern Med* 2004;141(10):781–788.

41. Ioannidis JP, Lau J. "Completeness of safety reporting in randomized trials: an evaluation of 7 medical areas." *JAMA* 2001;285(4):437–443.

42. Carrasco-Labra A, Brignardello-Petersen R, Yanine N, Araya I, Guyatt G. "Secondary versus primary closure techniques for the prevention of postoperative complications following removal of impacted mandibular third molars: a systematic review and meta-analysis of randomized controlled trials." *J Oral Maxillofac Surg* 2012;70(8):e441–e457.

43. Sun X, Ioannidis JP, Agoritsas T, Alba AC, Guyatt GH. "Advanced topics in systematic reviews: how to use a subgroup analysis (Chapter 25.2)." In: Guyatt G, Rennie D, Meade MO, Cook DJ, eds. *Users' Guides to the Medical Literature: A Manual for Evidence-Based Clinical Practice.* 3rd ed. New York, NY: McGraw-Hill; 2015.

44. ISIS-2 (Second International Study of Infarct Survival) Collaborative Group. "Randomised trial of intravenous streptokinase, oral aspirin, both, or neither among 17,187 cases of suspected acute myocardial infarction: ISIS-2." *Lancet* 1988;2(8607):349–360.

45. Kim AJ, Lo AJ, Pullin DA, Thornton-Johnson DS, Karimbux NY. "Scaling and root planing treatment for periodontitis to reduce preterm birth and low birth weight: a systematic review and meta-analysis of randomized controlled trials." *J Periodontol* 2012;83(12):1508–1519.

A version of this chapter originally appeared in the December 2015 edition of *JADA* (Volume 146, Issue 12, Pages 919–924). It has been reviewed and updated for accuracy and clarity by the editors of *How to Use Evidence-Based Dental Practices to Improve Your Clinical Decision-Making.*

Chapter 11. What Is the Difference between Clinical and Statistical Significance?

Romina Brignardello-Petersen, D.D.S., M.Sc., Ph.D.; Alonso Carrasco-Labra, D.D.S., M.Sc., Ph.D.; Prakeshkumar Shah, M.Sc., M.B.B.S., M.D., D.C.H., M.R.C.P.; and Amir Azarpazhooh, D.D.S., M.Sc., Ph.D.

Introduction

Investigators in a study published in 2010 compared the efficacy of nimesulide with that of meloxicam (two nonsteroidal anti-inflammatory drugs) in the control of postoperative pain, swelling, and trismus after extraction of impacted mandibular third molars.[1] Among their conclusions, the authors stated that "[nimesulide] was more effective than [meloxicam] in the control of swelling and trismus following the removal of impacted lower third molars."[1] This conclusion was supported by the results observed in their randomized clinical trial. The authors reported that after the third molar surgical extraction, patients experienced a reduction in mouth opening, but that this reduction was significantly larger at 72 hours after surgery when patients had received meloxicam than when patients had received nimesulide. The authors reported a P value of 0.03 for the difference in the mean reduced mouth opening of 1.39 centimeters in the nimesulide group versus 1.7 cm in the meloxicam group. This difference of 3.1 millimeters was the basis for the authors' claim of the superiority of nimesulide. However, from a clinical perspective, this difference does not seem large. How can we know if these numbers show that the reduction in mouth opening is significantly larger when patients received meloxicam therapy, as the authors report? What do the authors mean when they use the expression "significantly larger"? Is a P value < 0.05 sufficient to claim that there is a significant difference?

In this chapter, we aim to clarify and differentiate the concepts of statistical significance and clinical significance, as well as provide guidance on how to interpret research results to determine whether an observed difference is clinically meaningful.

Statistical Significance

It is not feasible to conduct a study in which investigators study all potential patients. Thus, researchers have to base their conclusions on a sample of people and then determine the probability that a conclusion made on the basis of an analysis of data from this sample will hold true when applied to the population as a whole.[2]

Researchers have used statistical significance for many years as a means to assess the effects of interventions in clinical research and to show that observed differences likely are not due to chance.[3] Usually, the claim of statistical significance depends on obtaining a specific P value after conducting a statistical significance test, as in the earlier example.

A P value is the probability of obtaining a mean difference that is at least as far from a specified value (null value) as the mean observed in the study, given that this specified value is the true value.[4] In the example above, if we assume that the true difference in mouth opening reduction between nimesulide and meloxicam is 0 mm, what the authors found was a 3% probability of observing the 3.1-mm difference (or larger) that they detected. Because the probability of that happening is so small, it is unlikely that the differences they observed were due to chance; thus, they could claim that there are real and statistically significant differences between the two treatments.

As stated earlier, the P value is obtained when conducting statistical hypothesis testing. To perform this test, we start by assuming that the result of interest (the mean or proportion of the outcome of the study) is equal to some specific value. This claim is called the null hypothesis. In the example, the null hypothesis was that there is no difference in mouth-opening reduction between the two drug groups. The investigators then construct an alternative hypothesis such that it contradicts the null hypothesis. In this case, the alternative hypothesis was that differences existed between the drugs with regard to mouth-opening reduction.[5] The next step is to compare the data obtained in the study with the value specified in the null hypothesis—using the probability theory—to attain a P value. The P value is related to how much the data contradict the null hypothesis. If a large P value is obtained, the data are consistent with the null hypothesis. Conversely, if a small P value is obtained, the data contradict the null hypothesis, and the results are unlikely to have occurred if the null hypothesis actually were true. However, the investigators must decide whether the P value is sufficiently small to reject the null hypothesis. Although it is arbitrary, a P value of 0.05 has been the conventionally accepted value for level of significance.[6]

Type I Error

The level of significance reflects the probability of committing a type I error—that is, rejecting the null hypothesis when it actually is true.[7] In other words, it is the probability of falsely claiming that there is a difference in mouth-opening reduction when there is not. According to the earlier description, the P value is not the probability that the null hypothesis is true. This is a common misconception. A large P value does not mean that the null hypothesis is true; at best, it implies that the study results are inconclusive. Likewise, a small P value does not mean that the alternative hypothesis is true; at best, it implies that the data are incompatible with the null hypothesis being true.[5]

Type II Error

On the other hand, a probability exists of not rejecting the null hypothesis when it is false, which is known as a type II error. A type II error occurs when researchers fail to observe a difference between interventions even though a true difference does exist.[8] For example, imagine a study in which the researcher wants to determine whether the incidence of cleft lip and palate is larger in one of two towns. Let us assume that a difference between the towns truly exists, and that the true incidence in town A is five in 1,000 newborns, whereas in town B, it is one in 1,000 newborns. If the researcher observes only 50 newborns in each town, it is likely that he or she will not find an infant with cleft lip and palate in either town. At the end of the study, the data will suggest that the incidence of this malformation is 0 for both towns. Therefore the researcher will claim falsely that no difference exists between the two towns with regard to the incidence of cleft lip and palate, because he or she failed to find any infant with the malformation. This is an issue of "power" of the study.

Study Power

The power of a study is its capacity to detect differences that truly exist, and it is defined as the probability of rejecting the null hypothesis when it is false.[5] Power is the opposite of a type II error; higher power implies a smaller probability of committing a type II error, and vice versa. Thus, our hypothetical study of the incidence of cleft lip and palate in two towns was underpowered. Also, as this example illustrates, the power of a study depends, in part, on the sample size (the number of newborns observed) and the effect size (the difference in the incidence of the malformation between the groups).

Issues Pertaining to Statistical Significance

Understanding statistical significance requires thinking in terms of probability. At the completion of a statistical significance test, there are two possible outcomes: reject the null hypothesis or fail to reject the null hypothesis. This qualitative result often is used as a substitute for quantitative scientific evidence.[7] As illustrated in Tables 11.1 and 11.2, one issue of concern is that the results of statistical testing are influenced highly by the sample size and variability within the sample. Table 11.1 shows that increasing the sample size, while keeping everything else constant, results in a smaller P value's having been obtained in hypothesis testing. This leads to statistically significant results when the sample size is larger and to nonstatistically significant results when the sample size is smaller. Table 11.2 shows that, while keeping everything else constant, a smaller variation in the response to an intervention among participants in one group results in a smaller P value's having been obtained in statistical testing. Consequently, statistically significant results are obtained when the variability is smaller, and nonstatistically significant results are obtained when the variability is larger.

Therefore, studies in which the sample size is large, in which there is little variability within the sample, or both, are more likely to lead to statistically significant results compared with identical studies in which the sample sizes are smaller and the variability is greater. This is true even when the effect size (the difference between the groups) is the same, as shown in Tables 11.1 and 11.2.

Table 11.1. Relationship Between Sample Size and *P* Values (Assuming Constant Means and SDs*)†

Hypothetical Scenario	Mean (SD) Reduction in Mouth Opening at 72 Hours, in Centimeters		Sample Size	P Value‡	Statistical Significance
	Meloxicam	Nimesulide			
1	1.70 (0.6)	1.39 (0.75)	20	0.321	No
2	1.70 (0.6)	1.39 (0.75)	40	0.157	No
3	1.70 (0.6)	1.39 (0.75)	60	0.082	No
4	1.70 (0.6)	1.39 (0.75)	80	0.045	Yes
5	1.70 (0.6)	1.39 (0.75)	100	0.025	Yes
6	1.70 (0.6)	1.39 (0.75)	120	0.014	Yes

* SDs = standard deviations.
† This table illustrates the influence that sample size has on *P* values. When the mean of the outcome and its SD are constant, an increase in sample size leads to smaller *P* values.
‡ Two-sided unpaired *t* test; significance level ≤ 0.05. *P* values were calculated by using statistical software (The R Project for Statistical Computing, The R Foundation for Statistical Computing, Vienna).

Table 11.2. Relationship Between Variability Estimates and *P* Values (Assuming Constant Means and Sample Size)*

Hypothetical Scenario	Mean (SD†) Reduction in Mouth Opening at 72 Hours, in Centimeters		Sample Size	P Value‡	Statistical Significance
	Meloxicam	Nimesulide			
1	1.70 (0.40)	1.39 (0.55)	60	0.015	Yes
2	1.70 (0.45)	1.39 (0.60)	60	0.027	Yes
3	1.70 (0.50)	1.39 (0.65)	60	0.043	Yes
4	1.70 (0.55)	1.39 (0.70)	60	0.061	No
5	1.70 (0.60)	1.39 (0.75)	60	0.082	No
6	1.70 (0.65)	1.39 (0.80)	60	0.105	No

* This table illustrates the influence that sample variability has on *P* values. When the mean outcome value and sample size are constant, an increase in sample variability leads to higher *P* values.
† SD = standard deviation.
‡ Two-sided unpaired *t* test; significance level ≤ 0.05. *P* values were calculated by using statistical software (The R Project for Statistical Computing, The R Foundation for Statistical Computing, Vienna).

In the study in which De Menezes and Cury[1] compared the efficacy of nimesulide versus that of meloxicam for the control of postoperative pain, swelling, and trismus after extraction of impacted mandibular third molars,[1] let us imagine that the authors had measured the outcome pain as dichotomous (that is, the presence or absence of pain). In addition, let us suppose that after completing the trial, these authors observed that 85% of participants who received nimesulide therapy reported experiencing no postoperative pain, whereas 90% of participants allocated to the meloxicam group reported experiencing no postoperative pain. If we compare these two proportions in a trial in which researchers enrolled a total of 80 patients, the *P* value for the hypothesis testing would be .25. On the other hand, had researchers in the trial enrolled 800 participants, the P value for the same comparison would be .016. Although the difference in the proportion of patients with no postoperative pain in both trials was 5%, the conclusion drawn in the trial with the smaller sample size is that there was no statistically significant difference between the two drugs, whereas in the trial with the larger sample size, the authors could have made the opposite claim.

In light of the above, the main problem is that hypothesis testing can omit any differences that were observed in the study. Statistical testing indicates only the probability of the observed differences—without regard to the size of the differences—occurring by chance.[2] By using the hypothesis testing approach and claiming that there are differences in effects of interventions on the basis of a P value alone, we lose valuable information regarding the size of the effect.[9] This is illustrated in Table 11.3, which shows different effect sizes leading to the same conclusion: the results are or are not statistically significant.

Table 11.3. Relationship Between Effect Size Increase and Statistical Significance (Assuming Constant Mean in Meloxicam Group and Constant Standard Deviations in Both Groups)*

Hypothetical Scenario	Mean (SD[†]) Reduction in Mouth Opening at 72 Hours, in Centimeters		Difference in Mean Reduction in Mouth Opening, in Centimeters	Sample Size	Statistical Significance[‡]
	Meloxicam	Nimesulide			
1	1.70 (0.6)	1.39 (0.75)	0.31	40	No
2	1.70 (0.6)	1.34 (0.75)	0.36	40	No
3	1.70 (0.6)	1.29 (0.75)	0.41	40	No
4	1.70 (0.6)	1.24 (0.75)	0.46	40	Yes
5	1.70 (0.6)	1.19 (0.75)	0.51	40	Yes
6	1.70 (0.6)	1.14 (0.75)	0.56	40	Yes

* This table illustrates that when statistical hypothesis testing is used, the conclusion drawn (that is, whether differences are or are not statistically significant) does not reflect how much larger the effect of one intervention is compared with another. Even though the mean difference in outcomes across the scenarios is increasing, the conclusion derived from statistical hypothesis testing is exactly the same.
† SD = standard deviation.
‡ Two-sided unpaired t test; significance level ≤ 0.05. P values were calculated by using statistical software (The R Project for Statistical Computing, The R Foundation for Statistical Computing, Vienna).

Researchers can reach the same P value in many ways by combining different treatment effects, within-group variability, and sample sizes. Thus, the results of a statistical test cannot indicate whether a treatment effect is important enough to be useful for patients.[10] Moreover, some readers may erroneously interpret small P values as large effects,[11] when in fact, the P values actually represent only the probability of having observed what was observed in the study and indicate nothing about the effect size.

Clinical Significance

In 1984, Jacobson and colleagues[12] proposed the term "clinical significance" as a means of evaluating the practical value of a treatment. Although the literature contains many definitions of and discussions about this term,[9,13–18] most authors agree that a clinically significant result must fulfill the following criteria:

- A change in an outcome or a difference in outcome between groups occurs that is of interest to someone; patients, physicians, or other parties interested in patient care conclude that the effect of one treatment compared with another makes a difference.

- The change or difference between groups must occur in an important outcome. It can be any outcome that may alter a clinician's decisions regarding treatment of a patient, such as a reduction in symptoms, improvement in quality of life, treatment effect duration, adverse effects, cost-effectiveness, or implementation.

- The change or difference must be statistically significant. The difference must be greater than what may be explained by a chance occurrence.[9,13–18]

Minimal Important Difference

Jaeschke and colleagues[19] introduced the concept of "minimal important difference" (MID) to determine whether a difference between treatments is of interest. They defined the MID as "the smallest difference in score in the domain of interest which patients perceive as beneficial and which would mandate, in the absence of troublesome side effects and excessive costs, a change in the patient's management." Even though this definition reflects the patient's perspective, it can be applied readily to any party involved in the health care chain (such as clinicians, family members, policymakers, and hospital administrators).

Although each member of the health care team may have their opinion as to what constitutes an important difference, the patient's perspective should take priority.[10] Because this is a relevant topic for interpreting the results of clinical studies, investigators have made many efforts to provide guidance and to determine the MID for outcomes in many clinical areas, including dentistry.[20–25]

Perceptions regarding which outcomes are important will likely vary within and across cultures, as well as on the basis of the perspective being considered (such as the patient's or the clinician's).[26–28] An important outcome from the patient's perspective has been defined as one in which the patient, if he or she knew the outcome would be the only thing that would change with a treatment, would consider receiving this treatment even if it is associated with adverse effects, inconvenience, or cost.[29] For example, most patients with oral cancer consider mortality to be an important outcome, and many are willing to receive chemotherapy despite its adverse effects to reduce the chance of dying. However, other perspectives often are important as well. Thus the relative importance given to outcomes should reflect the perspectives of those affected.[30]

Patient-Reported Outcome Measures (PROMs)

This specific type of patient-important outcome provides direct information about a patient's status without additional interpretation from a third party.[30] Given the complexity of measuring a patient's experience, researchers have created PROM instruments (for example, questionnaires evaluating oral-health-related quality of life, pain, fatigue, and social independence) that when reliable, valid, and responsive, provide a framework for appropriately reflecting the construct of interest and measurement of the impact of a health care intervention on a patient's status. Although the value of PROMs is clear, their interpretation is not without challenges. How large is the magnitude of change (that is, negligible, small, moderate, large, or very large) in the quality of life a patient experiences when comparing receiving partial dentures to dental implants? Answering this question is essential for patients and clinicians to fully understand the perceived benefit of either option. MID estimates are particularly relevant in this case as thresholds that can be used to determine the extent to which the improvement or deterioration in a PROM reported by patients in a clinical trial, for example, corresponds to or exceeds a value that they consider important.[19]

Although little evidence exists to support any judgment about the outcomes that are important in dentistry, some guidance is found in other medical fields. For example, when ranking outcomes for assessing the effectiveness of a drug for treating renal failure, most patients would agree that mortality is the most critical outcome, whereas an adverse effect such as flatulence is of lower importance.[30] In addition, with regard to surrogate outcomes, researchers generally agree that because the evidence is associated with a surrogate measure, it is weaker and thus of lower importance.[30,31]

Surrogate Outcomes

According to Temple,[32] a surrogate endpoint in the context of a clinical trial is a laboratory measurement or a physical sign used as a substitute for a clinically meaningful endpoint that directly measures how a patient feels, functions, or survives. Changes induced by a therapy on a surrogate endpoint are expected to reflect changes in a clinically meaningful endpoint.

In other words, a surrogate outcome is an outcome that is measured in place of a biologically definitive or clinically most meaningful outcome.[33] An example of a potentially misleading surrogate outcome in dentistry is a significant reduction in salivary mutans streptococci as a substitute for the occurrence of caries lesions,[34–36] or measuring pocket depth as a surrogate outcome for tooth loss or for a patient's quality of life.[34] Other examples of potentially misleading surrogate outcomes are biomarkers that have not been validated, such as the use of components of gingival crevicular fluid[37] or venous blood,[38] which are ubiquitous in clinical trials in periodontics.[39] Such surrogate outcomes and biomarkers are trustworthy when they meet two criteria: there is a strong, independent, and consistent association between the surrogate measure and the clinically meaningful outcome it is trying to measure; and the evidence shows improvement in both the clinically meaningful outcome and the surrogate outcome. Because this does not happen frequently, surrogate outcomes are not considered important to patients.[40]

Interpreting Research Findings

To determine whether the results of a study are clinically significant, we need to consider the three criteria described earlier. In addition, we must take into consideration the fact that the results obtained in a study reflect the specific sample used in the study. Consequently, even if the study were replicated, the subsequent *P* value would be different from the first.

Confidence Intervals

The use of confidence intervals (CIs) helps researchers and clinicians interpret both statistical and clinical significance and is a way to estimate what the results would be in the population.[41] A CI can be defined as a range of values calculated from the data, within which the investigator believes a true parameter value will lie with some specific probability.[42] In other words, a CI is a plausible range of values within which the true value will actually lie given the data observed in a study.[43] For example, consider a hypothetical study in which investigators aim to estimate the percentage of successful short versus conventional dental implants. The study results show a 10% difference in favor of the conventional implants. The 95% CI is 2% to 18%, which means that we can be 95% confident that the true (but unknown) difference between the two types of implants is between 2% and 18%. A study's CI either includes the true population difference or it does not. Thus, CIs provide information about the magnitude of an effect and the uncertainty surrounding it, which may help us to evaluate the clinical significance of the effect.[41,44]

CIs and MID

Using the CI and the concept of MID, we find that a difference observed in a study will be clinically significant when its 95% CI is higher than the MID. If the 95% CI contains the MID, then no conclusions regarding the clinical significance of an effect can be made.[44] However, readers must be careful when using CIs to assess clinical significance, because the width of a CI is associated with the sample size. Let us suppose that the MID for the example above is 4%. Because the CI indicates that the true difference between the implant types likely will be between 2% and 18%, we cannot claim that the study results are clinically significant. However, if the sample size were tripled, the 95% CI of the difference would be 5% to 15%. This range would indicate that it is not plausible for the difference between the two implant types to be as small as 4%, making it a clinically significant difference.

Discussion

We have argued that any benefit in terms of improved health outcomes must be both clinically and statistically significant; if there is no benefit at the threshold of both clinical and statistical improvement, then the treatment should not be used for that purpose.

In their study of the effects of nimesulide versus meloxicam on trismus after tooth extraction, De Menezes and Cury[1] reported that a 3.1-mm difference between the groups at 72 hours was statistically significantly large. As discussed earlier, the statistical testing process they used to compare the two interventions correctly supports this claim. However, their study lacked a deeper examination of the issue of significance.

To reiterate, the three main characteristics of a clinically significant effect are that the change (that is, the difference between the results of the experimental group and those of the control group) is of interest to someone, the change occurred in an important outcome, and the change reached statistical significance. Limitations in mouth opening can have many negative consequences, such as problems in nutrition and speech. For healthy patients undergoing third molar extraction, it is probably an important complication to consider. Thus, the study finding by De Menezes and Cury[1] seems to fulfill two of the three criteria to be considered clinically important. However, to claim that a difference of 3.1 mm in trismus is of interest to clinicians or patients—which would meet the first criterion and make this result clinically significant—is questionable. Would a patient be willing to overcome adverse effects or bear higher costs to experience 3.1 mm less trismus? Whether the difference between two groups with regard to an observed outcome is of interest is a matter of debate in many cases. This reminds us of the major role that judgment gained through clinical experience plays in interpreting and applying research results.

Conclusion

It is important to realize that values for statistical significance alone cannot convey the complete picture of effectiveness of an intervention or a difference between two groups. Both clinical and statistical significance are important for interpretation of clinical research results and should complement each other.

References

1. De Menezes SA, Cury PR. "Efficacy of nimesulide versus meloxicam in the control of pain, swelling and trismus following extraction of impacted lower third molar." *Int J Oral Maxillofac Surg* 2010;39(6):580-584.

2. Norman G, Streiner D. "Elements of statistical inference." In: Norman G, Streiner D, eds. *Biostatistics: The Bare Essentials*. 3rd ed. Hamilton, Ontario, Canada: B.C. Decker; 2008:46-62.

3. Bhardwaj SS, Camacho F, Derrow A, Fleischer AB Jr, Feldman SR. "Statistical significance and clinical relevance: the importance of power in clinical trials in dermatology." *Arch Dermatol* 2004;140(12):1520-1523.

4. Greenland S, Rothman K. "Fundamentals of epidemiologic data analysis." In: Rothman K, Greenland S, Lash T, eds. *Modern Epidemiology*. 3rd ed. Philadelphia: Lippincott Williams & Wilkins; 2008:213-237.

5. Pagano M, Gauvreau K. "Hypothesis testing." In: Pagano M, ed. *Principles of Biostatistics*. 2nd ed. Pacific Grove, Calif.: Duxbury; 2000:232-258.

6. Gauvreau K, Pagano M. "Why 5%?" *Nutrition* 1994;10(1):93-94.

7. Hayat MJ. "Understanding statistical significance." *Nurs Res* 2010;59(3):219-223.

8. Koretz RL. "Is statistical significance always significant?" *Nutr Clin Pract* 2005;20(3):303-307.

9. LeFort SM. "The statistical versus clinical significance debate." *Image J Nurs Sch* 1993;25(1):57-62.

10. Sackett DL. "The tactics of performing therapeutic trials." In: Haynes RB, ed. *Clinical Epidemiology: How to Do Clinical Practice Research*. 3rd ed. Philadelphia: Lippincott Williams & Wilkins; 2006:107.

11. Cleophas TJ. "Clinical trials: renewed attention to the interpretation of the P values—review." *Am J Ther* 2004;11(4):317-322.

12. Jacobson NS, Follette WC, Revenstorf D. "Psychotherapy outcome research: methods for reporting variability and evaluating clinical significance." *Behav Therapy* 1984;15(4):336-352.

13. Hujoel PP, Armitage GC, Garcia RI. "A perspective on clinical significance." *J Periodontol* 2000;71(9):1515-1518.

14. Killoy WJ. "The clinical significance of local chemotherapies." *J Clin Periodontol* 2002;29(suppl 2):22-29.

15. Kingman A. "Statistical vs clinical significance in product testing: can they be designed to satisfy equivalence?" *J Public Health Dent* 1992;52(6):353-360.

16. Lindgren BR, Wielinski CL, Finkelstein SM, Warwick WJ. "Contrasting clinical and statistical significance within the research setting." *Pediatr Pulmonol* 1993;16(6):336-340.

17. Greenstein G. "Clinical versus statistical significance as they relate to the efficacy of periodontal therapy." *JADA* 2003;134(5): 583-591.

18. Hollon S, Flick S. "On the meaning of clinical significance." *Behav Assess* 1988;10:10.

19. Jaeschke R, Singer J, Guyatt GH. "Measurement of health status: ascertaining the minimal clinically important difference." *Control Clin Trials* 1989;10(4):407-415.

20. Greenstein G, Lamster I. "Efficacy of periodontal therapy: statistical versus clinical significance." *J Periodontol* 2000;71(4):657-662.

21. Allen PF, O'Sullivan M, Locker D. "Determining the minimally important difference for the Oral Health Impact Profile-20". *Eur J Oral Sci* 2009;117(2):129-134.

22. Ingram M, Choi YH, Chiu CY, et al. "Use of the minimal clinically important difference (MCID) for evaluating treatment outcomes with TMJMD patients: a preliminary study". *J Appl Biobehav Res* 2011;16(3-4):148-166.

23. Thomson WM. "Measuring change in dry-mouth symptoms over time using the Xerostomia Inventory." *Gerodontology* 2007;24(1):30-35.

24. Tsakos G, Allen PF, Steele JG, Locker D. "Interpreting oral health-related quality of life data". *Community Dent Oral Epidemiol* 2012;40(3):193-200.

25. Tsakos G, Bernabe E, D'Aiuto F, et al. "Assessing the minimally important difference in the oral impact on daily performances index in patients treated for periodontitis". *J Clin Periodontol* 2010;37(10):903-909.

26. Blackhall LJ, Murphy ST, Frank G, Michel V, Azen S. "Ethnicity and attitudes toward patient autonomy." *JAMA* 1995;274(10):820-825.

27. Klessig J. "The effect of values and culture on life-support decisions." West J Med 1992;157(3):316-322.

28. Ruhnke GW, Wilson SR, Akamatsu T, et al. "Ethical decision making and patient autonomy: a comparison of physicians and patients in Japan and the United States." *Chest* 2000;118(4):1172-1182.

29. Akl EA, Briel M, You JJ, et al. "LOST to follow-up Information in Trials (LOST-IT): a protocol on the potential impact. *Trials* 2009;10:40.

30. Guyatt GH, Oxman AD, Kunz R, et al. "GRADE guidelines: 2—framing the question and deciding on important outcomes". I 2011;64(4):395-400.

31. Schunemann HJ, Oxman AD, Fretheim A. "Improving the use of research evidence in guideline development: 6—determining which outcomes are important." *Health Res Policy Syst* 2006;4:18.

32. Temple RJ. *A Regulatory Authority's Opinion about Surrogate Endpoints*. New York City: John Wiley & Sons; 1995.

33. Piantadosi S. "Objectives and outcomes." In: *Clinical Trials: A Methodologic Perspective.* 2nd ed. Hoboken, N.J.: Wiley-Interscience; 2005:187-210.

34. Hujoel PP. "Endpoints in periodontal trials: the need for an evidence-based research approach." *Periodontol 2000* 2004;36:196-204.

35. Forgie AH, Paterson M, Pine CM, Pitts NB, Nugent ZJ. "A randomised controlled trial of the caries-preventive efficacy of a chlorhexidine-containing varnish in high-caries-risk adolescents." *Caries Res* 2000;34(5):432-439.

36. Sandham HJ, Brown J, Chan KH, Phillips HI, Burgess RC, Stokl AJ. "Clinical trial in adults of an antimicrobial varnish for reducing mutans streptococci." *J Dent Res* 1991;70(11):1401-1408.

37. Oringer RJ, Al-Shammari KF, Aldredge WA, et al. "Effect of locally delivered minocycline microspheres on markers of bone resorption." *J Periodontol* 2002;73(8):835-842.

38. Vidal F, Figueredo CM, Cordovil I, Fischer RG. "Periodontal therapy reduces plasma levels of interleukin-6, C-reactive protein, and fibrinogen in patients with severe periodontitis and refractory arterial hypertension." *J Periodontol* 2009;80(5):786-791.

39. Pihlstrom BL, Barnett ML. "Design, operation, and interpretation of clinical trials". *J Dent Res* 2010;89(8):759-772.

40. Bucher HC, Kunz R, Cook D, Holbrook A, Guyatt GH. "Surrogate outcomes." In: Guyatt GH, Rennie D, Meade MO, Cook D, eds. *Users' Guides to the Medical Literature: A Manual for Evidence-Based Clinical Practice.* 2nd ed. New York City: McGraw Hill; 2008:317-340.

41. Fethney J. "Statistical and clinical significance, and how to use confidence intervals to help interpret both". *Aust Crit Care* 2010;23(2):93-97.

42. Piantadosi S. "Notation and terminology." In: Piantadosi S, ed. *Clinical Trials: A Methodologic Perspective.* 2nd ed. Hoboken, N.J.: Wiley-Interscience; 2005:569-585.

43. Guyatt GH, Walter S, Cook D, Wyer P, Jaeschke R. "Confidence intervals." In: Guyatt GH, Rennie D, Meade MO, Cook D, eds. *Users' Guides to the Medical Literature: A Manual for Evidence-Based Clinical Practice.* 2nd ed. New York City: McGraw Hill; 2008:99-107.

44. Braitman LE. "Confidence intervals assess both clinical significance and statistical significance." *Ann Intern Med* 1991;114(6):515-517.

A version of this chapter originally appeared in the July 2013 edition of *JADA* (Volume 144, Issue 7, Pages 780–786). It has been reviewed and updated for accuracy and clarity by the editors of *How to Use Evidence-Based Dental Practices to Improve Your Clinical Decision-Making.*

Chapter 12. A Primer to Biostatistics for Busy Clinicians

Michael Glick, D.M.D., and Barbara L. Greenberg, Ph.D., M.Sc.

In This Chapter:

Research Design and Clinical Interpretation

- **Experimental Trial**

- **Observational Studies**

Measures of Association

- **Mean Difference**

- **Standard Mean Difference**

- **Absolute Risk**

- **Relative Risk**

- **Odds Ratio**

- **Absolute Risk Reduction and Relative Risk Reduction**

- **Hazard Ratio**

Hypothesis and Significance Testing

Confidence Intervals (CIs)

- **How to Interpret a CI**

Probability and the Normal Curve

- **Standard Deviation and Standard Error**

Sample Size Considerations

- **Why Is Sample Size Important?**

Introduction

Scientific literacy is about an understanding of appropriate use of statistics and statistical concepts, as well as recognition of incorrect use.[1] In today's world of rapidly communicated health information, among and by both health care professionals and the lay public, lack of understanding of statistical concepts is troubling and has even been equated to scientific illiteracy.[2]

Statistics has its jargon, a language that enables data to be translated into useful information and knowledge that can be communicated among health care professionals and between health care professionals and patients. Statistics also provides evidence that can inform patient care. It is important to realize that many statistical terms are the same as everyday words, but their connotation may be different. Successfully navigating the professional literature requires an understanding of basic statistical concepts. Although some of these concepts have previously been addressed in the oral health literature,[3] this chapter will provide a primer on commonly used statistical concepts and relevant research study design issues.

How to Use Evidence-Based Dental Practices to Improve Your Clinical Decision-Making   **185**

Research Design and Clinical Interpretation

Applied epidemiologic and clinical research can broadly be divided into experimental research, in which exposure is assigned to a participant, and observational research, in which exposure is not assigned but is instead "observed" as being present or absent (Figure 12.1).[4] If there is a comparison group in an observational study, it is characterized as *analytical,* and when no comparison group is included, as *descriptive.* The appropriate research design is a function of the question being asked and logistics. In some instances, it is constrained by available data and/or resources.

Exposure is a term used to describe a factor that is thought to be associated with or predictive of an *outcome,* such as a disease or a condition. For example, examining the association between sugar (the exposure) and the risk of developing caries (the outcome) may be the aim of a study.

Figure 12.1. Algorithm for Classification of Types of Clinical Research

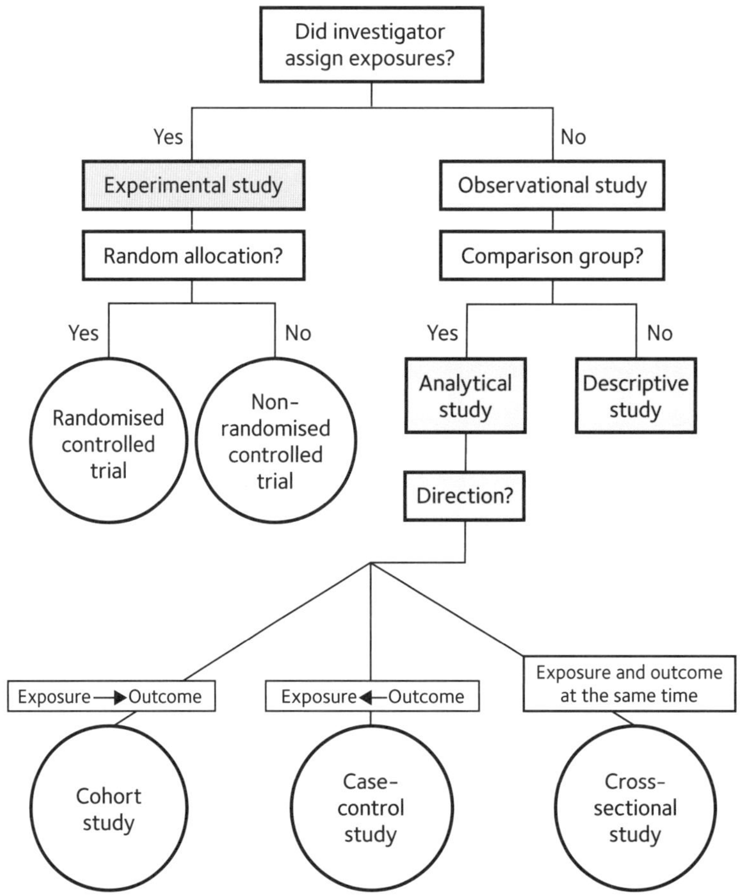

Adapted from Grimes DA, Schulz KF. "An overview of clinical research: the lay of the land." *The Lancet* 2002;359(9300):57-61

Experimental Trial

A *randomized controlled trial* (RCT) is considered the gold standard for answering questions of therapy (that is, determining the magnitude of the beneficial and harmful effects of health care interventions) and is the most rigorous study design. The hallmark of an RCT is the random allocation or assignment of study participants to treatment, intervention, or exposure groups. The main purpose of randomization (that is, randomly allocating trial participants) is to minimize *selection bias* on the part of the investigator (see Chapters 3 and 13). In addition, randomization increases comparability of the treatment groups for variables we can measure, as well as those we are not aware of or cannot measure, thus minimizing the impact of potential confounders. (A confounder is a factor that is associated with both the exposure and the outcome but does not lie in the causative pathway.) However, randomization does not ensure the study groups are indeed similar for all known confounders, and investigators should always assess comparability of the study groups at baseline for known relevant clinical and demographic characteristics (risk factors that are likely related to the exposure and outcome of interest). If the study groups are not comparable for all important risk factors that could affect the relationship of the exposure and the outcome, any observed association or difference could be due to a third factor, a confounder, that is linked to the exposure and the outcome. Another important design element of RCTs is *blinding* or masking. In this situation, study participants, clinicians, researchers, outcome adjudicators, and analysts can be unaware of which treatment group a particular patient has been assigned to. When both the investigators and the study participants are unaware of the group assignment, this is sometimes referred to as double blinding. Blinding is an important design strategy to reduce participant and investigator bias. A well-designed and implemented RCT can therefore minimize selection bias, information bias, and confounding (see Chapter 13). One of the advantages of an RCT is the certainty of the temporal relationship (which one comes first) between an exposure (for example, a treatment or an intervention) and an outcome. A potential concern with RCTs is the often-restrictive inclusion criteria for participant selection. RCT participant selection usually targets one specific condition among a select demographic who, other than the condition of interest, are considered healthy. Therefore, results from RCTs may sometimes be difficult to generalize or apply (external validity) to the total population from which the study participants were selected. The total population is likely to have many characteristics/ risk factors or other conditions that have not been eliminated in the study population, so the study results may or may not be applicable to the total population from which the study participants were selected. For example, it would represent a threat to applicability when a study that looks at the success rate of immediately versus nonimmediately placed dental implants uses exclusion criteria for the study population that could affect the outcome (success rate) by excluding based on factors that are commonly found in the general population, such as smoking, systemic diseases, medications, periodontal disease, or excluding certain genders or age groups.

Observational Studies

Analytical observational studies include cohort studies where a group of individuals with and without the exposure of interest are followed prospectively (forward in time), *case-control studies* where individuals with or without the outcome of interest (cases and controls, respectively) are traced backward in time to determine possible exposure, and *cross-sectional studies* where exposure and outcome are measured at the same time (Figure 12.1). Unlike RCTs, the exposure in observational studies is not assigned but is observed in groups of interest as it happens naturally.

Cohort studies are prospective in nature and compare outcomes in groups (cohorts) of participants with an exposure to a similar group of participants without an exposure (but having the same risk for developing the outcome). It is important to note that participants in the "exposed" group and the "unexposed" group need to be similar in all aspects except for their exposure (that is, they have the same characteristics). In this study design, it is also important to establish that the study participants are free of the disease or outcome of interest at the start of the study and to have a clear, measurable definition of the outcome. For example, two groups (cohorts) of children, one group that drinks sugar-sweetened beverages (SSBs, the exposure) and one group that does not drink SSBs, are followed forward in time. The two groups should be similar except for the fact that participants in the "exposure" group consume SSBs and participants in the control group do not consume SSBs. The outcome of interest is the development of caries, which will be assessed after a specific period (for example, two years). Because all participants are free of the outcome (caries) at the onset of the study, this type of study design can determine if the outcome was associated with the exposure based on the difference in incidence (the development of the disease [caries] over a specific time period) between the two groups. Cohort studies can determine incidence rates in the exposed and nonexposed groups.

In *case-control studies,* researchers will observe an outcome and then retrospectively try to determine the presence of past exposure. In this study design, the cases are those with the outcome of interest and the controls are a comparable group without the outcome of interest—but, it is important to note, with the same characteristics as the cases. Although the selection and source of cases and appropriate controls are critical elements in case-control studies, it is beyond the scope of this chapter to discuss this concern. Using a similar example to the one above, cases of children with caries (those with the outcome) are compared with children without caries (those without the outcome) to determine if an exposure, such as consumption of SSBs, is associated with the presence of caries. Information about prevalence rates or incidence rates cannot be determined by a case-control study design as the cases and the controls are not measured from a population-based sample and there is no information on the temporal relationship between exposure and outcome.

A *cross-sectional study* will assess the presence or absence of an exposure and the presence or absence of an outcome at a particular time (that is, the prevalence of the exposure and the prevalence of the outcome at the same point in time). Researchers may determine, at one particular time, the presence of children with or without caries who drink or do not drink SSBs. As this is a snapshot in time, it is not possible to know if the consumption of the SSBs occurred prior to the development of caries (a temporal relationship), and accordingly, it is not possible to determine whether drinking SSBs is associated with the development of caries. Cross-sectional studies cannot be used to claim any causative relationships and are generally used to help guide development of research questions.

Case reports and *case series* are purely descriptive and may, in a similar manner to other observational studies, generate hypotheses about exposure and outcomes that need to be tested with more complex study designs of greater rigor. Descriptive studies can be used to monitor the health of populations but cannot be used to assess associations.

Measures of Association

Measures of association quantify the relationship (an analysis of comparison) between exposure(s) and outcome(s) among groups. There are several different measures of association, such as *mean difference* (MD), *standardized mean difference* (SMD), *absolute risk* (AR), *relative risk* (RR), *odds ratio* (OR), and *hazard ratio* (HR). *Effect size* quantifies a measure of association as the size of the difference between groups (for example, the MD in number of teeth between two groups) or an estimate of a treatment's efficacy as a proportion of the reduction or increase in the outcome of interest in the intervention and control group (for example, the relative increase or decrease in developing caries after consuming or not consuming SSBs). An effect size can be standardized by dividing the measure of effect by the standard deviation (SD) of their difference (see below for a description of SD).

Mean Difference

The MD, or the "difference in means," measures the absolute difference between the mean values in two study groups. It quantifies the average of the means by which the study intervention changes the outcome in the study/treatment/intervention group compared with the means of the control group. Because this estimate is created by subtracting the mean from one group from the mean of the other group, an MD of 0 indicates no difference between the experimental and control groups.

Standard Mean Difference

The SMD is a summary statistic often used in meta-analyses when the studies all assess the same outcome but measure it in different scales (for example, measuring pain with two different types of visual analog scales). In this situation, the results of the different studies must be standardized to a uniform scale before they can be combined and compared and the results summarized. The SMD quantifies the intervention effect in each study relative to the variability observed in the particular study. In meta-analyses, the SMD is calculated for each study in the meta-analysis and then pooled to get an overall SMD. An SMD of 0 indicates there is no difference among groups.

Absolute Risk

Understanding the difference between probability and odds is essential in order to be able to interpret AR, RR, and OR. A probability is the chance of an event occurring as a ratio of all events. (For example, the probability of getting a 4 when tossing a six-sided die is the ratio of the event occurring [tossing a 4] to all possible events [tossing a 1, 2, 3, 4, 5, or 6], which equals 1/6). A probability can be any number between 0 and 1.

The *odds* is the chance that a particular event occurs versus the chance that it does not occur, or the ratio of the number with the event to the number without the event. For example, the odds of tossing a 4 is the ratio of the chance (probability) of getting a 4 (1/6) to the probability of not getting a 4 (5/6) [(1/6)/(5/6)], which equals 1/5. In other words, it is the probability of an event occurring to the probability of that event not occurring. Odds can be any number between 0 and infinity.

Risk in statistical terms suggests the probability, or the chance, that an event will occur, without any inference to whether it has a good or bad outcome. A measure of risk, or probability, is expressed as a number between 0 and 1, or as a percentage. Several different connotations of risk are used in biostatistics to describe different associations, specifically relationships between an exposure and an outcome.

As an example, we want to know the relationship between consuming SSBs and the development of caries. In a hypothetical study, one group of 1,000 children who are not consuming SSBs is followed for two years, and another group of 1,000 children, with the same risk factors for developing caries as the first group but who are consuming SSBs, is also followed for two years (Table 12.1). The AR is the number of children who develop caries in each group divided by the total number of children in the group during the designated study period (Table 12.1a). Using the data from Table 12.1, we can state that "not consuming SSBs is associated with an AR of developing caries of 15% (150 out of 1,000) at some point during two years" and "the AR of developing caries when consuming SSBs is 65% (650 out of 1,000) over a time span of two years."

Table 12.1. A Hypothetical Study Involving 2,000 Children—1,000 Who Drink Sugar-Sweetened Beverages (SSBs) and 1,000 Who Do Not Drink SSBs—Over a Time Period of Two Years

	Caries	No caries	Total
	a	b	a+b
Consuming SSBs	650	350	1,000
	c	d	c+d
Not Consuming SSBs	150	850	1,000
	a+c	b+d	a+b+c+d
	800	1,200	2,000

Table 12.1a. Absolute Risk and Absolute Risk Reduction Based on the Data Presented in the Hypothetical Study in Table 12.1

Absolute risk (AR) of developing caries **when drinking** SSBs (risk with exposure)

$$\frac{a}{a+b} = \frac{650}{1,000} = 0.65$$

AR of developing caries **when not drinking** SSBs (risk without exposure)

$$\frac{c}{c+d} = \frac{150}{1,000} = 0.15$$

Absolute risk reduction (ARR) (the risk reduction of developing caries when switching from drinking to not drinking SSBs)

$$a/(a+b) - c/(c+d) = 0.65 - 0.15 = 0.50$$

Relative Risk

The relative risk (RR), also known as the *risk ratio,* is the proportion of participants who developed the outcome in the cohort with the exposure as a ratio of the proportion of participants who developed the outcome in the cohort without the exposure (Table 12.1b). It can also be defined as the probability of an outcome occurring in a treatment, or intervention, group divided by the probability of an outcome occurring in a comparison, or control, group, or vice versa. In other words, the RR is the incidence of the outcome in the exposed group relative to the incidence of the outcome in the nonexposed group and provides a measure of the risk of developing disease if exposed. The RR is the measure of association for cohort studies and clinical trials (Table 12.2). Using the data and the formula in Table 12.1b, we can state, "There is an RR of developing caries of 4.33, over a period of two years, if consuming SSBs compared with not consuming SSBs," or, "People consuming SSBs have 4.33 times the risk of developing caries compared with those not consuming SSBs, over a period of two years," or conversely, "People not consuming SSBs have 0.23 times the risk of developing caries compared with those consuming SSBs, over a period of two years." An RR of 1 suggests no difference in risks, an RR of more than 1 indicates an increased risk, and an RR of less than 1 indicates reduced risk.

Table 12.1b. Relative Risk and Relative Risk Reduction Based on the Data Presented in the Hypothetical Study in Table 12.1

Relative risk (RR), or risk ratio, of developing caries **when drinking** SSBs compared with developing caries **when not drinking** SSBs =

$$\frac{\text{AR of developing caries } \textbf{when drinking } \textit{SSBs}}{\text{AR of developing caries } \textbf{when not drinking } \textit{SSBs}} = \frac{a/(a+b)}{c/(c+d)} = \frac{0.65}{0.15} = 4.33$$

Relative risk, or risk ratio, of developing caries **when not drinking** SSBs compared with developing caries **when drinking** SSBs =

$$\frac{\text{AR of developing caries } \textbf{when not drinking } \textit{SSBs}}{\text{AR of developing caries } \textbf{when drinking } \textit{SSBs}} = \frac{0.15}{0.65} = 0.23$$

Relative risk reduction (RRR) if not drinking SSBs =

$$\frac{\text{AR of developing caries } \textbf{when drinking } \textit{SSBs} - \text{AR of developing caries } \textbf{when not drinking } \textit{SSBs}}{\text{AR of developing caries } \textbf{when drinking } \textit{SSBs}} =$$

$$\frac{0.65 - 0.15}{0.65} = 1 - 0.23 = 0.77, \text{ or } 77\%$$

Odds Ratio

Because case-control studies do not have a true denominator of "at risk" individuals and the temporal relationship of exposure to an outcome is not clearly established, case-control studies cannot use the RR as a measure of association and will instead use the odds ratio (OR) as a measure of association (Table 12.2).

The OR in a case-control study is the ratio of the odds of individuals in the disease group having the exposure divided by the odds of individuals in the comparison group having the exposure (Table 12.1c); in other words, it is the odds of having the exposure in the cases compared with the odds of having the exposure in the controls.

When warranted, odds can be converted to risks and subsequently to RR (Table 12.3). An OR approximates an RR when the prevalence of disease is low, typically below 10%.[5] (This is illustrated in Table 12.3, where it is noticeable how low odds approximates the risk.) An RR is an inappropriate measure in a case-control study.

Cohort studies can also use an OR as the measure or association; in this case, the OR is the odds of experiencing the outcome or disease in the group exposed to a risk factor compared with the odds of experiencing the outcome or disease in the group not exposed to the same risk factor (Table 12.1.c). Results from RCTs are usually reported as an RR or as an OR. In RCTs, ORs are interpreted similarly to ORs in cohort studies (Table 12.2).

Table 12.1c. Odds and Odds Ratios Based on the Data Presented in the Hypothetical Study in Table 12.1

Case-Control Study

Odds of **having** caries when drinking SSBs $= \dfrac{a}{c} = \dfrac{650}{150} = 4.33$

Odds of **not having** caries when drinking SSBs $= \dfrac{b}{d} = \dfrac{350}{850} = 0.41$

Odds ratio (OR) $= \dfrac{\text{odds of having caries } \textbf{when drinking } SSBs}{\text{odds of having caries } \textbf{when not drinking } SSBs} = \dfrac{a/c}{b/d} = 10.52$

Cohort Study

Odds of developing caries **when drinking** SSBs $= \dfrac{a}{b} = \dfrac{650}{350} = 1.86$

Odds of developing caries **when not drinking** SSBs $= \dfrac{c}{d} = \dfrac{150}{850} = 0.18$

Odds ratio (OR) $= \dfrac{\text{odds of developing caries } \textbf{when drinking } SSBs}{\text{odds of developing caries } \textbf{when not drinking } SSBs} = \dfrac{a/b}{c/d} = 10.52$

Table 12.2. Interpretation of Relative Risk and Odds Ratio in Different Study Designs

	Relative Risk	Odds Ratio
Experimental Studies		
Randomized Trial (for comparing treatments or interventions)	The risk of developing disease among those who are exposed relative to the risk of developing disease among those who are not exposed; the ratio of the incidence of new disease among the exposed relative to the non-exposed. An RR > 1 suggests the exposure is a risk factor for developing the disease, an RR < 1 suggests an exposure is protective against developing the disease, and an RR = 1 suggests there is no association between the exposure and disease.	The odds that an exposed person develops disease relative to the odds that a non-exposed person develops disease. An OR > 1 suggests the exposure is positively associated with the disease, an OR < 1 suggests the exposure is negatively associated with the disease, and an OR = 1 suggests no association between exposure and disease.
Observational Studies		
Cohort Study	The risk of developing disease among those who are exposed relative to the risk of developing disease among those who are not exposed; the ratio of the incidence of new disease among the exposed relative to the non-exposed. An RR > 1 suggests the exposure is a risk factor for developing the disease, an RR < 1 suggests an exposure is protective against developing the disease, and an RR = 1 suggests there is no association between the exposure and disease.	The odds that an exposed person develops disease relative to the odds that a non-exposed person develops disease. An OR > 1 suggests the exposure is positively associated with the disease, an OR < 1 suggests the exposure is negatively associated with the disease, and an OR = 1 suggests no association between exposure and disease.
Case-Control Study	Cannot be calculated directly	The odds of those with disease having been exposed relative to the odds of those without disease having been exposed. An OR > 1 suggests the exposure is positively associated with the exposure, an OR < 1 suggests the exposure is negatively associated with the disease, and an OR = 1 suggests no association.
Cross-Sectional Study	Cannot be calculated	Cannot be calculated unless there is a comparison group; in that case, similar to interpretation for a case-control study.
Case Report/ Case Series	Cannot be calculated	Cannot be calculated.

Table 12.3. Converting Odds to Risk and Risk to Odds

Odds	Ratio		Ratio	Risk
9.00	9:1	or	9:1	0.90
4.00	4:1	or	8:2	0.80
2.33	2.33:1	or	7:3	0.70
1.50	1.50:1	or	6:4	0.60
1.00	1:1	or	5:5	0.50
0.67	0.67:1	or	4:6	0.40
0.43	0.43.1	or	3:7	0.30
0.25	0.25:1	or	2:8	0.20
0.11	0.11:1	or	1:9	0.10
0.05	0.05:1	or	5:95	0.05

$$risk = \frac{odds}{odds + 1} \qquad odds = \frac{risk}{1 - risk}$$

Absolute Risk Reduction and Relative Risk Reduction

Understanding the difference between AR and RR, and *absolute risk reduction* (ARR) and *relative risk reduction* (RRR), is important in order to make appropriate clinical decisions. In the example in Table 12.1, there is a different AR for having caries among children who do not consume SSBs compared with the AR for having caries among children who consume SSBs. The ARR is the difference of the AR in the test group and the control group. As seen from the data in Table 12.1a, not consuming SSBs is associated with an ARR of having caries of 0.50 (0.65 minus 0.15), or stated differently, "not consuming SSBs will reduce the AR for having caries from 650 in 1,000 (65%) to 150 in 1,000 (15%)" or "500 fewer cases of caries can be expected among 1,000 patients who do not consume SSBs compared with 1,000 patients who consume SSBs over a period of two years."

Looking again at Table 12.1, there is a relationship between the two ARs that can be quantified with RR: the proportion, or relative change, between the AR for caries among children who do not consume SSBs and the AR among children who consume SSBs (Table 12.1b).

In the hypothetical study depicted in Table 12.1, the RRR is the risk reduction for developing caries associated with not consuming SSBs (Table 12.1b). As the RR of not consuming SSBs compared with consuming SSBs is 0.23, the RRR of not consuming sugar is 77% (1 minus 0.23), or a 77% reduction in the risk of developing caries in the group that is not consuming SSBs compared with the group that is consuming SSBs.

Although the RRR was 77%, the ARR was 50% (65% minus 15%). The difference between the RRR and the ARR is more dramatic when the prevalence of a disease is low. For example, if the AR for developing caries is 1.6% and a particular diet would decrease this risk to 1%, there is an RRR of 37.5% but an ARR of only 0.6%. Both of these concepts will inform practice, but in different ways.

Hazard Ratio

The HR is another measure of association that deals with time-to-event data, also known as survival data. Hazard is the instantaneous event rate, which is expressed as the probability for an individual to have an event of interest at a particular time (assuming they are event-free up to that time). The HR quantifies risk as the ratio of hazards in the treatment group and the control group at a particular point in time. It is the hazard of developing an event in the intervention group relative to the hazard of developing the event in the control group at any particular time along the follow-up period. An HR of 1.0 means the event rates are the same in both groups; an HR of 2.0 means that, at any particular time during the study follow-up, twice as many patients in the treatment group are having an event proportionally to the control group. An HR of 0.5 means that, at any particular time, half as many patients in the treatment group are experiencing the event proportionally to the controls. In a hypothetical clinical study, the reported HR is 0.45, which means that patients in the treatment group at any point in time along the follow-up are 55% less likely to experience the event. Although the HR takes into account not only the total number of events but also the timing of each event (that is, the event rate), the RR measures the cumulative risk over the total time period of interest.

Hypothesis and Significance Testing

When researchers are trying to determine whether an association exists between two factors (for example, consuming or not consuming SSBs), or between patients' characteristics (for example, patients with low education levels or high education levels), and the presence of an outcome, the ideal situation would be to recruit the whole population to whom the results would be applied to into the study. It is not difficult to understand that such an approach would have serious implementation issues, and a massive amount of resources and time would need to be allocated. As a way to solve this conundrum, researchers take a sample, a portion of the whole population, expecting that this sample will provide good representation of the individuals, factors, or characteristics under study. Extrapolating the study sample findings to the whole population is called *inferential statistics*. ("Population" is a term used in statistics to describe the entire "universe" of individuals from which researchers draw their study sample.) Inferential statistics differ from *descriptive statistics,* where collected data are only used to describe the study sample without making inferences to a population.

Users of the dental literature will find that there are two types of hypotheses: the null hypothesis (H_0) and the research (or alternative) hypothesis (H_a). The null hypothesis states that there is no (that is, null) association between the predictor or exposure and outcome variable, or therefore there is no difference in the outcome between the study groups, and further, any observed difference is due to chance alone (Box 12.1 and Figure 12.2).

Box 12.1. Examples of Hypotheses

Null hypothesis (H_0)

The incidence of caries in the group of children consuming sugar-sweetened beverages (SSBs) compared with those children not consuming SSBs is the same.

Research (or alternative) hypothesis (H_a)

1. The incidence of caries in the group of children consuming SSBs compared with those children not consuming SSBs is different.

2. The incidence of caries in the group of children consuming SSBs is higher compared with those children not consuming SSBs.

3. The incidence of caries in the group of children consuming SSBs is lower compared with those children not consuming SSBs.

Figure 12.2. Hypothesis Testing

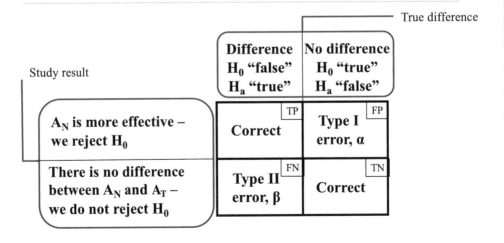

Study to ascertain the efficacy of a new anesthetic.
A_N = new anesthetic; A_T = traditional anesthetic

Hypothesis (H_a) = A_N is more effective than A_T
Hypothesis (H_0) = There is no difference in efficacy between A_N and A_T

TP = true positive; FP = false positive; FN = false negative; TN = true negative

The null hypothesis is the basis for statistical testing because researchers only have to test to one value, a 0% difference; the question is whether the observed study data are consistent with the null hypothesis, which states that there is no difference. The alternative hypothesis can be nondirectional and just state there is an association (or a difference) or directional (better or worse, higher or lower) (Box 12.1 and Figure 12.2).

Statistical significance testing is the method used to support or reject inferences based on observed sample data. In other words, from the observed study sample, can researchers infer what is "true" for the population? In terms of hypothesis testing, the purpose of statistical testing is to determine whether the observed study data support (warrant) rejecting or not rejecting the null hypothesis. Failure to reject the null hypothesis is not exactly the same as accepting the null hypothesis; the correct conclusion is that there is not enough evidence to reject the null hypothesis of no association/difference. Nonsignificant results mean that there is not enough evidence to reject the null hypothesis and suggest that there is an association/difference. ("Enough" is quantified by a predetermined value or level called the alpha level [see more about the alpha level below]). If the results of a study to assess if there is an association/difference are not significant, concluding that the two groups under comparison are the same or equivalent is incorrect and a typical misunderstanding. If the statistical testing suggests the study observations are consistent with the null hypothesis of no association/difference, the null hypothesis is not rejected and one cannot state that there is a difference between the groups. If the statistical significance testing indicates that it is unlikely that the study results are consistent with the null hypothesis (that is, it is unlikely that there is a difference), the null hypothesis is rejected and we proceed with the alternative hypothesis, or we reject the null hypothesis in favor of the alternative hypothesis.

Significance testing is based on a designated, or predetermined, *alpha level* and calculated *probability (P) values*. The alpha level is the probability chosen by the investigator to be the threshold of statistical significance, or stated differently, the predetermined threshold of confidence to reject or not reject the null hypothesis. It is an arbitrary value, but the accepted convention for most studies is to set the alpha at 0.05. The alpha level is also the probability of committing a type I error given the null hypothesis is true—concluding that there is a statistically significant difference when in fact there is not a statistically significant difference, also known as a false-positive result (Figure 12.2). An alpha of 0.05 suggests that 5% of the time the investigator will conclude that there is an association or difference, when in fact there is not a real association/difference and the observed results are merely due to chance. Another way of interpreting an alpha of 0.05 is to say one is willing to accept a 5% risk of committing a type I error (getting a false-positive result), or that 5% of the time you will falsely conclude there is a difference when in fact there really is no true difference (Figure 12.2).

A *P* value less than alpha is considered statistically significant, and the null hypothesis is rejected in favor of the alternative hypothesis; a *P* value equal to or greater than alpha is not considered statistically significant, and based on the study data, the null hypothesis is not rejected. The *P* value is the probability that an outcome (result) as extreme (or as unusual), or even more extreme (or more unusual), as that obtained from the study could have occurred by chance alone assuming the null hypothesis is true. The *P* value is the measure of evidence for or against the null hypothesis (no association/difference) and indicates the observed results are either statistically significant or not statistically significant. It is a binary, yes or no, outcome; for this reason, it is incorrect to say that there is a trend toward statistical significance or results are marginally significant. For example, *P* values of 0.03 and 0.04 are both statistically significant, but one is not more significant than the other. Also, a *P* value above but close to 0.05 should not be interpreted as "marginally statistically significant" or a "trend toward significance."

Although the *P* value is frequently used, it is often misinterpreted.[6] Therefore, it is important to be aware of what it does not tell you. The *P* value does not provide any indication of the direction (decreased or increased) or magnitude of the association/difference; it also does not indicate the potential clinical or practical significance of the results (see Chapter 11). Furthermore, the *P* value does not indicate the probability that the null hypothesis is true, how true the study results are, or how likely the results are to be true. There is a consensus in the scientific community that the *P* value is often misinterpreted and that when using a *P* value, it should always be accompanied by confidence intervals. CIs provide information about the statistical significance along with information about the direction and strength of the association or magnitude of effect (see the following section on CIs).

Confidence Intervals (CIs)

When faced with clinical choices, patients and clinicians would like as much information as possible in order to make an informed decision. Consider an example of a clinician talking to a patient about placing an implant, in which the patient wants to know if this procedure is associated with any marginal bone loss (MBL). In a hypothetical example, a study shows that the mean MBL, using the particular implant offered to the patient, was 5 mm. This is important information, but even more informative would be to know the range of MBL reported in the study. The 95% CI in the study ranged from 1 to 9 mm, or the mean ±4 mm. Thus, although the mean MBL was 5 mm, the expected MBL could be as much as 9 mm and as little as 1 mm. Knowing this information, the patient may decide that the risk of 9 mm MBL is too much, or decide to accept the risk and agree to have the implant placed as there is also a chance that the MBL will be much less (as little as 1 mm). Thus, a CI will provide additional information to evaluate the clinical relevance of the study findings (see Boxes 12.2 and 12.3).

The level of confidence is the certainty that a range, or interval of values, contains the "true" or accurate value of a population that would be obtained if the experiment were repeated multiple times. In other words, a 95% CI purports that if a CI is calculated for numerous samples (experiments), we would expect that the true population value (mean, proportion, etc.) be included in 95% of the sampled CIs. A 95% CI is commonly used in clinical and applied research, but if more confidence is desired, researchers can use a CI larger than 95%, such as 99%. A CI can only be correctly interpreted if we use a random sample, if the samples are selected independently of each other, if the data are accurately measured, and if the variable being measured is the right one to make an inference about the population. For example, we cannot use a measure of bone loss from numerous samples to make an inference about implant failure in the population. As an aside, it is not correct to state that "there is a 95% probability that the population mean is contained within a specific 95% CI." Such a statement would imply that the population mean could be different depending on which CI we examine. However, we have only one "true" population mean, which does not change, but we have several different samples, with CIs, that may or may not contain the population mean. Thus, the 95% probability is about the CIs and not about the fixed, or "true," population mean, or stated correctly, "There is a 95% probability that this sample's specific 95% CI contains the population mean."

How to Interpret a CI

A CI provides information about both the direction and magnitude of a treatment effect, which provides more information on the clinical importance than the *P* value, as a *P* value can only provide a "yes" or "no" answer on whether to reject or not reject the null hypothesis (see the section on *P* value). All CIs are reported around a *point estimate* (a specific sample mean, mean difference, etc., which is computed from the data of the experiment and is the best estimate for the observed data) and lower and upper limits (confidence limits or boundaries).

The width of a CI may be determined by several different factors. The obvious one is the sample size (Table 12.4a). Increasing the number of participants would increase our confidence that the "true" effect is closer to our measured (observed) effect. The outcome of an experiment with only four participants would provide us with a measure that may be close to the "true" effect, but enrolling 100 participants would enhance our confidence that our observed result is even closer to the "true" effect. However, there may be other factors that could affect the width of a CI.

If researchers conducted experiments to compare implant failures using an experimental technique to a failures using a conventional technique, they can calculate the ARR and RRR to determine which technique is associated with a better or worse outcome. If the ARR (the difference between the AR in the experimental group and the AR in the control group) increased, yet the sample size in all experiments remained the same, the RRR might not change but the width of the CI will narrow (Table 12.4b). The difference between the AR in the experimental and the control group will determine the width of the CI (that is, the precision). In this case, it is the ARR and not the sample size that will determine the width of the CI, where a higher ARR will provide a more precise CI. Thus, both sample size and the number of events observed are key determinants of the width of a CI.

Table 12.4a. Sample Size and Width of a Confidence Interval (CI)

Experimental Group			Control Group			Absolute Risk Reduction (ARR)	Relative Risk Reduction (RRR)	RRR; 95% CI
Implant Failures	Total Number of Implants	Absolute Risk	Implant Failures	Total Number of Implants	Absolute Risk			
8	20	0.40	10	20	0.50	0.10	0.20	0.20; −60 to 60%
16	40	0.40	20	40	0.50	0.10	0.20	0.20; −31 to 51%
32	80	0.40	40	80	0.50	0.10	0.20	0.20; −13 to 43%
128	320	0.40	160	320	0.50	0.10	0.20	0.20; 5 to 33%
320	800	0.40	400	800	0.50	0.10	0.20	0.20; 11 to 28%

The five different studies above illustrate that an increase in sample size will result in a more narrow confidence interval constructed around the relative risk reduction (RRR) (that is, provide more confidence that the "true" RRR for the implant failure rate is close to our observed 10% absolute risk reduction and 20% RRR).

Table 12.4b. Absolute Risk Reduction and Width of a Confidence Interval (CI)

Experimental Group			Control Group					
Implant Failures	Total Number of Implants	Absolute Risk	Implant Failures	Total Number of Implants	Absolute Risk	Absolute Risk Reduction (ARR)	Relative Risk Reduction (RRR)	RRR; 95% CI
8	100	0.08	10	100	0.10	0.02	0.20	0.20; −94 to 67%
24	100	0.24	30	100	0.30	0.06	0.20	0.20; −26 to 49%
40	100	0.40	50	100	0.50	0.10	0.20	0.20; −9 to 41%
56	100	0.56	70	100	0.70	0.14	0.20	0.20; 7 to 36%
72	100	0.72	90	100	0.90	0.18	0.20	0.20; 8 to 30%

The five different studies above show that although the sample size and the relative risk reduction (RRR) remained the same, the width of the confidence interval (CI) constructed around the RRR changed. This is due to an increase in the absolute risk reduction (the difference between the absolute risk in the control group and the absolute risk in the experimental group), which will result in a narrower, and thus more precise, CI. Accordingly, in this scenario, the number of events, and not the sample size, affected the width of the CI.

There are several other factors that impact the width of the CI. The width of the CI decreases as the sample size increases; an increase in the SD will increase the width of the CI; and, all variables remaining equal, increasing the level of confidence desired from 95% to 99% will increase the width of the CI. Another factor that can impact the width of the CI is the level of significance; as the significance level decreases (for example, 0.05 to 0.01) with all other variables being equal, the width of the CI increases.

Treatment effect can be measured by an RR or OR among other measures of association (see the section on measures of association). If the CI constructed around an RR or OR includes 1, the result is not statistically significant as 1 is the null value for a ratio (Table 12.5), indicating that the "true" difference may be 1, which for a ratio indicates no difference between the two groups compared. This could also raise questions about the potential clinical importance of the finding. If we are comparing means, an MD (the mean of one study group minus the mean of the other study group) of 0 is the null value and would suggest no difference. A CI surrounding the MD that crosses the null value of 0 is considered not statistically significant. This concept applies to differences of SMD, ARR, HR, and other measures of association. Statistical significance can thus be assessed using both *P* values and CIs.

For more information on the calculation of CIs, see Box 12.2, and for more discussion on CIs, significance, and clinical implications, see Box 12.3.

 Treatment effect can be measured by an RR or OR among other measures of association (see the section on measures of association).

Table 12.5. Assessing Statistical Significance Using Confidence Intervals and *P* Values

Parameter	Null Value	Assessing Significance Using the Confidence Interval (CI)	Assessing Significance Using the Corresponding *P* Value
Difference: mean difference, standardized mean difference, risk difference, rate difference	0	CI contains 0 = non-significant	$P \geq 0.05$
		CI does not contain 0 = significant	$P < 0.05$
Ratio: relative risk, odds ratio, risk ratio	1	CI contains 1 = non-significant	$P \geq 0.05$
		CI does not contain 1 = significant	$P < 0.05$

Probability and the Normal Curve

The use of statistical testing is meant to quantify the probability of getting the observed results if they were due solely to random variation, also referred to as chance. It does so by comparing observed outcomes with theoretical outcomes that would be expected because of random variation. An illustrative way to think about this is a coin toss experiment. What is the probability of obtaining nine heads and one tails after tossing a coin 10 times? We can calculate this probability with available formulas, and we can conduct an experiment. After comparing the observed result in the experiment to the calculated probability (the expected result), we can make a statement about the chance of the coin being a fair or biased coin.

The experiment consists of tossing a coin 10 times and observing the results (the proportion of heads compared with tails). Every 10 coin tosses is a trial, and every trial will not result in the same proportion of heads to tails. But the more trials we conduct, the more our certainty of what the proportion of heads to tails truly is will increase. After plotting the outcome of each trial, for example as a histogram, a certain pattern will emerge. The pattern of values of a measured quantity, in this case the outcome of each 10 coin tosses, is in statistics called a *distribution.* The *normal distribution,* or normal sample distribution curve, is the shape most commonly used to model expected probabilities under the null hypothesis (Figure 12.3). (The word "normal," when used to describe this particular curve, does not have the same meaning as in everyday language and is used in statistics to denote this particular curve.) The normal curve is used both in inferential and descriptive statistics and is also referred to as the *bell-shaped* or *Gaussian curve.* The area under the normal curve between different data points corresponds to a probability that can be calculated or obtained from tables found in most textbooks on statistics (Figure 12.3). Thus, by plotting our observed results from our trials of 10 coin tosses, we can calculate the probability of the result we observed and then compare our observed probability with our expected probability. For example, if our expected probability of obtaining nine heads and one tails after 10 coin tosses is 1%, and our observed probability of getting nine heads and one tails after having conducted our trials of 10 coin tosses was 4.5%, we need to determine if the difference between our expected result and our observed result could inform whether we tossed a fair or biased coin.

Figure 12.3. Normal Sample Distribution Curve with Standard Deviations and Areas Under the Curve

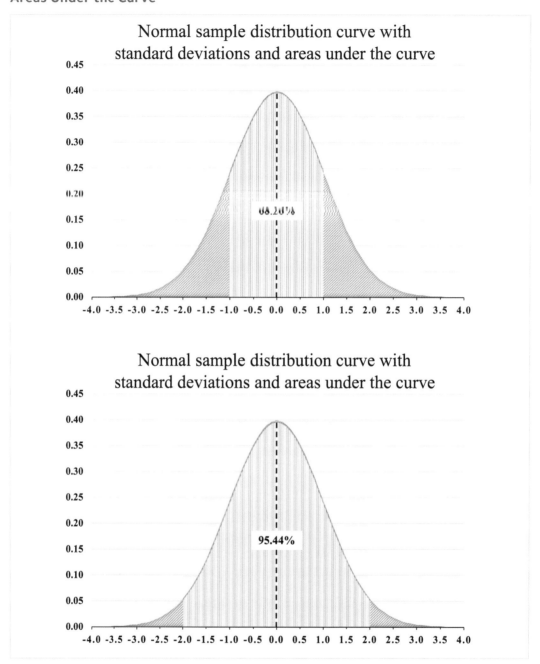

The mean in a normal sample distribution is usually the midpoint of the X-axis. In the examples above, the mean is 0. The standard deviation (SD) is evenly distributed around the mean.

The area under the curve between −1 SD and +1 SD is always ≈68.26%, the area between −2 SDs and +2 SDs is always ≈95.44%, and the area between −3 SDs and +3 SDs is always ≈99.72%.

Conversely, an area of 99% under the curve corresponds to ≈2.58 SDs; an area of 95% under the curve corresponds to ≈1.96 SDs; and an area of 90% under the curve corresponds to ≈1.65 SDs.

Figure 12.4. The Observed Result of a Study of Marginal Bone Loss after Placement of Dental Implants

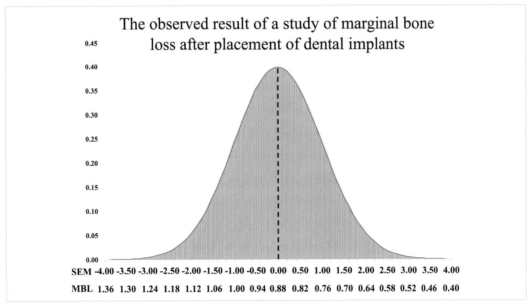

See Box 12.3 for more explanations.

The mean marginal bone loss (MBL) in this study was 0.88 mm, with a standard error of the mean (SEM) of 0.12 mm. The margin of error (ME) is ±0.24 mm associated with a 95% confidence interval (CI). Thus, the 95% CI constructed around the observed mean is 0.88 ± 0.24 mm, written as **mean 0.88; 95% CI, 1.12 to 0.64.**

One of the important attributes of the normal curve is that it can be described by two parameters, the *mean* and *standard deviation* (SD) (Figures 12.3 and 12.4). The SD is a measure of the variability of the observations or a measure of the spread of the data around the mean of a sample. Although there are an infinite number of "normal curves" depending on the mean and SD, all have the same property: The calculated area under the curve is proportional to a probability. Any observation that follows a normal distribution can be located on the normal curve based on the number of SDs it is from the mean, or center, of the curve. All normal curves have another shared characteristic: 68% of the area under the curve lies between the mean ± 1 SD, 95% of the area under the curve lies between the mean ± 2 SD, and 2.5% of the area under the curve lies in each respective tail of the curve beyond the mean ± 2 SDs (Figure 12.3). The area under the curve in the tails is the probability of an outcome as extreme as or more extreme than that observed if the null hypothesis is true. For example, if an alpha level of 5%, or 0.05, is chosen, any observation that lies beyond 95% of the curve (that is, 2.5% under each tail of the curve, which is interpreted as less than a 5% chance of obtaining our result if the null hypothesis is "true") will be considered not statistically significant and the null hypothesis will be rejected.

Standard Deviation and Standard Error

If we could repeat an experiment many, many times on different samples with the same number of subjects, the resultant sample statistic would not always be the same (because of variability in the samples, or dispersion, or chance). Two measures of sampling variability are the standard deviation (SD) and the standard error (SE). "Deviation" refers to the difference between the observed values and the estimated values, while the connotation of "error" is variability. It is important to understand the distinction between these two measures.

The SD is a measure of variation used with interval or ratio data. Interval data have no true zero, such as in the case of measures of temperature in a Fahrenheit or Celsius scale. As there is no true zero, it is not possible to say that 25°F is half as hot as 50°F. Ratio data has a true zero, such as in the case of weight, where 50 lb is twice as heavy as 25 lb. The SD is a measure of the variability in the observations in a given study sample. The SD is a measure of the spread of the observations around the study sample mean. In a given study, the SD indicates, on average, how much the individual observations differ from the study mean. The SD also defines the shape of the normal curve; a larger SD indicates more scatter about the mean and indicates worse precision, while a smaller SD indicates less scatter about the mean and better precision. This is reflected in the width of the normal curve, which increases with a larger SD and decreases with a smaller SD.

The SE refers to the mean of a study sample and quantifies the variation of the sample mean compared with the population mean. It indicates how reliable the study sample mean is as an estimate of the true population mean. Because the SE is calculated by taking the SD and dividing it by the square root of the study sample size (SE = SD/$\sqrt{}$(*sample size*)), the SE is always smaller than the SD. Thus, the SE depends on the study sample size (n) and the variability in the population from which the study sample was drawn (SD). A larger sample size will decrease the SE, while a population with a lot of individual variability for the given measurement of interest will increase the SE. The size of the SE gives an indication of the precision of the parameter estimate (an estimate of a population variable) and is the primary basis for calculating the CI used in statistical inference. To summarize, the SD quantifies the variability of the observations in a study sample, while the SE quantifies the variability of the sample mean from the true population mean. It is not correct to report the SE to indicate the variability of observations in a given study, although some investigators find it tempting as the SE is always smaller than the SD.

Sample Size Considerations

When a clinician is reading a research study, the *level of power* for the specific study is critical to interpreting the results; the investigator should always indicate the power of the study in the methods section. The level of power is the probability of finding a difference when one truly exists (that is, the probability of a true-positive finding). The desired level of power is, by convention, at least 80%. Increasing the level of power (for example, from 80% to 90%) for a treatment effect of interest when mortality is the outcome (a quite infrequent event) will require a markedly larger sample size. As the concepts of study power and sample size are directly related, sample size calculations are also referred to as *power analysis*. With a large enough sample, even a very small effect can be found to be statistically significant, although it would not necessarily be clinically relevant.

The calculated sample size is a function of the desired power of the study, which is directly related to the designated *beta level* (Figure 12.2). The beta level is the probability of committing a type II error (concluding that there is no association/difference when in fact there really is one, or a false-negative result) (Figure 12.2). The chosen beta level is based on the investigator's degree of willingness to accept making a type II error. This is analogous to choosing an alpha level based on the investigator's degree of willingness to accept a type I error, or false-positive result. Power is equal to 1-beta and is the probability of observing an effect in the study sample that reflects a "true" effect (the effect found in the population, the true-positive finding) as large as or larger than the observed effect. The convention is to set beta at 20%, which means the investigator is accepting that there is a one in five chance of missing a true difference (that is, of getting a false-negative result). A beta of 20% represents a power of 80% (an 80% probability of finding a "true" effect), which is the minimum acceptable power level to consider that a study was adequately powered. If it is particularly important to avoid a type I error (for example, making a false-positive diagnosis of cancer that requires therapeutic choices with potentially dire side effects), alpha can be set at a lower value such as 0.01; if, on the other hand, it is particularly important to avoid a type II error (for example, missing a diagnosis of a disease that is highly contagious and can affect a large number of people), beta can be set lower to, for example, 10%.

A priori determining the expected treatment effect can be the most difficult aspect of sample size planning. The desired treatment effect can be determined using data from other studies in the literature that report a statistically significant and clinically meaningful effect or using pilot data to make an informed estimate. In some instances, there are no data available to use, so the investigator will use their best judgment and experience to identify a clinically meaningful effect for a given outcome of interest. For example, if a study is designed to examine changes in the caries rate after consuming SSBs, the researcher has to predetermine what level of change in the caries rate would be relevant. The relevance may be decided upon by the cost of a potential intervention. Although a change of 1% might not be considered important, any change of 10% or more may be considered enough to decide to implement a specific caries-preventive intervention. The smaller the magnitude of the expected treatment effect, the larger the sample that is needed to show a statistically significant difference at alpha = 0.05 and power of 80%. Thus, all other factors being the same, to find a 1% difference requires a larger sample size than what would be required to find a 10% difference. When considering the expected magnitude of a treatment effect, it is critical to pay attention to clinical importance.

It is critical that, for each study, the elements used to conduct the sample size calculation are clearly specified and the power of the study is at least 80%. A study that has less than 80% power to detect the desired or observed effect is underpowered, and the results are not considered reliable. From a statistical standpoint, a study that does not find statistical significance is referred to as a "negative study." It is unclear if the nonstatistically significant result is valid or just the result of a lack of power due to an inadequate sample size. In this case, money and time (the investigator's and participants') have been wasted.

Why Is Sample Size Important?

An adequate sample size is essential to producing informative study results. The larger the sample size, the smaller the magnitude of a treatment effect that can be detected as statistically significant. For a given study, there should be sufficient power (at least 80% power) to detect a difference if there really is a difference. Studies that do not have adequate samples to attain at least 80% power are considered underpowered and may produce results that lack validity from a study design perspective and precision from a statistical perspective. For example, if there is an underpowered study of the efficacy of drug A compared with drug B and the results indicate that the effect of drug A is not statistically significantly different from the effect of drug B, the question is whether that is due merely to the fact that the study sample was not large enough to detect a difference. Did the investigator commit a type II error? Did the investigator conclude there was no difference and fail to reject the null hypothesis when in fact there was a real difference (Figure 12.2)? Increasing the sample size makes the hypothesis testing more sensitive by making it more likely that the null hypothesis will be rejected when, in fact, it is false. The sample size also impacts the magnitude of the SE and the width of the CI, two essential estimates in research for making statistical inferences (the larger the sample size, the smaller the SE and the greater precision, which in turn produces a narrower CI).

Box 12.2. Confidence Interval Constructed around a Mean

Knowing how a confidence interval (CI) is constructed is helpful for the interpretation. Let's suppose we want to know the average marginal bone loss (MBL) around single implants placed by every dentist in New York City. There is no way we can measure the bone loss of all the placed implants. Instead, we measure bone loss around a *random sample* of implants (for example, a *sample size* of 100). We find that the average mean bone loss is 0.88 mm, and the *standard error of the mean* (SEM) is 0.12 mm.

The empirical rule states that for a normal sample distribution, 95% of the possible sample means will fall within two (or more accurately $\approx$1.96) SEMs of the population mean. In other words, the length of the interval that contains this 95% is 1.96 SEMs above and 1.96 SEMs below the population mean (Figure 12.4); $\pm$1.96 SEM is also known as the margin of error (ME). The value 1.96 is sometimes called the "confidence coefficient" for the 95% CI; the confidence coefficient for the 90% CI is 1.65; the confidence coefficient for the 99% CI is 2.58. We can now use the "length" of this interval to construct a CI. If we construct an interval around any given sample mean, will the upper and lower bound include the population mean? It will do so 95% of the time. We can "move" this interval along the number line (the *X* axis), and wherever we place it, we are confident that 95% of the time this interval will contain the population mean; 2.5% of the time, this interval will have a sample mean that is more than 1.96 SEMs above the population mean (and thus not contain the population mean), and 2.5% of the time, this interval will have a sample mean that is more than 1.96 SEMs below the population mean (and thus not contain the population mean). We can therefore state that we are 95% confident that the population mean is between the lower and upper bound of the interval.

The ME is the amount of error we expect between the population mean or parameter of interest that we want to infer and the study sample estimate of that mean or parameter of interest. If we are calculating a 95% CI, we know from the discussion above that we have to multiply our SEM with 1.96 to get the ME for a 95% CI. In our example above, we will get 1.96 x SEM = 1.96 x 0.12 = 0.24 (the ME) (Figure 12.4). As this is the distance above and below the mean, the upper boundary of the CI will be 0.88 + 0.24 = 1.12, and the lower boundary will be 0.88 − 0.24 = 0.64. This can be expressed as "mean 0.88; 95% CI, 1.12 to 0.64." We can now state that "we are 95% confident that the mean MBL for all single implants placed by dentists in NYC is between 0.64 and 1.12 mm." It is up to the clinician to decide if a bone loss between 0.64 and 1.12 mm is clinically relevant.

Box 12.3 Significance and Clinical Implication

Does providing fluoride to children over a period of two years reduce the decayed, missing, and filled teeth (DMFT) index?

We performed a study in which 100 children received fluoride (the treatment group, or group A) and 100 children did not receive fluoride (the comparison group, or group B). All children were randomly assigned (allocated) to group A or group B, had the same initial DMFT score, and had the same risk for developing caries at the start of the study.

Our study results showed that, after two years, children in the treatment group had an added mean DMFT score of 3.50, with a standard deviation (SD) of 1.40, while the control group had an added mean DMFT score of 5.10, with an SD of 1.60. Given these results, could we infer what the "true" mean change of the DMFT score would be if we provided the entire population of children with fluoride for two years? This is not possible, but we could calculate a 95% confidence interval (CI) around the mean difference (MD) between the DMFT scores for which we would be able to state that "there is a 95% probability that this interval contains the true population mean or difference in DMFT."

Our study showed an MD (5.10 less 3.50) of 1.60 DMFT score between the groups.

As we are assuming a normal sampling distribution, we can calculate, or look up in a table, the number of SDs that match 95%. As alluded to earlier, 95% is 1.96 SDs away from the mean. Our margin of error (ME) can now be calculated, ±1.96 x 0.21 (where 0.21 is the "combined" standard error of the mean calculated from both samples), which equals ±0.41. Thus, our 95% CI constructed around the MD in our example is 1.60 ± 0.41. This can be expressed as *mean difference 1.60; 95% CI, 1.19 to 2.01.*

We can now state that we are 95% confident that if we provided fluoride to the entire population of children for two years, we would be able to reduce the mean DMFT score to between 1.19 and 2.01 for any group of 100 children. As this interval did not include 0, our result is statistically significant, but a clinician must determine whether this result is clinically important. For example, our result would not be clinically important (or clinically significant) if a clinician determined that only an MD of at least 2.50 would be clinically important.

References

1. Glick M, Carrasco-Labra A. "Misinterpretations, mistakes, or just misbehaving." *J Am Dent Assoc* 2019;150(4):237-9

2. Glick M, Greenberg BL. "The need for scientific literacy." *J Am Dent Assoc* 2017;148(8):543-5

3. Greenberg BL, Kantor ML. "The clinician's guide to the literature." *J Am Dent Assoc* 2009;140(1):48-54

4. Grimes DA, Schulz KF. "An overview of clinical research: the lay of the land." *The Lancet* 2002;359(9300):57-61

5. Sedgwick P. "What are odds?" *BMJ* 2012;344:e2853

6. Best AM, Greenberg BL, Glick M. "From tea tasting to *t* test: a *P* value ain't what you think it is." *J Am Dent Assoc* 2016;147(7):527-9

Chapter 13. Issues of Bias and Confounding in Clinical Studies

Elliot Abt, D.D.S., M.S., M.Sc.; Jaana Gold, D.D.S., M.P.H., Ph.D., C.P.H.; and Julie Frantsve-Hawley, Ph.D., C.A.E.

In This Chapter:

Confounding

- Control of Confounding

Bias

- Bias in Therapy Studies
- Bias and Prognostic Studies
- Bias in Diagnostic Test Studies

Conclusion

Introduction

Bias and confounding are two phenomena that can distort the results of a study, thus lowering validity (internal validity) and applicability (external validity). Bias is a systematic error in the design, conduction, or data analysis that leads to an incorrect assessment of the true effect of an exposure (or intervention) on an outcome.[1] Confounding, on the other hand, is the presence of a third factor that can alter the association between an exposure and an outcome.

Investigators may make wrong conclusions about the beneficial or harmful effects of a tested treatment, and it is important for clinicians to understand how bias can impact study results.[2] Bias can be intentional—which is considered unethical and one should expect that this not be done—or unintentional, as a result of poor methodology.

It is important to note that one cannot assess the absolute impact that bias has on a study. However, one can and should assess the potential or the risk that bias could have impacted results and conclusions. Bias can also cause associations to be either larger (overestimation) or smaller (underestimation) than the true associations.[3] Oftentimes, little can be done when bias has occurred as there are no statistical tests that can control for bias. However, it can be minimized when a study is carefully designed and conducted.[4] Potential sources of bias can differ among study designs. Conversely, confounding can be minimized in the design and/or analysis phase of a study.

Specific concerns about confounding and the different types of biases found in clinical trials, prognostic studies, and diagnostic test studies will be discussed in more detail in this chapter.

Confounding

Confounding occurs when a variable is associated with both an exposure (or intervention) and the outcome of interest.[1] A true confounder must be associated with the exposure and be an independent risk factor for the outcome of interest without being in the causal pathway between exposure and outcome. Additionally, a confounder must be distributed unequally among study groups. Issues of confounding are problematic because they can distort true associations between exposure and outcome by either exaggeration or minimization. That is, confounding can bias the association away from the null (positive confounding) or toward the null (negative confounding), and the magnitude of such confounding can be small, moderate, or large.

Age and smoking are common confounders. An association between diabetes and periodontal disease may be confounded by age if not controlled for in either the study design or statistical analysis. One might find an association between coffee drinking (exposure) and cardiovascular disease (outcome). This association should raise suspicion for confounding, as there is little evidence linking exposure and outcome. Smoking may be confounding this relationship if coffee drinkers are more likely to smoke than nonsmokers, because smoking is a known risk factor for cardiovascular disease. This would be an example of positive confounding if further analysis found that coffee drinking has no effect on cardiovascular disease.

Diseases that share several risk factors can be confounded in poorly designed or analyzed studies. Studies assessing the relationship between periodontal disease and coronary heart disease can be confounded with common risk factors such as age, smoking, stress, socioeconomic status, and obesity.[5]

Control of Confounding

Confounding can be controlled for in the design phase, the analysis phase, or a combination of both. In the study design phase, randomization, restriction, and stratification can be used in randomized trials, whereas matching is often done in observational studies. In the analysis stage, statistical methods such as stratification of analysis (adjusting) and multiple (or logistic) regression analyses are commonly employed.

The single best method to control for confounding is randomization, a powerful tool that controls for all known and unknown confounders (see Chapter 3). However, randomization may not ensure that potential confounders are distributed equally among study groups. For example, appropriate randomization could result in unequal numbers of smokers in control and treatment groups. This is when stratification or restriction can be employed. Stratification of randomization calls for randomizing smokers separately from nonsmokers to ensure equal distribution among groups. Restriction would involve preventing smokers from meeting the inclusion criteria for participation, thus eliminating smoking as a potential confounder. The disadvantage of restriction is that the effect of an intervention among smokers would be unknown.

Observational studies are highly affected by confounding as true randomization is not employed (see Chapter 4). In a case–control study, a patient with a particular condition or disease (case) is matched with another person without the condition (control) who is similar in age, gender, ethnicity, and/or socioeconomic status. The goal is to mimic randomization by having groups as similar as possible to each other to minimize potential confounding factors.

In the analysis phase, stratification of analysis refers to separately analyzing groups. Thus, for coffee drinking/cardiovascular disease, separate 2 x 2 tables (see Chapter 12) would be done for smokers and nonsmokers. This stratification provides an *adjusted* result, which may or may not be different from a *crude* (unadjusted) result. Although many criteria exist, if the results of the stratified analysis differ from the crude result by more than 10%, confounding may be present. In the above example, if the crude risk ratio is 2.5 and the adjusted risk ratio is 1.1, clearly the association between coffee drinking and cardiovascular disease has been positively confounded by smoking. That is, smoking has exaggerated the effects of the exposure on the outcome.

If multiple potential confounders are suspected, rather than numerous 2 x 2 tables being employed, multiple (or logistic) regression analysis can be performed. This is a statistical technique whereby the effect of many potential confounders, termed "input variables," can be measured on a single "outcome variable." Regression is an effective statistical tool to simultaneously observe whether multiple variables are or are not confounding an outcome. An example of the effects of confounding is provided in Box 13.1.

Box 13.1. Example of Confounding in Dentistry

Study: "Periodontitis Increases the Risk of a First Myocardial Infarction: A Report from the PAROKRANK Study." Rydén et al., 2016.[6]

Study Design: Case-control study of 805 patients with myocardial infarction (MI) (cases) matched with 805 patients without MI (controls). All patients were given a periodontal assessment, which included a panoramic radiograph, and periodontal status was classified as healthy, mild-moderate disease, or severe disease based on percentage of alveolar bone loss.

Results: Crude odds ratio (OR) = 1.49 (95% confidence interval [CI], 1.21 to 1.83), and an adjusted OR = 1.28 (95% CI, 1.03 to 1.60). This means that patients with MI had 49% greater odds of having periodontal disease, but when adjusted for potential confounders including smoking and diabetes, this percentage dropped to 28%.

Appraisal: As both the crude and adjusted odds ratios were statistically significant, the authors claimed a relationship exists between periodontal disease and MI independent of confounding. However, the change in odds ratio from crude to adjusted was greater than 10%, which suggests that there was confounding present, pushing the association between outcome and exposure further away from the null value of 1, reducing the strength of the association. This is an example of positive confounding, where potential confounding variables exaggerated the relationship between outcome and exposure. Thus, it appears likely that potential confounders such as smoking and diabetes were distorting the relationship between periodontal disease and MI. Additionally, the reader should consider the magnitude of the effect. From case-control studies, odds ratios greater than 4 are generally needed to overcome the potential effects of bias and confounding.[7] With odds ratios only slightly greater than the null, this magnitude is not generally impressive enough to support causal inference. A scientific statement from the American Heart Association does not support a causal relationship between periodontal disease and cardiovascular disease.[8]

Bias

Bias in Therapy Studies

Clinicians are often interested in the effectiveness of a treatment, therapy, or preventive intervention. A therapy or treatment can be defined as any intervention—which may include prescribing drugs, performing surgery, or counseling—that is intended to improve the course of or prevent the onset of disease.[9] Randomized controlled trials (RCTs) (see Chapter 3) and systematic reviews (see Chapter 6) of RCTs are the best study designs to provide evidence for clinicians in their decisions on therapeutic interventions.[4,10] Again, randomization controls for (but may not eliminate) all known and unknown confounders. In an RCT, study subjects are randomly allocated into two or more groups, usually treatment and control groups, and then followed for a certain time period to assess how the treatment affects the selected outcome(s). When critically appraising therapy studies, the reader needs to assess the following domains: sequence generation (selection bias), allocation concealment (selection bias), blinding of participants and personnel (performance bias), blinding of outcome assessment (detection bias), incomplete outcome data (attrition bias), selective outcome reporting (reporting bias), and other potential sources of bias (Figure 13.1).

Selection bias refers to systematic errors in how study groups were derived.[11] Study subjects should be reflective of the general population from which the study sample is intended to be generalized, and a potential for bias can occur when efforts are not made to ensure that this is in fact the case. When separate criteria are used to recruit and enroll patients into different study groups, selection bias can result. In clinical trials, selection bias can occur if patients with better anticipated outcomes are allocated to a treatment group and those with worse outcomes are allocated to the control group. An example of selection bias can be identified in a coronary artery surgery study in which coronary bypass surgery was compared with medical therapy.[12] The groups differed in the degree of baseline coronary artery disease. The medical therapy group had more extensive baseline coronary artery disease, which ultimately biased the results.

Selection bias can also occur when people who volunteer and agree to participate in a study are different than "regular" control subjects or from those who do not participate. This bias, sometimes called response bias, may favor the treatment group if volunteers are more motivated and concerned about their health. For example, in an oral hygiene study, people with better oral hygiene practices may be more likely to respond and agree to participate in the study.

Clinicians can identify studies where the impact of selection bias was minimized or reduced by evaluating how randomization was implemented, which consists of sequence generation and allocation concealment.[11] Sequence generation refers to how the randomization schedule is achieved; this is best accomplished by drawing lots or using a computer to generate numbers. However, even a well-prepared (typically, computer-generated) randomization schedule does not ensure random allocation. Examples of inappropriate sequence generation would be randomization via alternation (that is, one patient goes to the intervention arm, the next one is allocated to the control arm, the third one back to the intervention arm, and so on), date of birth, or last-name alphabetization. Allocation concealment, in which the investigators do not know the treatment allocation prior to the start of a study, lowers the risk of selection

Figure 13.1. Bias Elements for Therapy Studies

Selection Bias	**Are there systematic errors in how study groups were derived?** *Consider:* Whether study subjects' characteristics are representative of the general population, probabilistic equivalence of study subjects in the treatment group compared with the control group, using appropriate sequence generation and allocation concealment
Performance Bias	**Are there systematic errors in how researchers implement the interventions under investigation?** *Consider:* Whether the control group and treatment group receive similar care except for the intervention/exposure, the use of blinding
Detection Bias	**Are there systematic differences in how the outcomes are measured and evaluated?** *Consider:* Blinding of those assessing outcomes
Attrition Bias	**Is there something about the study conduct, or the intervention/exposure, that is influencing subjects' continuation in the study?** *Consider:* Whether there was excessive loss to follow-up, fundamental differences in the reason or percentage of dropouts exist between study arms, intention-to-treat analysis
Reporting Bias	**Are there systematic errors in reporting study results?** *Consider:* Whether all results are reported as planned, evidence of publication bias, trial preregistration

 Clinicians can identify studies where the impact of selection bias was minimized or reduced by evaluating how randomization was implemented, which consists of sequence generation and allocation concealment.[11]

bias. Lack of proper allocation concealment can lead to spurious study results. Schulz et al.[13] reported that trials in which allocation concealment was either inadequate or unclear can exaggerate treatment effects as much as 40%.

Performance bias refers to systematic errors in how researchers implement the interventions under investigation.[4,11] For RCTs, both the control group and the treatment group should receive similar care except for the intervention or exposure being studied. Any additional differences in treatments between groups could alter the study results. For example, groups or individuals are treated unequally if some receive more or different oral health education or more treatment visits than others. Additionally, knowledge of the interventions or therapy by the participants, study personnel, or investigators can be reduced by blinding, which can reduce performance bias. However, blinding is not always possible, because of the nature of the therapy or treatment. For example, in clinical trials comparing composite to amalgam restorations, blinding of both investigators and participants would not be possible.[14]

Detection bias refers to systematic differences in how the outcomes are measured and evaluated.[4,11] In clinical trials, the concern is that detection bias can influence the study results by over- or underestimating the treatment effect. That is, investigators may be aware of the specific therapy provided and may assign a more favorable outcome to the participants from one group compared with those from the other group. Blinding of outcome assessors (that is, those assessing or adjudicating an outcome) is one way to overcome this issue. This is especially important when assessing subjective outcomes, such as postoperative pain.[11] In clinical studies in which the outcome is very different between groups and is clinically visible or recognizable, it may be impossible to blind those assessing clinical outcomes. For example, trials of silver diamine fluoride would reveal black-stained arrested dentinal lesions.[15] However, even in these circumstances, nonclinical personnel analyzing data can often be blinded.

Attrition bias can occur when loss to follow-up is significant within an entire study and/or when fundamental differences in the reason for or percentage of dropouts exist between study arms. This brings into question whether something about the study conduct, or the intervention/exposure, is influencing subjects' continuation in the study. For example, if patients with adverse effects are more likely to drop out of a study, the resultant data from the retained patients is likely to be distorted. Patients may become unavailable for examinations during the study period because they no longer want to participate (noncompliance) or cannot be contacted. In a clinical trial, patients could withdraw from the treatment group if the treatment is causing side effects, is not tolerated well, or causes other symptoms. Loss of participants can affect the validity/results of a study. It has been suggested that even less than a 5% loss can lead to a small bias; however, greater loss can be a threat to the validity of the study.[16]

 Attrition bias can occur when loss to follow-up is significant within an entire study and/or when fundamental differences in the reason for or percentage of dropouts exist between study arms.

To preserve the prognostic balance afforded by randomization, all randomized patients should be included in the final analysis and in their original groups. The analysis should be performed according to the intention-to-treat (ITT) principle in which the primary outcome is recorded for all randomized patients throughout the follow-up period. An ITT analyzes data "as randomized,"[17] and it ignores noncompliance, protocol deviations, withdrawal, and anything that happens after randomization. A numerical example of the importance of ITT would be if 20 patients were originally in a study arm and five patients experienced success; the success rate would be 5/20, or 25%. However, if 10 patients dropped out of the study and their data was not analyzed, success would then be 5/10, or 50%. Thus, failure to employ an ITT principle would double the success rate. An ITT approach was used in a study by Weintraub et al.[18] on fluoride varnish efficacy in preventing caries in young children, which showed a beneficial effect of fluoride varnish in caries incidence. The primary analysis included data from all children regardless of their adherence to the study protocol.

Reporting bias refers to systematic errors in reporting study results. This may occur when only those results that support the intervention under testing and/or statistically significant results are reported. When researchers, sponsors, and editors prefer to publish only positive or significant results and leave studies with nonsignificant findings unpublished, this is referred to as **publication bias.**[3,10,19–22] Publication bias has been a problem in health research for many years. Studies with statistically significant results are more likely to be published, published multiple times, or published in higher-impact journals (see Chapter 14). Efforts have been made to address this bias by requiring that clinical trial methods be preregistered with organizations such as *ClinicalTrials.gov* to ensure that analyses are determined a priori and reported as planned. With clinical trials, withholding negative results from publication could have a major impact on the quality and safety of our health care system.[20,22] Publication bias can exaggerate results of systematic reviews and meta-analyses, which can impact scientific validity.[19,20] One of the most commonly used tests to detect publication bias in systematic reviews is the funnel plot.[20] Unfortunately, a trend for a significant increase in publication bias over the years has been reported[22] and evidence on publication bias in the dental literature is limited.[19]

Systematic reviews of randomized trials should have strict inclusion/exclusion criteria as well as an assessment of the quality of included studies. Reviews that include studies at high risk of bias can overestimate treatment effects by 40%.[23] In a Cochrane review by Rasines Alcaraz et al.,[14] all seven included trials were at high risk of bias because of significant issues with the reporting, and the final analysis included only two studies. The authors concluded that there was low-quality evidence on the risk of recurrent caries with resin composites as compared with amalgam restorations. Many Cochrane reviews have similar conclusions because of the high risk of bias in individual RCTs. For example, a Cochrane review by Riley et al.[24] included 10 RCTs assessing the effects of xylitol on dental caries with seven studies assessed at high risk of bias. However, readers need to remember that insufficient evidence from systematic reviews does not mean a particular therapy is not working or that treatment is not effective. An example of assessing bias in a therapy study from the dental literature is provided in Box 13.2.

Box 13.2. Example of Assessing Bias in a Dental Therapy Study

Study: "Treatment of Deep Caries Lesions in Adults: Randomized Clinical Trials Comparing Stepwise vs. Direct Complete Excavation, and Direct Pulp Capping vs. Partial Pulpotomy," Bjørndal et al., 2010[25]

Study Design: Multicenter randomized controlled trial of 314 patients with deep carious lesions that received partial caries removal, followed by complete excavation at a later date (treatment group) or complete caries excavation. The two primary outcomes measured were pulpal exposure and maintenance of pulp vitality.

Results: Partial or stepwise caries removal resulted in a lower risk of pulp exposure (risk difference = 11.4%; 95% confidence interval [CI], 1.2 to 21.3) and an increased odds of success, defined as maintaining vitality at one year, of 74% (odds ratio=1.74; 95% CI, 1.03 to 2.94).

Appraisal: Selection bias was avoided by having sequence generation performed by computer-generated numbers, and allocation concealment was achieved by central telephone randomization. Adequate randomization controls for but does not always eliminate confounding, as baseline differences between groups may persist. To lower this risk, the investigators stratified the randomization scheme by creating different strata (in this case, for pain, age, and location) whereby randomization is performed within each stratum.[1] That is, patients with and without pain, greater or less than 50 years of age, and being treated at one of six centers were done in blocks of six to more equally distribute these prognostic variables between control and treatment groups. Performance bias was minimized by blinding patients and treating both groups equally, apart from the intervention. Although investigators cannot be blinded, those evaluating radiographs and statistical analyses were unaware of group assignment, thus lowering the risk of detection bias. Attrition bias also appeared to be minimal, as only 7% of patients were lost to follow-up and the numbers were similar for both groups. Although it was unclear if an intention-to-treat analysis was performed, there was no evidence of reporting bias.

From a methodological standpoint, this randomized controlled trial was well done as close attention was paid to the multiple factors that can lead to bias, which can negatively impact the validity of an investigation. Understanding the domains of quality in randomized trials can help readers of the dental literature develop good critical appraisal skills.

Bias and Prognostic Studies

Prognostic studies are important for medicine and dentistry because they allow for prediction between baseline health or exposure and risk of future outcomes.[26,27] Knowing risks allows practitioners and patients to implement treatments and/or behaviors to mitigate risks, or if risks cannot be changed, allows for active surveillance.[28,29] Prognostic studies tend to be observational in nature, especially when the outcome of concern is rare. Study designs that may be employed include prospective cohort, retrospective cohort, case-control, and cross-sectional studies. Although long-term cohort studies may be the design of choice for prognostic studies, it is important to realize that case-control studies may be the most pragmatic option for very rare outcomes because sufficient numbers of patients with the outcome of interest are not available to conduct studies of other designs (see Chapter 4).

There are several potential biases in prognostic studies, and it is important that these potential biases be considered and assessed. The biases include selection, attrition, prognostic factor measurement, outcome measurement, and confounding (Figure 13.2).[30–32]

Figure 13.2. Bias Elements for Prognostic Studies

Selection Bias	**Is the study sample similar enough to the population so as to have minimal bias in the study results?** *Consider:* Key population characteristics (age, gender, etc.), recruitment method, inclusion/exclusion criteria, the proportion of eligible subjects who participate in the study, recruitment at similar disease state
Attrition Bias	**Does the loss to follow-up rate (rate of study subject dropouts) compromise validity of the study?** *Consider:* Dropout rates between study groups, reasons for loss to follow-up, potential differences in characteristics among dropouts compared with those retained in the study
Prognostic Factor Measurement	**Are the prognostic factors measured in a similar way, using valid and reliable methodology, for all study subjects?** *Consider:* Whether a consistent methodology was used, whether measurements were blinded to the extent possible
Outcome Measurement	**Are the outcomes measured in a similar way, using valid and reliable methodology, for all study subjects?** *Consider:* Whether the outcome was clinically relevant, blinded to the extent possible, measurements were performed by calibrated clinicians, and inter-rater reliability was assessed
Confounding	**Do factors other than the prognostic factor have the potential to influence the outcome of interest?** *Consider:* Potential confounders should be identified a prioi, reliably measured in all subjects, and assessed in multivariate analyses

Selection bias occurs when a study's population does not represent the general population from which the subjects are selected. This is of concern because selection bias may influence the study's outcome. In assessing the study's selected population for potential bias, one needs to consider if the study sample is similar to the larger population from which the sample was selected. The characteristics of study subjects to consider include key population characteristics (for example, age and gender), recruitment method, inclusion/exclusion criteria, the proportion of eligible subjects who participate in the study, and whether the subjects were recruited at similar disease state.[30-33] For example, if patients for the exposure group are selected from a hospital and controls selected from the general population with different exposures and variables, researchers may create selection bias. If these characteristics result in a study population that is significantly dissimilar from the general population intended to be analyzed, then there may be challenges in interpreting the results and applying them to a broader population. In this instance, we say that the results are not generalizable to other populations. Ideally, a study should have a high participation rate, with study group characteristics similar to that of the source population.

Attrition refers to the loss of follow-up data throughout a study.[30-33] Ideally, there should be little to no loss to follow-up. If loss to follow-up does occur, it is important to determine if the attrition rate is similar among all groups. If this is not the case, then there is a possibility that study factors may have influenced dropout rates differentially among the groups. When assessing attrition bias, it is important to consider three factors: 1) dropout rates among study groups, 2) reasons for loss to follow-up, and 3) potential differences in characteristics between dropouts compared with those retained in the study.

A prognostic factor is an element that is associated with a disease outcome. Examples of prognostic factors in dentistry include the location for dental implants[34]—where the anterior maxilla has a higher rate for implant loss and the anterior mandible has an increased rate for implant success—and metastases and molecular markers for oral cancer.[35,36] **Prognostic factor measurement** should be performed in a similar way for all study subjects using valid and reliable measurement tools.[30-32] Biases can enter into the prognostic measurement if measurements are not taken with consistent methodology and in blinded and independent ways.[31,37]

As with prognostic factors, the **outcome measurement** should be conducted in a similar way for all study subjects using valid and reliable measures and be determined a priori.[30-33] The outcome should be clinically relevant and have blinded assessment whenever possible. In circumstances where the outcome may be subjective (requiring clinical judgment), such as caries or periodontal disease severity, outcome measurements should be performed by calibrated clinicians, and inter-rater reliability should be assessed.

Confounding refers to the potential of factors other than the prognostic factor to influence or contribute to the outcome of interest.[30-32] Potential confounders should be identified a priori and should be reliably measured in all subjects. The impact of potentially confounding factors should be assessed in multivariable analyses.[32]

An example of assessing bias in a dental prognostic study is provided in Box 13.3.

Box 13.3. Example of Assessing Bias in a Dental Prognostic Study

Study: "Dental X-rays and Risk of Meningioma," Claus et al., 2012.[38]

Study Design: A case-control study that included 1,433 case subjects with meningioma diagnosed at ages 20 to 79 years and a control group of 1,350 control subjects. The study objective was to assess a potential association between meningioma and self-reported bitewing, full-mouth, and panoramic dental X-rays.

Results: Cases were more likely than controls to report having ever had a bitewing examination over a lifetime (odds ratio [OR], 2.0; 95% confidence interval [CI], 1.4 to 2.9) or panoramic films at ages greater than 10 years (OR, 4.9; 95% CI, 1.8 to 13.2).

Appraisal: A critical analysis of this study identifies a number of potential biases. In regard to the participation criteria, both the case and control groups appear to have been matched in terms of age, gender, and geography (state of residence). No information was provided as to the willingness of subjects to participate in the study or differences in participation rates between groups. Additionally, for the case patients, physician approval was required before subjects were contacted, and approval criteria were not disclosed, which increases the risk of selection bias.

As a case-control study, 2,228 eligible case subjects and 2,604 eligible control subjects were identified. Sixty-five percent of case subjects and 52% of control subjects participated in the interview. The reason for attrition within each group is presented, but no rationale for the differences between groups is presented in the study.

Significant concerns exist about the prognostic factor measure employed in the study. Information about dental radiograph exposure up to five decades prior to meningioma diagnosis was obtained through phone interviews of all individuals in both groups rather than examination of dental records. This represents a significant risk of recall bias, as patients' accuracy of recalling actual dental radiograph exposure over a five-decade period, especially distinguishing among bitewing, full-mouth, and panoramic radiographs, is questionable. The study authors identified the possibility of the over- or underreporting of dental radiographs as a potential study flaw.

Because case-control studies start with the outcome and measure differences in exposure, differences in odds of dental radiographs between groups were reported as ORs. In this case, an OR is defined as the odds of dental radiographs in the case group divided by odds of radiographs in the control group. An OR = 1 represents the null, indicating that there is no difference in odds between the case and control groups. Because of inherent bias in case-control studies, ORs less than four are not considered clinically relevant,[7] and CIs that touch or cross the null value of 1 are not statistically significant. Among the 53 unique measures of the association between dental radiographs and meningioma presented in the manuscript, only one represented statistically significant and clinically relevant results: ever having had a panoramic at an age greater than 10 years (OR = 4.9, CI = 1.8–13.2). The remainder of the reported outcomes were either statistically significant but not clinically relevant with ORs <4 (*n* = 12) or not statistically significant (*n* = 29) or the ORs were not presented (*n* = 11).

Although not under the umbrella of bias/confounding, the authors did not take into account the potential effect of multiple statistical tests on study results, known as the problem of multiplicity or the multiple testing problem.[39] With a *P* value typically set at <0.05 as a threshold for statistical significance, as more statistical tests are conducted, there is an increased chance of finding a statistically significant result by random chance.[40-43] This problem can be addressed by adjusting the *P* value upward to reduce the likelihood of finding a false statistical significance, or simply minimizing the number of measured outcomes.[44] Given the 53 unique outcome measures and tests of statistical significance conducted in the meningioma study, there is a very real likelihood that the problem of multiplicity provided a source of bias in the results.

It is unclear if all measures were reported, but based on the methods provided in the manuscript, no discrepancies in reporting are evident. In interpreting the results, the authors did not address the lack of dose response in the presented data. This is significant because full-mouth radiographs have significantly higher exposure levels than bitewings or panoramic films.

Bias in Diagnostic Test Studies

The prior two sections demonstrated the effects of bias in dealing with studies on therapy (RCTs) and prognosis (observational studies). Diagnostic test studies can have several different designs, and ideally, RCTs should be employed to compare one diagnostic test to another (see Chapter 5). Unfortunately, randomized trials for diagnosis are rather uncommon. Most often, diagnostic test studies are observational in nature and are typically cross-sectional or consecutive series but can occasionally be a case-control design. These (observational) studies start with a group of patients thought to be at risk for a particular disease, yet there is uncertainty as to the presence or absence of disease. A diagnostic test, often referred to as an index test, is used to help rule in or rule out the diagnosis, and the results of the index test are then compared with a reference standard, which is considered to be the most ideal method to establish a diagnosis. How well the index test performs in relation to the reference standard can then be measured by calculating estimates of their sensitivity, specificity, predictive values, or likelihood ratios.

Bias in diagnostic test studies exists in several domains and can alter the results, most often making the index test appear to be more accurate than it truly is. Biases in diagnostic test studies include spectrum, verification, and review bias (Figure 13.3).

Diagnostic test studies can have several different designs, and ideally, RCTs should be employed to compare one diagnostic test to another (see Chapter 5).

Figure 13.3. Bias Elements for Diagnostic Tests

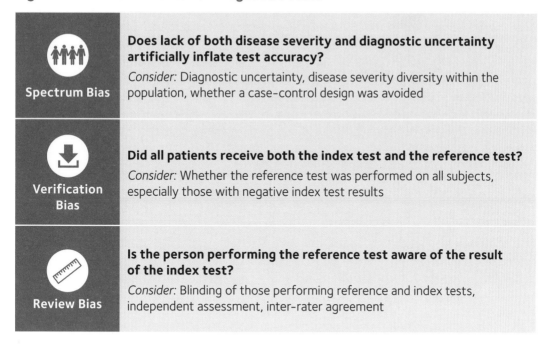

Spectrum Bias

Does lack of both disease severity and diagnostic uncertainty artificially inflate test accuracy?
Consider: Diagnostic uncertainty, disease severity diversity within the population, whether a case-control design was avoided

Verification Bias

Did all patients receive both the index test and the reference test?
Consider: Whether the reference test was performed on all subjects, especially those with negative index test results

Review Bias

Is the person performing the reference test aware of the result of the index test?
Consider: Blinding of those performing reference and index tests, independent assessment, inter-rater agreement

One of the first things to consider in any study, and certainly in a diagnostic test study, is the study design and population or sample that was used. In the context of diagnostic tests, case-control studies are suboptimal, and the study population should represent a broad spectrum of disease severity and other conditions with similar symptoms. Otherwise **spectrum bias** can occur, where the lack of both disease severity and diagnostic uncertainty can artificially inflate test accuracy. For example, investigators may want to assess the accuracy of a caries detection device where the cases were financially disadvantaged and control patients were affluent. This is a case-control design, and the caries device will tend to look very accurate as caries rates tend to be much higher in areas of low socioeconomic level. In fact, in this scenario, one could argue that a diagnostic test is not needed, as the differences between cases and controls might be clear to a seasoned clinician. Therefore, dental practitioners should view diagnostic test studies with a case-control design with extreme caution, and a study population where there is diagnostic uncertainty is needed to avoid this type of spectrum bias.

Another characteristic of the study population is disease severity.[45] That is, with more severe disease, diagnostic test accuracy can also be artificially inflated, which is why index tests can be more accurate in specialty clinics than in general medical/dental practices. To protect against this, a population with differing severity of disease, including patients under real clinical uncertainty from a diagnostic perspective, will provide a more truthful representation of populations in which a clinician might actually choose to use a diagnostic test. Therefore, readers of diagnostic test studies should look for study populations where the diagnosis is uncertain and that include other conditions with similar symptoms and a broad range of disease severity. Additionally, there should also be a similar range/balance of age and gender among study participants.

Another important issue in diagnostic test studies is making sure that all patients received both the index test and the reference test. Patients, especially ones who have a negative result with an index test, must also have the reference test performed. Some diagnostic studies will not have patients who test negative undergo a reference test, assuming (falsely) that the index test represents a true-negative result. In reality, the result could represent a false negative, and this will improve both sensitivity and specificity. This phenomenon is commonly referred to as **verification bias** and is easily avoided if all patients receive both the index test and the reference standard.

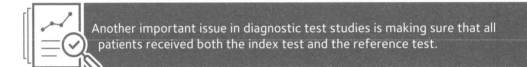

Another important issue in diagnostic test studies is making sure that all patients received both the index test and the reference test.

Review bias is another type of bias that can affect diagnostic test studies. Review bias can occur when the person performing the reference test is aware of the result of the index test for a particular patient or group of patients. If, for example, the reference standard is a biopsy, and the pathologist is aware of the results of an index test, that knowledge can influence the result of the reference standard, which would, again, artificially inflate the overall accuracy of a diagnostic test. Therefore, an important feature in diagnostic studies is the blinding of those performing reference tests from those performing index tests. Additionally, those performing index and reference tests should be independent of each other, and if multiple individuals are performing reference tests, they should have good agreement with each other. This is often measured with a Kappa statistic, which measures chance-corrected inter-rater agreement. Pathologists occasionally do not agree with themselves, and if so, they should be replaced by someone with good intra-rater agreement.

An example of assessing bias in a dental diagnostic study is provided in Box 13.4.

Box 13.4. Example of Assessing Bias in a Dental Diagnostic Study

Study: "Adjuncts for the Evaluation of Potentially Malignant Disorders in the Oral Cavity: Diagnostic Test Accuracy Systematic Review and Meta-analysis—a Report of the American Dental Association," Lingen et al., 2017.[46]

Study Design: Systematic review/meta-analysis of diagnostic tests for oral cancer and potentially malignant disorders.

Results: Pooled sensitivity and specificity of adjuncts ranged from 0.39 to 0.96 for the evaluation of innocuous lesions and from 0.31 to 0.95 for the evaluation of suspicious lesions. Cytologic testing used in suspicious lesions appears to have the highest accuracy among adjuncts (sensitivity, 0.92; 95% confidence interval [CI], 0.86 to 0.98; specificity, 0.94; 95% CI, 0.88 to 0.99).

Appraisal: This systematic review included many studies at high risk of bias. One such study evaluated the effectiveness of brush biopsy in the diagnosis of oral leukoplakia.[47] Twenty-four patients participated in the study, which reported sensitivity of 73% and specificity of 92% (low certainty of the evidence). The authors concluded that brush biopsy may have high sensitivity and specificity, which would make it a good tool for monitoring oral leukoplakia, but biopsy remains the most reliable method to confirm a diagnosis.

There were a number of significant issues with bias in this study, which can affect the study results. The authors incorrectly stated that they conducted a controlled clinical trial, when in fact it was either a consecutive series or a cross-sectional study. While there were equal numbers of men and women, no information was given on ethnicity, socioeconomic status, or risk factors. It was also unclear as to any range of disease severity. This represents spectrum bias, where uncertainty exists with variation in disease severity. Additionally, disease prevalence was 46%, which may be a gross overestimation of prevalence in most dental settings, although this generally does not affect sensitivity/specificity.[33] A lack of clarity also existed as to what constitutes a negative versus a positive biopsy, and failure to disclose a threshold for positivity can affect both sensitivity and specificity.

Another source of bias with this study is that the same investigator performed both the index test and the reference standard. This means there is no blinding or independence of those assessing outcomes from those performing diagnostic tests. This represents reporting bias, and it should be apparent that knowledge of the brush biopsy can easily influence results of the reference standard, oftentimes improving both sensitivity and specificity. Additionally, there was no mention of intra-rater agreement, as only one investigator performed the histologic analysis.

In addition to issues of bias, there would be a subtle, yet significant, issue with the interpretation of the statistical analysis in this study. In a general dental practice, prevalence of oral cancer would generally be quite low, and the objective for practitioners in such an environment is to rule out disease. To do so, one needs a negative result with an index test that has good sensitivity; a sensitivity of 73% would likely be inadequate to rule out disease.

While it is unclear whether verification bias has occurred, the results of this study should be interpreted with caution because of the abovementioned biases. Unfortunately, this is all too common in diagnostic test studies. Thus, readers of these types of papers should carefully examine the methods sections to ensure that study authors adhered to the dimensions of quality in diagnostic test studies to assess the validity of the results. One method of doing so is the QUADAS-2 tool,[48] which is a checklist for adhering to quality in diagnostic test studies.

Conclusion

Both bias and confounding can distort study results and are threats to internal and external validity. Typically, biases tend to exaggerate results, whereas confounding can either over- or underestimate results. Bias can be avoided if investigators plan properly and use good methodology in the design, execution, and analysis phases of scientific studies. Confounding can occur when a known or unknown variable affects the relationship between exposure and outcome. Confounding can be controlled in either the design or analysis phases of a study but may be difficult to eliminate, especially in observational studies. Ignoring bias and confounding could lead to biased and poor treatment decisions. Identifying bias and confounding helps in critically appraising evidence, and readers of the dental literature need to identify the source of bias, assess its strength, and determine its direction.

References

1. "Bias, Confounding, and Effect Modification." Penn State Eberly College of Science; Stat 507; Section 3.5; *https://newonlinecourses.science.psu.edu/stat507/node/34/*. Accessed June 3, 2018.

2. Gerhard T. Bias: "Considerations for Research Practice." *Am J Health Syst Pharm* 2008;65(22):2159-68.

3. Pannucci CJ, Wilkins EG. "Identifying and Avoiding Bias in Research." *Plast Reconstr Surg* 2010;126(2):619-25.

4. Higgins JP, Altman DG, Gotzsche PC, et al. "The Cochrane Collaboration's Tool for Assessing Risk of Bias in Randomised Trials." *BMJ* 2011;343:d5928.

5. Hujoel PP, Drangsholt M, Spiekerman C, DeRouen TA. "Periodontal Disease and Coronary Heart Disease Risk." *JAMA* 2000;284(11):1406-10.

6. Rydén L, Buhlin K, Ekstrand E, et al. "Periodontitis Increases the Risk of a First Myocardial Infarction: A Report from the PAROKRANK Study." *Circulation* 2016;133(6):576-83.

7. S.E. S, W.S. R, P. G, R.B. H. *Evidence-Based Medicine: How to Practice and Teach It*. 4th Edition ed: Churchill Livingstone; 2010.

8. Lockhart PB, Bolger AF, Papapanou PN, et al. "Periodontal Disease and Atherosclerotic Vascular Disease: Does the Evidence Support an Independent Association? A Scientific Statement from the American Heart Association." *Circulation* 2012;125(20):2520-44.

9. *Clinical Epidemiology: The Essentials*. 4th Edition ed. Baltimore, MD Lippincott Williams & Wilkins; 2005.

10. Brignardello-Petersen R, Carrasco-Labra A, Yanine N, et al. "Positive Association between Conflicts of Interest and Reporting of Positive Results in Randomized Clinical Trials in Dentistry." *J Am Dent Assoc* 2013;144(10):1165-70.

11. Higgins JPT, Altman DG, Sterne JAC, on behalf of the Cochrane Statistical Methods Group and the Cochrane Bias Methods Group "Chapter 8: Assessing Risk of Bias in Included Studies." *https://handbook-5-1.cochrane.org/chapter_8/8_assessing_risk_of_bias_in_included_studies.htm*. Accessed March 17, 2019.

12. Berger VW, Exner DV. "Detecting Selection Bias in Randomized Clinical Trials." *Control Clin Trials* 1999;20(4):319-27.

13. Schulz KF, Chalmers I, Hayes RJ, Altman DG. "Empirical Evidence of Bias. Dimensions of Methodological Quality Associated with Estimates of Treatment Effects in Controlled trials." *JAMA* 1995;273(5):408-12.

14. Rasines Alcaraz MG, Veitz-Keenan A, Sahrmann P, et al. "Direct Composite Resin Fillings versus Amalgam Fillings for Permanent or Adult Posterior Teeth." *Cochrane Database Syst Rev* 2014(3):CD005620.

15. Gold J. "Limited Evidence Links Silver Diamine Fluoride and Caries Arrest in Children." *J Evid Based Dent Pract* 2017;17(3):265-67.

16. Sacket DL, Richardson WS, Rosenberg WM. *Evidence-Based Medicine: How to Practice and Teach EBM* New York, NY: Churchill Livingstone; 1997.

17. Fisher LD, Dixon DO, Herson J, et al. "Intention to Treat in Clinical Trials." In: *Statistical Issues in Drug Research and Development*. New York, NY: Marcel Dekker, Inc.; 1990.

18. Weintraub JA, Ramos-Gomez F, Jue B, et al. "Fluoride Varnish Efficacy in Preventing Early Childhood Caries." *J Dent Res* 2006;85(2):172-6.

19. Coleman BG, Johnson TM, Erley KJ, et al. "Preparing Dental Students and Residents to Overcome Internal and External Barriers to Evidence-Based Practice." *J Dent Educ* 2016;80(10):1161-69.

20. Crawford JM, Briggs CL, Engeland CG. "Publication Bias and Its Implications for Evidence-Based Clinical Decision Making." *J Dent Educ* 2010;74(6):593-600.

21. Dickersin K. "The Existence of Publication Bias and Risk Factors for Its Occurrence." *JAMA* 1990;263(10):1385-9.

22. Joober R, Schmitz N, Annable L, Boksa P. "Publication Bias: What Are the Challenges and Can They Be Overcome?" *J Psychiatry Neurosci* 2012;37(3):149-52.

23. Kunz R, Oxman AD. "The Unpredictability Paradox: Review of Empirical Comparisons of Randomised and Non-randomised Clinical Trials." *BMJ* 1998;317(7167):1185-90.

24. Riley P, Moore D, Ahmed F, Sharif MO, Worthington HV. "Xylitol-Containing Products for Preventing Dental Caries in Children and Adults." *Cochrane Database Syst Rev* 2015(3):CD010743.

25. Bjørndal L, Reit C, Bruun G, et al. "Treatment of Deep Caries Lesions in Adults: Randomized Clinical Trials Comparing Stepwise vs. Direct Complete Excavation, and Direct Pulp Capping vs. Partial Pulpotomy." *Eur J Oral Sci* 2010;118(3):290-7.

26. Hemingway H, Croft P, Perel P, et al. "Prognosis Research Strategy (PROGRESS) 1: A Framework for Researching Clinical Outcomes." *BMJ* 2013;346:e5595.

27. Matino D, Chai-Adisaksopha C, Lorio A. "Systematic Reviews of Prognosis Studies: A Critical Appraisal of Five Core Clinical Journals." *Diagnostic and Prognostic Research* 2017;1(9):2-10.

28. Iorio A, Spencer FA, Falavigna M, et al. "Use of GRADE for Assessment of Evidence about Prognosis: Rating Confidence in Estimates of Event Rates in Broad Categories of Patients." *BMJ* 2015;350:h870.

29. Spencer FA, Iorio A, You J, et al. "Uncertainties in Baseline Risk Estimates and Confidence in Treatment Effects." *BMJ* 2012;345:e7401.

30. D'Amico G, Malizia G, D'Amico M. "Prognosis Research and Risk of Bias." *Intern Emerg Med* 2016;11(2):251-60.

31. Hayden JA, Cote P, Bombardier C. "Evaluation of the Quality of Prognosis Studies in Systematic Reviews." *Ann Intern Med* 2006;144(6):427-37.

32. Hayden JA, van der Windt DA, Cartwright JL, Cote P, Bombardier C. "Assessing Bias in Studies of Prognostic Factors." *Ann Intern Med* 2013;158(4):280-6.

33. G. G, D. R, M.O. M, D.J. C. *Users' Guides to the Medical Literature: A Manual for Evidence-Based Clinical Practice.* 3rd Edition: McGraw-Hill Education/Medical, 2014.

34. Geckili O, Bilhan H, Geckili E, et al. "Evaluation of Possible Prognostic Factors for the Success, Survival, and Failure of Dental Implants." *Implant Dent* 2014;23(1):44-50.

35. Mielcarek-Kuchta D, Paluszczak J, Seget M, et al. "Prognostic Factors in Oral and Oropharyngeal Cancer Based on Ultrastructural Analysis and DNA Methylation of the Tumor and Surgical Margin." *Tumour Biol* 2014;35(8):7441-9.

36. Montoro J, Hicz HA, de Souza L, et al. "Prognostic Factors in Squamous Cell Carcinoma of the Oral Cavity." *Braz J Otorhinolaryngol* 2008;74(6):861-66.

37. Donders AR, van der Heijden GJ, Stijnen T, Moons KG. "Review: A Gentle Introduction to Imputation of Missing Values." *J Clin Epidemiol* 2006;59(10):1087-91.

38. Claus EB, Calvocoressi L, Bondy ML, et al. "Dental X-rays and Risk of Meningioma." *Cancer* 2012;118(18):4530-7.

39. Ahlbom A. *Biostatistics for Epidemiologists.* Boca Raton, FL: Lewis Publishers; 1993.

40. Bland JM, Altman DG. "Multiple Significance Tests: the Bonferroni Method." *BMJ* 1995;310(6973):170.

41. Greenhalgh T. "How to Read a Paper. Statistics for the Non-statistician. I: Different Types of Data Need Different Statistical Tests." *BMJ* 1997;315(7104):364-6.

42. Ludbrook J. "Multiple Comparison Procedures Updated." *Clin Exp Pharmacol Physiol* 1998;25(12):1032-7.

43. Tukey JW. "Some Thoughts on Clinical Trials, Especially Problems of Multiplicity." *Science* 1977;198(4318):679-84.

44. Feise RJ. "Behavioral-Graded Activity Compared with Usual Care after First-Time Disk Surgery: Considerations of the Design of a Randomized Clinical Trial." *J Manipulative Physiol Ther* 2001;24(1):67-8.

45. Sackett DL, Haynes RB. "The Architecture of Diagnostic Research." *BMJ* 2002;324(7336):539-41.

46. Lingen MW, Tampi MP, Urquhart O, et al. "Adjuncts for the Evaluation of Potentially Malignant Disorders in the Oral Cavity: Diagnostic Test Accuracy Systematic Review and Meta-analysis—A Report of the American Dental Association." *J Am Dent Assoc* 2017;148(11):797-813 e52.

47. Seijas-Naya F, Garcia-Carnicero T, Gandara-Vila P, et al. "Applications of OralCDx(R) Methodology in the Diagnosis of Oral Leukoplakia." *Med Oral Patol Oral Cir Bucal* 2012;17(1):e5-9.

48. Whiting PF, Rutjes AW, Westwood ME, et al. "QUADAS-2: A Revised Tool for the Quality Assessment of Diagnostic Accuracy Studies." *Ann Intern Med* 2011;155(8):529-36.

Chapter 14. What Is Certainty of the Evidence, and Why Is It Important to Dental Practitioners?

Alonso Carrasco-Labra, D.D.S., M.Sc., Ph.D.; Olivia Urquhart, M.P.H.; Malavika P. Tampi, M.P.H.; Lauren Pilcher, M.S.P.H.; Jeff Huber, M.B.A.; Anita Aminoshariae, D.D.S., M.S.; Douglas Young, D.D.S., Ed.D., M.S., M.B.A.; Satish S. Kumar, D.M.D., M.D.Sc., M.S.; Carlos Flores-Mir, D.D.S., M.Sc., D.Sc.; and Gordon H. Guyatt, M.D., M.Sc.

In This Chapter:

Introduction

Dental practitioners often encounter clinical recommendations addressing the potential effects of a number of interventions. It is important for clinicians to be aware of not only the best estimates of anticipated net benefits, but how much trust they can place in those estimates.[1] The need for an explicit assessment of the trustworthiness of the evidence supporting recommendations became apparent in the early 2000s. In fact, by 2002, more than 100 systems to evaluate the quality of clinical research were available.[2] This large number of frameworks created confusion, inconsistencies, and frustration for practicing clinicians and patients making health care decisions.[3,4]

To address this issue, in the early 2000s a group of methodologists and guideline developers created a common, transparent, and sensible process to assess the certainty of the evidence and grade strength of recommendations: the Grading of Recommendations Assessment, Development, and Evaluation (GRADE) approach.[5] GRADE is currently the most accepted approach to assess the certainty of the evidence and formulate recommendations. It has been adopted by more than 100 organizations around the world, including the World Health Organization, Cochrane, the American Academy of Pediatric Dentistry (AAPD), and the American Dental Association (ADA).

When selecting the most appropriate treatments, patients and clinicians have a variety of interventions from which they can choose. Consider, for example, choosing among different nonrestorative treatments for arresting carious lesions.[6,7] The dentist's task is to determine whether the incremental benefit expected from implementing a nonrestorative approach to manage carious lesions is worthy of the additional costs (for example, additional visits, possible progression of carious lesions to a more severe stage requiring more invasive treatment, and additional testing including dental radiographs). In doing so, a dentist considers issues such as the severity of the disease, the patient's specific characteristics, the most important outcomes informing the decision, the underlying body of evidence informing each outcome, the balance between the desirable and undesirable consequences among all interventions, the certainty of the evidence, and the management of limited resources. Clinical practice guidelines and systematic reviews, presented in a succinct and convenient format, are frequently available to support patients and clinicians in addressing the issues presented above (see Chapters 6 and 7).

In this chapter, we summarize how GRADE can help clinicians to assess the certainty of the evidence in systematic reviews and clinical practice guidelines and inform health care decision making.

Certainty of the Evidence

In 2016, the ADA and the AAPD published a clinical practice guideline addressing pit-and-fissure sealants on the occlusal surfaces of primary and permanent molars in children and adolescents.[8] The guideline panel recommended "the use of sealants compared with nonuse in permanent molars with both sound occlusal surfaces and noncavitated occlusal carious lesions in children and adolescents." This recommendation was graded as a strong recommendation based on moderate certainty of the evidence. What did the ADA-AAPD guideline panel mean by moderate certainty of the evidence?

In the context of recommendations from clinical practice guidelines (for example, sealants for preventing and arresting carious lesions), the certainty of the evidence reflects "the extent of [the guideline panel's] confidence that the estimates of an effect are adequate to support a particular decision or recommendation."[9] This means that overall, considering all patient-important outcomes, the panel has moderate certainty that pit-and-fissure sealants applied to occlusal surfaces reduce the incidence of carious lesions sufficiently to outweigh potential downsides, including lack of sealant retention, costs, and other burdens.

When guideline panels need to formulate recommendations, they usually focus on various aspects of care. Questions of therapy are quite common in most guidelines; however, it is not unusual to see questions related to diagnosis,[10] screening,[11] and prognosis. To inform these decisions, panels identify key patient-important outcomes. The evidence supporting the effect of interventions on these outcomes come from different types of study designs.

In GRADE, evidence from randomized controlled trials (RCTs) starts as high certainty of the evidence; however, serious or very serious limitations in the body of evidence from this type of study design can reduce certainty to moderate, low, or very low. Observational studies, on the other hand, although starting as low certainty, can, under specific circumstances, be rated up to moderate or high certainty.

Criteria to Rate Down the Certainty of the Evidence

Risk of Bias

Guideline panels need to evaluate the extent to which the studies included in the guideline or systematic review may be affected by methodological issues to the point that those flaws may seriously increase the chance of misleading results.[12] Different study designs may be associated with different types of bias. Some of the most common limitations in RCTs are 1) an inappropriate randomization strategy, 2) a lack or poor implementation of allocation concealment, 3) a lack of blinding, 4) the presence of important missing participant data, and 5) selective outcome reporting (see Chapters 3 and 13). For observational studies, issues related to eligibility criteria, flawed measurement of exposure and outcomes, inappropriate control for confounding, and incomplete follow-up are among the most common limitations (see Chapters 4, 5, and 13). When using GRADE, panels and reviewers first assess the risk of bias at an individual study level across outcomes and then consolidate the assessment into one judgment that reflects to what extent the methodological flaws across different studies (that is, the body of evidence) informing an outcome were serious enough to merit rating down the certainty of the evidence. In the case of the 2016 ADA-AAPD sealants guideline, the certainty of the evidence for the outcome "caries incidence," although informed by nine RCTs, was rated down from high to moderate certainty because of the risk of bias stemming from serious concerns about the implementation of allocation concealment and blinding.[8,13]

Inconsistency

When examining a group of studies informing a particular outcome, guideline panels or reviewers are more certain of evidence when results are similar across studies (that is, most studies tell a "similar story") than when they differ. Differences that cannot be explained are referred to as unexplained heterogeneity in the magnitude of effect from different studies (that is, studies telling "different stories" without finding a plausible reason for those differences).[14] When assessing inconsistency, there are four criteria to consider for rating down:

1. Point estimates vary widely across studies, showing dissimilar treatment effects.

2. Confidence intervals (CIs) show minimal to no overlap.

3. Heterogeneity testing proves significant, which means a low P value (<0.1) that rejects the null hypothesis that all studies in the meta-analysis have a similar magnitude of effect.

4. The I^2 statistic is large, which means a large proportion of variability in point estimates due to between-study differences. Usually, an "I^2 of less than 40% is low, 30–60% may be moderate, 50–90% may be substantial, and 75–100% is considerable."[14]

Figure 14.1. Meta-Analysis Comparing Antibiotic Prophylaxis versus Placebo and the Effect on Pain (Presence or Absence) on the Sixth- and Seventh-Day Post-Dental Extraction, Including Subgroup Analysis for Pre-, Post-, and Pre- and Post-Operative Administration

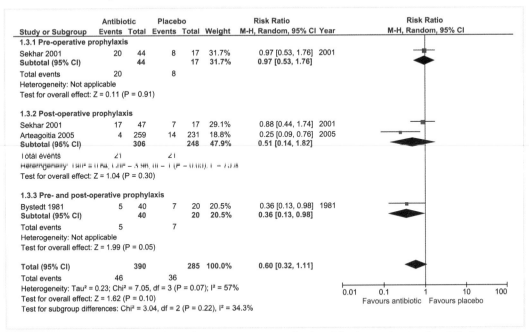

Source: Lodi G, Figini L, Sardella A, et al. "Antibiotics to prevent complications following tooth extractions." *Cochrane Database of Systematic Reviews* 2012, Issue 11 ArtNo:CD003811 DOI: 10.1002/14651858.CD003811.pub2.

Consider Figure 14.1. This forest plot compares the effect of antibiotic prophylaxis versus placebo on pain (presence or absence) on the sixth- and seventh-day post-dental extraction. The authors defined a *priori* hypotheses to explain any heterogeneity that they may have found and conducted subgroup analysis for pre-, post-, and the combination of pre- and post-operative administration of antibiotics.[15] When applying the four criteria described above, we see that the point estimates vary across studies (relative risks of 0.97, 0.88, 0.36, and 0.25); there is only a small overlap of CIs; the test for heterogeneity results in a *P* value of 0.07, which means that chance is unlikely to explain the difference among studies; and the I^2 statistic is 57%, suggesting substantial heterogeneity. The authors conducted subgroup analysis and explored whether the antibiotic prophylaxis regimen provided in the different studies (pre-, post-, and the combination of pre- and post-operative administration) can explain the inconsistency. Unfortunately, chance easily explains the apparent differences among the subgroups in Figure 14.1 (*P* = 0.22), and differences among subgroups are only moderate in magnitude (I^2 = 34%), leaving the heterogeneity unexplained and therefore requiring rating down certainty of the evidence for inconsistency.

Imprecision

When assessing imprecision in the context of clinical practice guidelines, the primary criterion is to determine to what extent the true effects represented by the 95% CIs across a set of outcomes lie in a particular range or on one side of a threshold that may incline a guideline panel to conclude that it is worthwhile to recommend for a specific intervention.[9] Outcomes can be separated into those that reflect benefit of the intervention relative to a comparator and those that reflect harm. In isolation, each outcome and its 95% CI can inform the effect of a specific intervention, but only for that particular outcome. Guideline panels, clinicians, and patients interested in defining the best course of action for a given condition need to consider all outcomes simultaneously to then determine whether they can establish the net benefit (overall, after looking at both subsets of outcomes, benefits and harms).

For example, the ADA-AAPD clinical practice guideline addressing the use of pit-and-fissure sealants versus nonuse of sealants evaluated the impact of this intervention in reducing caries incidence (desirable outcome) while also addressing sealants' lack of retention and other adverse effects (undesirable outcomes).[8] The systematic review and meta-analysis informing this guideline reported a pooled estimate of absolute reduction on caries incidence (after three years for a moderate-risk population: 30% baseline risk) of 21% in patients receiving sealants, with a 95% CI of 23–19% when compared with patients not receiving sealants. The review also suggests that approximately one in three sealants (30%) will lose retention after 3.5 years of application.[13] Sealants are known for presenting no serious adverse effects, minimal burden for patients beyond the expected regular visits for a dental check-up, and costs that seem to be worth the benefit, especially in children and adolescents.[8,16-18] When we consider imprecision, we ask ourselves how small the benefit would have to be before use of sealants would still outweigh the cost and burden of monitoring?

Let's assume that a threshold of 10% reduction in caries incidence is the minimum threshold we are willing to accept in order to recommend the use of sealants (that is, if the absolute benefit is less than a reduction of 10%, we would not use sealants). Because the entire 95% CI (23–19%) represents benefits greater than the 10% threshold, excluding a benefit smaller than the threshold, this means that we are confident that the true effect lies above the threshold, the precision of the estimate is sufficient to support a recommendation in favor of using sealants compared with not using them, and rating down because of imprecision is not warranted (Figure 14.2, Scenario 1).

 Guideline panels, clinicians, and patients interested in defining the best course of action for a given condition need to consider all outcomes simultaneously to then determine whether they can establish the net benefit.

Figure 14.2. Use of a Threshold to Determine Precision of an Estimate to Inform a Recommendation

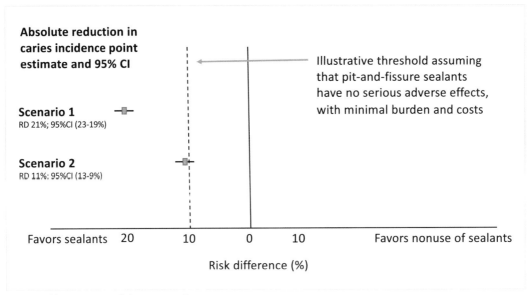

RD: risk difference, CI: confidence interval

Using the same 10% threshold, consider now a hypothetical scenario in which the pooled estimate of the absolute reduction in caries incidence is 11%, with a 95% CI of 13–9%. The point estimate is suggesting that the effect of sealants may be above the threshold (10%), which means that a recommendation in favor of sealants may still be appropriate. However, the 95% CI crossing the 10% threshold is imprecise: The CI tells us that the true effect is plausibly as little as 9%, below our threshold for sealant use. In this situation, we would therefore rate down our certainty of the evidence for imprecision (Figure 14.2, Scenario 2).

The decision about where to set these thresholds "requires a judgment regarding the relative desirability of"[9] the beneficial outcomes while considering, simultaneously, the harm outcomes or undesirable consequences associated with the implementation of the intervention. Such judgment about the relative desirability of certain outcomes over others is informed by patients' values and preferences.[19,20]

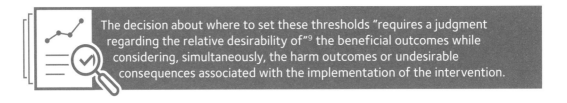

The decision about where to set these thresholds "requires a judgment regarding the relative desirability of"[9] the beneficial outcomes while considering, simultaneously, the harm outcomes or undesirable consequences associated with the implementation of the intervention.

Indirectness

Indirectness, or applicability/generalizability, is another domain to consider when assessing the quality of the evidence. When we have direct evidence that closely matches our clinical question, we can be more confident in our results. If the population, interventions, or outcomes differ from those in which we are interested, we may lose certainty in the evidence.[21]

- *Population.* The underlying characteristics of the populations enrolled in the relevant studies—characteristics such as gender, setting, and age—may differ from those in which the guideline panel is interested. For example, a guideline targeted for general practitioners may address the ability of light-based adjuncts to detect, during routine dental examinations, potentially malignant disorders in the oral cavity. A systematic review[10] addressed the accuracy of these adjuncts in secondary and tertiary care settings such as oral medicine clinics and oral and maxillofacial surgery and pathology units in hospitals. The prevalence of oral cancer in these specialized clinics is much higher than in a general practice dental office (primary care), and the severity of presentations may also differ—therefore, the properties of the tests may also differ. Applying the results to general practice may warrant skepticism, and a guideline panel may therefore rate down the certainty of the evidence because of indirectness.

- *Intervention or diagnostic test strategy.* When searching the literature for evidence regarding a specific intervention, guideline panels may find studies in which the mode of delivery, dosage, frequency of administration, or molecular configuration of the intervention differs from the one in which they are interested. If this is the case, the panel should consider whether the difference in the intervention will influence the outcome of interest. For example, if clinicians want to know the effect of antibiotic prophylaxis on reducing infectious complications post-dental extraction, they can find a systematic review to inform this question.[15] This review, although initially focused on determining the effect of antibiotic prophylaxis for any dental extraction, identified only studies in which the intervention was evaluated in third-molar extractions. There is evidence suggesting that patients undergoing surgical removal of third-molar extraction are at a much higher risk for infection because they usually have a surgical wound and require osteotomy.[22] Thus, when comparing other conventional dental extractions, antibiotics may work differently.

  Another aspect to consider is how the intervention or test is administered. A light-based adjunct may work better in the hands of specialists in oral pathology and oral medicine than in the hands of general dentists. This could be because, given the nature of their specialty, specialists are likely to see more patients with potentially malignant disorders than general dentists, who may see just a few cases in their career.[10]

- *Outcome.* Sometimes, the outcomes in which patients and clinicians are interested are not reported in the literature. Rather, only "surrogate outcomes" are available. These surrogate outcomes, although they may be in the causal pathway from the intervention to the patient-important outcome of interest, are not themselves of interest to patients.[23] Picture a situation in which you want to know whether a patient with a prosthetic heart valve would benefit from receiving prophylactic antibiotics to prevent infective endocarditis (IE). You find a recent systematic review addressing this question.[24] All of the included trials reported the incidence of bacteremia, a surrogate outcome, and not the incidence of IE (the important outcome to answer your question). None of the trials measured IE, and because bacteremia is thought to be a precursor to IE (in the causal pathway), it is the best available surrogate outcome, although indirect in relation to the posed clinical question. The time frame, or follow-up times that the primary studies considered before measuring the outcome, is also a potential source for issues of indirectness.

After identifying any one of the three aforementioned sources of indirectness, one must not only assess whether they are present, but also how likely they are to modify the effect of treatment, and thus represent indirectness serious enough to rate down the certainty of the evidence.

Publication Bias

Publication bias is the tendency to submit or accept research to be published based on the direction or strength of the study findings, including statistical significance.[25] This tendency may result in a biased estimate of the effect of an intervention, potentially overemphasizing positive effects and/or underestimating negative ones.[26]

Publication bias is the result of what may appear, or not appear, in journals. For example, RCTs with positive findings or statistical significance tend to be published more frequently and more rapidly than trials with negative findings or without statistical significance.[25] Thus, positive studies that are published earlier are particularly suspect, especially if the studies are small.

Publication bias can occur at several levels, including during the decision to submit a study report for publication. Authors may believe their results are not likely to be of interest to prominent journals because the results fail to achieve statistical significance, and as a result, they may fail to submit their research. Authors may also fail to resubmit a manuscript because it was rejected in the past and they anticipate future rejection. Research sponsored by industry can be vulnerable to pressures to withhold, delay, or influence the journal to which the research is submitted.[19,27,28] A positive association between the reporting of positive findings in RCTs and conflicts of interest in a study's authors was also found in dentistry (odds ratio, 2.40; 95% CI, 1.16–5.13).[29]

Publication bias can also result when systematic review authors and guideline developers fail to conduct a thorough search for studies. For example, if a positive study is published promptly and a negative study is delayed and missed by review authors, it may lead to an overestimation of benefits and an underestimation of harms. The omission of studies by systematic review authors due to delayed publication is referred to as lag bias.[30] Some studies are missed because they are published in less-desired journals or not listed on major databases. Many reviews do not include searches in non-English journals. Negative studies are sometimes published in the gray literature (for example, abstracts, theses, and textbook chapters; see Chapter 2) and missed in systematic reviews.[31] Regardless of the cause, if systematic review authors and guideline developers fail to identify studies (whether obscurely published or unpublished), it may lead to an unrepresentative sample of studies. If negative studies are not published and identified and are not included in meta-analysis, this could result in substantial inflation of estimates of effect.

Small studies (which some define as those including fewer than 1,000 patients[32]) tend to show greater treatment effects than larger studies (see Chapter 10).[33,34] This phenomenon is called small-study effects. Lower methodological quality, between-trial heterogeneity, and reporting bias (including publication bias) can all contribute to small-study effects.[33,34] However, a small study could also demonstrate a large effect size for reasons other than small-study effects, such as more careful patient selection or study researchers using intervention procedures that align with their areas of expertise.[35]

Small-study effects and publication bias can be evaluated based on the pattern of data using a funnel plot. The funnel plot is a visual tool that plots effect estimates on the horizontal axis against sample/study size on the vertical axis.[36] A symmetrical funnel plot suggests the absence of publication bias, while an asymmetrical appearance indicates possible publication bias. Missing data points from one quadrant of a funnel plot are often caused by small negative studies not being published (Figure 14.3).

Figure 14.3. Funnel Plot Presenting Two Hypothetical Scenarios: Left, Symmetrical Funnel Plot Suggesting No Issues of Publication Bias. Right, Asymmetrical Funnel Plot Suggesting that Small Studies Showing No Benefits are Missing

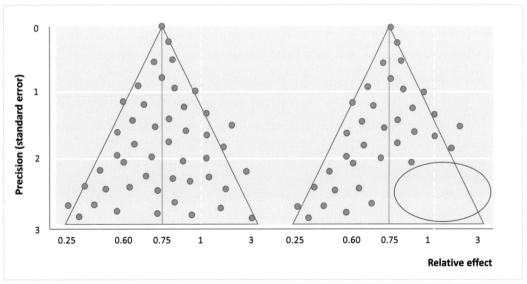

Data adapted from Wright JT, Tampi MP, Graham L, et al. "Sealants for preventing and arresting pit-and-fissure occlusal caries in primary and permanent molars: A systematic review of randomized controlled trials-a report of the American Dental Association and the American Academy of Pediatric Dentistry." *J Am Dent Assoc* 2016;147(8):631-45.e18.

In addition to a visual assessment, there are other statistical methods to evaluate funnel plot asymmetry, such as Egger's linear regression method,[36] Begg and Mazumdar's rank correlation test,[37] Duval and Tweedie's trim-and-fill method,[38] and Rosenthal's fail-safe N.[39,40] Any of these empirical methods may suggest publication bias, but all have substantial limitations and should be interpreted with caution.

In 2015, Papageorgiou and colleagues investigated topics in pediatric dentistry to determine whether publication bias was present and to what extent.[41] Out of 46 meta-analyses including 882 studies, 39 provided enough evidence to be reanalyzed qualitatively. Publication bias was assessed using contour-enhanced funnel plots, Egger's linear regression method, Begg and Mazumdar's rank correlation test, Duval and Tweedie's trim-and-fill method, and Rosenthal's fail-safe N. The results indicated that small-study effects and publication bias in pediatric dentistry existed and only a few meta-analyses adequately assessed publication bias. The funnel plots indicated asymmetry, which was confirmed in 33% of the meta-analyses evaluated with Egger's method and 18% evaluated with Begg-Mazumdar's test. Papageorgiou and colleagues concluded that because small-study effects and publication bias were present in pediatric dentistry, the influence of small or missing trials on estimated treatment effects should be routinely assessed in future systematic reviews.[42]

Authors of systematic reviews and guidelines should determine how likely it is that the body of evidence suffers from publication bias, particularly when collecting evidence from a number of small commercially funded studies. Because it is never possible to ascertain completely whether a guideline developer or a systematic reviewer retrieved all available studies answering a clinical question, GRADE is particularly explicit about this and uses the word "suspected" to describe potential publication bias issues and the word "undetected" when no evidence of this issue is apparent.

Criteria to Upgrade the Certainty of the Evidence

As described previously, in GRADE, a body of evidence informed by observational studies (see Chapters 4 and 13) starts as low certainty. However, there are three situations where certainty may be upgraded:[43]

- A large-magnitude treatment effect or strong association is identified.

- A dose-response gradient is present.

- All plausible residual confounders or biases would reduce a demonstrated effect or suggest a spurious effect when results show no effect.

As of the date of the publication of this book, we have identified no systematic review or clinical practice guideline in the dental literature that warrants upgrading a body of evidence for the reasons presented in the three bullet points above.

Conclusion

In GRADE, the certainty of the evidence reflects "the extent of our confidence that the estimates of an effect are adequate to support a particular decision or recommendation."[9] "Adequate," in this context, means determining how confident we are that the true effect lies within a particular range or on one side of a defined threshold.

References

1. Guyatt GH, Oxman AD, Kunz R, et al. "What is 'quality of evidence' and why is it important to clinicians?" *BMJ* 2008;336(7651):995-8.

2. West S, King V, Carey TS, et al. "Systems to Rate the Strength of Scientific Evidence: Summary." AHRQ Evidence Report Summaries. Rockville (MD): Agency for Healthcare Research and Quality (US); 1998-2005. 47. Available from: *https://www.ncbi.nlm.nih.gov/books/NBK11930/; 2002.*

3. Djulbegovic B, Guyatt GH. "Progress in evidence-based medicine: a quarter century on." *Lancet* 2017;390(10092):415-23.

4. Atkins D, Eccles M, Flottorp S, et al. "Systems for grading the quality of evidence and the strength of recommendations I: critical appraisal of existing approaches The GRADE Working Group." *BMC Health Serv Res 2004;4(1):38.*

5. Atkins D, Best D, Briss PA, et al. "Grading quality of evidence and strength of recommendations." *BMJ* 2004;328(7454):1490.

6. Slayton RL, Urquhart O, Araujo MWB, et al. "Evidence-based clinical practice guideline on nonrestorative treatments for carious lesions: A report from the American Dental Association." *J Am Dent Assoc* 2018;149(10):837-49.e19.

7. Urquhart O, Tampi MP, Pilcher L, et al. "Nonrestorative Treatments for Caries: Systematic Review and Network Meta-analysis." *J Dent Res* 2019;98(1):14-26.

8. Wright JT, Crall JJ, Fontana M, et al. "Evidence-based clinical practice guideline for the use of pit-and-fissure sealants: A report of the American Dental Association and the American Academy of Pediatric Dentistry." *J Am Dent Assoc* 2016;147(8):672-82.e12.

9. Hultcrantz M, Rind D, Akl EA, et al. "The GRADE Working Group clarifies the construct of certainty of evidence." *J Clin Epidemiol* 2017;87:4-13.

10. Lingen MW, Abt E, Agrawal N, et al. "Evidence-based clinical practice guideline for the evaluation of potentially malignant disorders in the oral cavity: A report of the American Dental Association." *J Am Dent Assoc* 2017;148(10):712-27.e10.

11. Moyer VA. "Screening for oral cancer: U.S. Preventive Services Task Force recommendation statement." *Ann Intern Med* 2014;160(1):55-60.

12. Guyatt GH, Oxman AD, Vist G, et al. "GRADE guidelines: 4. Rating the quality of evidence—study limitations (risk of bias)." *J Clin Epidemiol* 2011;64(4):407-15.

13. Wright JT, Tampi MP, Graham L, et al. "Sealants for preventing and arresting pit-and-fissure occlusal caries in primary and permanent molars: A systematic review of randomized controlled trials-a report of the American Dental Association and the American Academy of Pediatric Dentistry." *J Am Dent Assoc* 2016;147(8):631-45.e18.

14. Guyatt GH, Oxman AD, Kunz R, et al. "GRADE guidelines: 7. Rating the quality of evidence—inconsistency." *J Clin Epidemiol* 2011;64(12):1294-302.

15. Lodi G, Figini L, Sardella A, et al. "Antibiotics to prevent complications following tooth extractions." *Cochrane Database Syst Rev* 2012, Issue 11. Art.No.:CD003811. DOI: 10.1002/14651858.CD003811.pub2.

16. Akinlotan M, Chen B, Fontanilla TM, Chen A, Fan VY. "Economic evaluation of dental sealants: A systematic literature review." *Community Dent Oral Epidemiol* 2018;46(1):38-46.

17. Bhuridej P, Kuthy RA, Flach SD, et al. "Four-year cost-utility analyses of sealed and nonsealed first permanent molars in Iowa Medicaid-enrolled children." *J Public Health Dent* 2007;67(4):191-8.

18. Dasanayake AP, Li Y, Kirk K, Bronstein J, Childers NK. "Restorative cost savings related to dental sealants in Alabama Medicaid children." *Pediatr Dent* 2003;25(6):572-6.

19. Ioannidis JP. "Effect of the statistical significance of results on the time to completion and publication of randomized efficacy trials." *JAMA* 1998;279(4):281-6.

20. Guyatt GH, Oxman AD, Kunz R, et al. "GRADE guidelines: 2. Framing the question and deciding on important outcomes." *J Clin Epidemiol* 2011;64(4):395-400.

21. Guyatt GH, Oxman AD, Kunz R, et al. "GRADE guidelines: 8. Rating the quality of evidence—indirectness." *J Clin Epidemiol* 2011;64(12):1303-10.

22. Bouloux GF, Steed MB, Perciaccante VJ. "Complications of third molar surgery." *Oral Maxillofac Surg Clin North Am* 2007;19(1):117-28, vii.

23. Guyatt GH, Rennie D, Meade MO, Cook DJ, eds. *Users' Guides to the Medical Literature: A Manual for Evidence-Based Clinical Practice.* 3rd ed. United States of America: McGraw-Hill Companies, Inc; 2015.

24. Cahill TJ, Harrison JL, Jewell P, et al. "Antibiotic prophylaxis for infective endocarditis: a systematic review and meta-analysis." *Heart* 2017;103(12):937-44.

25. Hopewell S, Loudon K, Clarke MJ, Oxman AD, Dickersin K. "Publication bias in clinical trials due to statistical significance or direction of trial results." *Cochrane Database Syst Rev* 2009(1):Mr000006.

26. Guyatt GH, Oxman AD, Montori V, et al. "GRADE guidelines: 5. Rating the quality of evidence—publication bias." *J Clin Epidemiol* 2011;64(12):1277-82.

27. Melander H, Ahlqvist-Rastad J, Meijer G, Beermann B. "Evidence b(i)ased medicine—selective reporting from studies sponsored by pharmaceutical industry: review of studies in new drug applications." *BMJ* 2003;326(7400):1171-3.

28. Lexchin J, Bero LA, Djulbegovic B, Clark O. "Pharmaceutical industry sponsorship and research outcome and quality: systematic review." *BMJ* 2003;326(7400):1167-70.

29. Brignardello-Petersen R, Carrasco-Labra A, Yanine N, et al. "Positive association between conflicts of interest and reporting of positive results in randomized clinical trials in dentistry." *J Am Dent Assoc* 2013;144(10):1165-70.

30. Hopewell S, Clarke M, Stewart L, Tierney J. "Time to publication for results of clinical trials." *Cochrane Database Syst Rev* 2007(2):Mr000011.

31. Hopewell S, McDonald S, Clarke M, Egger M. "Grey literature in meta-analyses of randomized trials of health care interventions." *Cochrane Database Syst Rev* 2007(2):Mr000010.

32. Cappelleri JC, Ioannidis JP, Schmid CH, et al. "Large trials vs meta-analysis of smaller trials: how do their results compare?" *JAMA* 1996;276(16):1332-8.

33. Sterne JA, Egger M, Smith GD. "Systematic reviews in health care: Investigating and dealing with publication and other biases in meta-analysis." *BMJ* 2001;323(7304):101-5.

34. Sterne JA, Gavaghan D, Egger M. "Publication and related bias in meta-analysis: power of statistical tests and prevalence in the literature." *J Clin Epidemiol* 2000;53(11):1119-29.

35. Cuijpers P, Smit F, Bohlmeijer E, Hollon SD, Andersson G. "Efficacy of cognitive-behavioural therapy and other psychological treatments for adult depression: meta-analytic study of publication bias." *Br J Psychiatry* 2010;196(3):173-8.

36. Egger M, Davey Smith G, Schneider M, Minder C. "Bias in meta-analysis detected by a simple, graphical test." *BMJ* 1997;315(7109):629-34.

37. Begg CB, Mazumdar M. "Operating characteristics of a rank correlation test for publication bias." *Biometrics* 1994;50(4):1088-101.

38. Duval S, Tweedie R. "Trim and fill: A simple funnel-plot-based method of testing and adjusting for publication bias in meta-analysis." *Biometrics* 2000;56(2):455-63.

39. Dwan K, Altman DG, Arnaiz JA, et al. "Systematic review of the empirical evidence of study publication bias and outcome reporting bias." *PLoS One* 2008;3(8):e3081.

40. Dwan K, Gamble C, Williamson PR, Kirkham JJ. "Systematic review of the empirical evidence of study publication bias and outcome reporting bias - an updated review." *PLoS One* 2013;8(7):e66844.

41. Papageorgiou SN, Dimitraki D, Coolidge T, Kotsanos N. "Publication bias & small-study effects in pediatric dentistry meta-analyses." *J Evid Based Dent Pract* 2015;15(1):8-24.

42. Sterne JAC, Egger M, Moher D, (editors). "Chapter 10: Addressing reporting biases." In: Higgins JPT, Green S (editors). *Cochrane Handbook for Systematic Reviews of Intervention*. Version 5.1.0 (updated March 2011). The Cochrane Collaboration, 2011. Available from *www.handbook.cochrane.org*.

43. Guyatt GH, Oxman AD, Sultan S, et al. "GRADE guidelines: 9. Rating up the quality of evidence." *J Clin Epidemiol* 2011;64(12):1311-6.

Chapter 15. Strategies for Teaching Evidence-Based Dentistry

Cheryl L. Straub-Morarend, D.D.S.; Jaana Gold, D.D.S., M.P.H., Ph.D., C.P.H.; Kelly C. Lemke, D.D.S., M.S.; Parthasarathy Madurantakam, D.D.S., M.D.S., Ph.D.; David M. Leader, D.M.D., M.P.H.; Richard Niederman, D.M.D., M.A.; and Teresa A. Marshall, Ph.D., R.D.N./L.D.N., F.A.N.D.

In This Chapter:

Introduction

Health information is rapidly generated and communicated through nontraditional avenues in contemporary society. Patients are invested in their health care, seek information, and, at times, question their providers. The clinician versed in evidence-based practice (EBP) skills is best equipped to address patients' queries and maintain a cutting-edge practice. EBP is defined as the integration of the best available scientific evidence, clinician expertise, and patient values and preferences during the clinical decision-making process.[1] EBP is often confused with the academic practice of critiquing science; however, EBP involves more than just a critical appraisal of the literature. It is equally inclusive of clinician expertise and patient values and preferences.

Dental organizations have recognized the importance of EBP in dentistry (known as evidence-based dentistry, or EBD) and made concerted efforts to educate clinicians through workshops, resource centers, and publications.[1,2,3] Concurrently, the importance of providing dental students with the skill set needed to practice EBD has been noted by the American Dental Education Association (ADEA), the Commission on Dental Accreditation (CODA), and the American Dental Association (ADA). Accreditation Standard 2-21 of CODA's Accreditation Standards for Dental Education Programs states, "Graduates must be competent to access, critically appraise, apply, and communicate scientific and lay literature as it relates to providing evidence-based patient care."[3] EBD instruction provides dental students with the skill sets they need to independently identify the best science and integrate that evidence with their expertise and patient values and preferences during clinical decision-making. EBP requires critical thinking skills and, combined with competency in EBD, provides future dental practitioners with the tools to make better-informed treatment decisions and become lifelong learners.

Although EBD is considered an important component of dental education and continuing education (CE) for clinicians, few resources are available to guide dental faculty, CE providers, or journal club leaders on how to educate their respective learners in EBD. The objective of this chapter is to identify curricular content and approaches for teaching EBD to dental learners in a variety of educational environments.

EBD hinges on the following five-step process:

1. Asking an answerable question;

2. Searching for the best evidence;

3. Critically appraising the evidence;

4. Applying the evidence in practice; and

5. Evaluating the impact of implementation on health outcomes.

This chapter addresses the first three steps of this process and includes three different approaches to EBD training, each of which addresses the objectives of the ADA CODA requirements for EBD.

Curricular Outcomes

The first step in designing a curriculum or educational program is to identify the desired curricular outcomes: what do you want the learner to gain from the experience? Although the desired overall outcome might be for the learner to practice EBD, it is important to identify specific knowledge and skills that you hope a learner will gain by the end of their instruction. Such identification helps to facilitate curricular development and outcome measurement. The learner audience, the time allotted for instruction, and the educational environment should also be considered when identifying outcomes. Examples of curricular outcomes for EBD might include the following:

Upon course completion, the learner will be able to:

a. Define EBD

b. Identify the components of EBD's five-step process

c. Apply each step of the five-step process

d. Describe the rationale for practicing EBD

Curricular Content

After identification of curricular outcomes, the content necessary to achieve those outcomes is defined. This content can be categorized into knowledge, scientific evidence, and behavior.

Knowledge

To practice EBD, learners must be able to define EBD and identify the components of its five-step process. To ask a question (that is, the first step of the five-step process), learners must be able to identify gaps in their knowledge and both describe and identify a PICO (population, intervention, comparison, outcomes) question (see Chapter 2). To search for the best evidence (the second step of the five-step process), learners must be able to identify appropriate resources (for example, critical summaries, clinical practice guidelines, and primary and secondary resources) and describe steps to obtain those resources (see Chapter 2). To appraise a resource (step three), the learner must be able to identify research study designs, describe the EBP evidence hierarchy, identify expected research study components, assess the validity of the research methodology used, identify potential sources of bias, and interpret the results (see Chapters 12, 13, and 14). Once the learner masters components of the appraisal process, the learner is then able to critique the quality of the science in question and assess applicability.

Foundational knowledge can be taught through lecture, problem-based learning, or online activities. In an ideal situation, foundational knowledge acquisition occurs prior to or during clinical experiences, given that predoctoral students must be prepared to apply this knowledge once they initiate clinical activities. The context for EBD may be premature during early didactic (that is, preclinical) instruction because of a lack of clinical maturity in the learners involved. For such instances, case-based instruction is useful to communicate relevance.

Scientific Evidence

EBP relies on the integration of high-quality contemporary scientific evidence into clinical decision-making. As such, curricular approaches for instruction in EBP must first equip learners with a knowledge of research study design and the evidence hierarchy, including an introduction to quantitative and qualitative primary and secondary research.

Foundational knowledge of scientific evidence includes the ability to identify the appropriate type of evidence to seek for the PICO question being asked. Learners must be trained in search strategies to efficiently and effectively identify key scientific evidence to address clinical questions. Training in the identification of scientific evidence should include the presentation and differentiation of the resources available to the learner in their current and future practice settings to assist in the acquisition of the highest level of evidence (see Chapter 2).

Strategies to identify evidence aim to first identify secondary preappraised sources of evidence (see Chapters 6 and 7) in order to minimize the time needed for critical appraisal as well as to overcome learners' lack of statistical knowledge and/or confidence in the critical appraisal process. If secondary resources are not available to address the question posed, then high-quality primary science should be sought. Critical appraisal checklists can be used to appraise research studies. Guided completion of critical appraisal checklists facilitates development of prioritization and interpretation skills in a structured process.

Behavior

Application
EBP behavior includes the assimilation of evidence-based principles and their application to patient care. Learners must possess the skills necessary to determine the relevance of scientific evidence for patient care, the feasibility of treatment, and the balance between benefits and harms while articulating explicit patient-centered outcomes.

Professionalism
Throughout the process of EBP instruction, learners develop the qualities of professionalism as they discover the value of practicing EBD, develop the skills needed for lifelong learning, and observe the modeling of professional behavior in an environment that mirrors current or future practice.

Communication
EBP is observed when learners use patients' values, preferences, and circumstances to effectively communicate evidence to patients and integrate evidence in the clinical decision-making process. Ongoing observation of learners' evidence-based communication with patients and colleagues, followed by structured feedback, helps guide the development of learners' skills and proficiency in EBP.

Instructional Methods

EBD can be taught using various methods of didactic learning, application, and clinical activity.

Didactic Learning

The rationale for didactic or preclinical instruction is to equip learners with the knowledge and skills needed to practice EBP while, at the same time, supporting the growth of the fundamental behaviors needed to one day apply didactic concepts to clinic experiences.

Didactic content lays the foundation so that learners can effectively practice EBP in the future. Foundational knowledge can be delivered through lectures, readings, online tutorials, self-directed learning, problem-based learning, flipped classrooms, and/or Process Oriented Guided Inquiry Learning (POGIL). Writing assignments for groups and individuals, combined with guiding questions and structured reflections, provide insight into how learning is progressing. Scaffolding content and experiences enables students to acquire the knowledge and skills essential for competence in EBP.

Application

EBP is a behavior requiring repetition and application. Application of EBD's five-step process begins with the didactic presentation of scenarios, followed by instruction through preclinical or clinical interactions, and, finally, the integration in real time of evidence to patient care. Instructional strategies for the integration of EBP center on diagnosis, treatment planning, patient education, and outcome assessment. The use of guiding questions during the presentation of information, patient cases, student reports, team presentations, formal case presentations, and reflection activities supports the advancement and application of desired EBP skills.

Clinical Activity

EBP clinical instruction integrates an authentic environment while refining EBD's five-step approach and skills through real-world experiences. Clinical instruction guides the integration of scientific evidence with clinician expertise and patient values and preferences. The learning process evolves from an instructor-guided treatment planning process to a learner-initiated process where learners defend their treatment rationale by using the best available evidence and assessing outcomes of evidence-based interventions. Self-assessment and formative and summative feedback are integral pieces of clinical instruction in EBP.

Real-World Examples

Here we present three contemporary examples of programs in academic institutions that have successfully implemented EBP into their dental curriculums.

Virginia Commonwealth University School of Dentistry

The EBD program at the Virginia Commonwealth University (VCU) School of Dentistry provides students with the skills necessary to practice EBD upon graduation. EBD instruction is layered over three semesters, beginning in the second semester. The courses are strategically positioned to allow seamless integration of EBD in year 3 (D3) and year 4 (D4) treatment planning clinical courses.

In the first course, students are introduced to the concepts of EBP in a large classroom setting. Using interactive role-playing sessions, students are presented with real-life examples of how "good" scientific information can be misreported by public media (for example, TV, newspapers, and internet outlets) and/or how "bad" science can be published in reputable professional journals. Students learn to challenge assumptions, verify study validity, and question conclusions. Students acquire the skills needed to navigate the scientific literature in a hands-on workshop taught by the School of Dentistry's library liaison. Additionally, students learn the basic concepts of biostatistics, the evidence pyramid, and study designs and how to frame clinical questions using the PICO format. Student performance is evaluated using a digital response system in class and written midterm and final exams.

During the second semester, students apply their acquired critical appraisal knowledge when evaluating peer-reviewed scientific manuscripts. Small groups present their critical appraisal of a systematic review or a primary study article addressing a PICO question. The students frame questions that stimulate critical thinking among their peers in the audience and are assessed by the quality of questions and in-class presentation. Student performance is evaluated based on the presentation, written quizzes, and a written final exam.

Knowledge and application of EBD are assessed using a modified POGIL group project in addition to an individual paper during the third course. POGIL is based on the philosophy that teaching is enabling, knowledge is understanding, and learning is active construction of subject matter.[4] POGIL activities encourage a deeper understanding of core concepts while developing higher-order process skills including critical thinking, problem-solving, and communication through cooperation and reflection. Additionally, POGIL improves self-assessment and helps students identify areas of limited understanding.

At VCU, each class is divided into 12 groups of approximately eight students, and each group facilitates one POGIL session. The presenting group is given a clinical scenario one week in advance, and the members work together to develop a worksheet. After constructive feedback from faculty on the draft worksheet, the students refine the content. Prior to the session, the presenting group and faculty finalize the questions and responses. To ensure the success of the POGIL session, the presenting group is instructed not to divulge the contents of the worksheet to their peers.

At the beginning of the POGIL session, the case scenario is revealed and the class divides into small groups for discussion. Each group is assigned a student facilitator to guide discussion as the team addresses the worksheet questions. The groups have the freedom to work on the questions at their own pace; however, if the conversation stalls or deviates greatly from the topic, the student facilitator redirects attention to the topic. The student facilitator uses the completed template to guide discussion. At the end of the session, individual groups turn in their worksheets and the student facilitators meet to reflect on their experience and prepare a two-page summary of the experience.

The worksheets are the foundation of the modified POGIL activity and require hours of preparation. An effective worksheet (1) starts with a realistic clinical scenario with sufficient background information on the topic of interest, (2) contains open-ended questions to encourage problem-solving during student deliberation and discussion, and (3) is based on students' prior knowledge. Although it is important to challenge students, questions should be within reach.

University of Texas Health Science Center San Antonio School of Dentistry

Foundations

At the University of Texas Health Science Center San Antonio (UTHSCSA) School of Dentistry, the EBP program is designed to educate students on the traditional EBD approach with an emphasis on "just in time" learning.[5,6] This approach was developed in response to the need for clinicians to stay up-to-date over the course of their careers while faced with a constant flood of new biomedical information and products.

In the just-in-time model, when faced with a clinical treatment or care dilemma, students are taught to (1) formulate a focused clinical question and then quickly (2) search the biomedical research literature (for example, via PubMed or the Trip Database) for the most recent and highest level of evidence, (3) critically evaluate that evidence, and (4) make a clinical judgment about the applicability of that evidence for their patient. These techniques and the skills required for execution are taught to predoctoral dental students in graded didactic courses during the first two years of training.

Critically Appraised Topics (CATs)

After didactic training, students apply these just-in-time skills when preparing a concise one-page Critically Appraised Topic (CAT)[5,7] on a focused clinical question under the guidance of a faculty mentor. The student and faculty mentor work together to refine the CAT, and the faculty mentor is listed as coauthor of the CAT.

A separate faculty member serves as the CAT's editor, providing a secondary level of editing and peer review. Both the CAT's editor and faculty mentor are ultimately responsible for the quality and accuracy of the CAT. A key component of the UTHSCSA School of Dentistry EBP/CAT initiative has been a formal faculty development program on EBD, with an emphasis on the skills needed to prepare CATs and mentor their student authors.

Completed CATs are published in a searchable online CAT library.[8] The content and structure of a CAT mirrors EBD's five-step process. For students in the preclinical stage of learning, a CAT's focused clinical question is usually formulated based on the student's area of interest or a classroom encounter, rather than an actual patient encounter. Once students progress to the clinical phase of their training and are faced with a clinical dilemma, they are encouraged to apply the CAT protocol to locate, evaluate, and identify the strongest evidence relevant to a patient's problem.

Evidence-Based Case Presentations

To achieve the goal of integrating EBP skills into all levels of the curriculum and especially into direct patient care, skills are further reinforced in the context of formal case presentations during the final two years of clinical training. A student's general practice group provides the forum for these presentations, which document the comprehensive care of a patient, including the peer-reviewed evidence base for treatment.

Graduate-Level EBD Training Strategy

The same EBP/CAT skills are taught in the majority of the school's residency programs. Each resident is required to write a CAT as part of their course or residency requirements. Graduate-level students may choose to write their CAT based on their area of research or on a clinical encounter. As with the undergraduate students, these CATs are coauthored by a faculty mentor and formally reviewed by the CATs editor.

FAST CATs Program: Academic Detailing

The FAST CATs (Faculty, Alumni, Student, Team: Critically Appraised Topics) Program provided dental students the opportunity to serve as academic detailers.[6] In academic detailing, a trained "detailer" meets face-to-face with a practitioner in the practitioner's office and provides evidence-based information about patient care topics. In the FAST CATs Program, dental students served as the detailers.

After a two-and-a-half-day workshop, students visited general dentists and presented CATs in person during the students' summer breaks. Students received credit for this selective course, and the dentist received one hour of CE credit. This program was designed to reinforce the EBP teaching program, to facilitate the flow of information from scientific literature to dental practitioners, and to obtain the opinion of experienced practitioners on the practicality of new interventions in real-world settings. Students reported that their participation in the project reinforced their commitment to EBP, and the detailing was well received by the dentists involved.[9] FAST CATs was a pilot program funded by a National Institutes of Health (NIH) Education Grant (R25) for several years.

Impact of the UTHSCSA School of Dentistry EBD/CATs Program

The impact of the EBD/CATs program on students, residents, and faculty was evaluated using the Knowledge, Attitudes, Access, and Confidence Evaluation (KACE) questionnaire.[10] The KACE questionnaire assessed individuals' understanding of EBP, attitudes toward EBP, evidence-searching methods, and comfort with critical appraisal. Scores across these four dimensions were compared before and after EBP/CATs courses. Among students and residents, all scores, except resident attitudes toward EBP, increased significantly. What's more, post-training EBD knowledge scores for dental students and residents equaled or surpassed those of faculty.

Challenges

Full implementation and integration of an evidence-based teaching program is not without its challenges. The CATs were piloted with an ADA Foundation grant, subsequently developed and supported by an NIH R25 grant, and then supported in part by a U.S. Health Resources and Services Administration grant. Grants are, of course, a self-limited source of funding. Moreover, the success of a fully implemented EBD program depends on faculty who serve as not only mentors but also as valued collaborators for evidence-based care in the clinic. Investigating clinical problems, locating and appraising the evidence base for treatment, and reporting back to the general practice group requires a time commitment on the part of faculty, which takes time away from patient treatment. State budget cuts—and therefore dental school budget cuts—have added to the challenge of full clinical integration of EBD.

University of Iowa College of Dentistry

Overview

The University of Iowa College of Dentistry (UI COD) EBD instructional track is designed to prepare graduates with the skills and experience necessary to independently apply EBD principles to clinical practice.[11] The instructional track includes educational content within EBD, professionalism, and lifelong learning domains, while the types of learning include knowledge (for example, facts and concepts) and behavior (for example, application, practice, and assimilation).[12] The curriculum is designed to bring consistency to EBD across departments and throughout the four predoctoral years so as to help manage student expectations.

Assessment

Each curricular component incorporates a learning guide that serves as the foundation for assessment. Outcome assessment is both formative, to guide students during the learning process, and summative, to document outcome achievement. Assessment of knowledge is relatively straightforward; however, assessment of behavior is difficult. Better or worse responses in the context of differing environments with differing confounders necessitate a subjective assessment process. Assessment confounders (including the student's knowledge base, clinical maturity, technical skills, ethical maturity, and faculty guidance) result in students acquiring skills at different points in their clinical training. Formative feedback is individualized to support each student's growth at the time of evaluation.

Year 1 (D1)

Students are introduced to primary literature with an emphasis on study design, statistical principles, and critical appraisal. Fundamental knowledge is presented didactically; students apply their new knowledge when appraising primary literature in small groups. Knowledge (for example, statistical facts and concepts) is assessed summatively through written exams, while application (for example, appraisal) is assessed formatively through group presentations.

Year 2 (D2)

Students are introduced to EBD concepts, principles, and professionalism. Students complete short online assignments designed to introduce or reinforce EBD knowledge and write arguments in response to EBD-related editorials and perspectives. The short assignments are considered low stakes; formative feedback is designed to guide students' thought process.

Students apply EBD's five-step process to four simulated and/or clinical scenarios (for example, exercises); expectations for the steps of asking an answerable question, searching for the best evidence, and critically appraising the evidence increase throughout the year. Assessment of the five-step exercises is considered high stakes; both formative and summative feedback are provided.

Year 3 (D3)

Students continue to be introduced to EBD principles and professionalism. Similar to the D2 year, students complete short, low-stakes online assignments designed to further develop their appraisal skills and/or introduce professionalism concepts. EBD content is integrated into clinical decision-making as part of patient care during the D3 year. Students apply EBD's five-step process to patient cases during four different clerkship rotations (that is, high-stakes exercises), and EBD content is included in student case presentations. Assessment of five-step exercises is both formative and summative.

Although lifelong learning is emphasized by faculty during the D1 and D2 years, students gain a new appreciation for the importance of lifelong learning during the D3 year as they assimilate new knowledge, clinical expertise, patient values and preferences, and alternative viewpoints during clinical decision-making.

Year 4 (D4)

During the D4 year, students are expected to assimilate the EBD knowledge and skills acquired during their D1 through D3 years within EBP to further develop lifelong learning skills. Throughout didactic activities, students utilize EBD's five-step process to support decision-making as they prepare for entry into independent practice. For example, students use EBD skills as a foundation for technology decision-making during group activities. In the clinical setting, students integrate EBD elements into comprehensive patient care in real time. Students formally present their application of EBD's five-step process to support their clinical decisions in a capstone case presentation. Students reflect on their patient care experiences and the impact of these experiences on their professional growth as part of lifelong learning. Assessment throughout the D4 year is both formative and summative, with feedback designed to support ongoing growth.

Summary

UI COD's EBD predoctoral curriculum is published and available for reference.[11] A companion manuscript describes the development and implementation of assessment strategies guiding student learning in EBD knowledge and behavior.[12] Although EBD competency is not universally defined, the UI COD team identified educational objectives for EBD's five-step process using Benjamin Bloom's knowledge and cognitive dimensions and Stuart and Hubert Dreyfus's model of skill acquisition.[13] UI COD student growth in EBD behavior has been evaluated utilizing this approach.[14]

Competency Assessment

Documentation of learner performance is an essential component of all educational programs. Currently, EBD competency does not have a clear definition, although several investigators have defined competency for research purposes.[12,14] Therefore, program faculty are charged with defining competency and designing assessment strategies for competency outcomes. Within a curriculum, educational activities must communicate the desired outcomes and impart the knowledge and behaviors necessary to achieve these outcomes. In general, documentation of competency includes identification of outcomes, design of assessment activities, and evaluation of student performance.[15]

For example, the objective of the UTHSCSA School of Dentistry EBD program is to provide students with lifelong learning skills that will enable them to provide the best patient care and remain up-to-date during their 30 to 40 years of dental practice. This approach entails learning the EBD skills needed to quickly find the latest scientific evidence related to a patient's specific problem at the point of care. In this context, EBD competency is defined as the demonstrated ability to apply those skills in both preclinical and clinical settings.

Consider the field of fixed prosthodontics, where students are presented with didactic instruction on the preparation of teeth for full-coverage crowns. Students apply this knowledge at the preclinical stage through preparation of typodont teeth. When a minimum level of competency has been achieved, the students transfer their knowledge of crown preparations to patient care in the clinic. They demonstrate their mastery of these skills through traditional assessment methods (for example, multiple-choice testing) as well as through formal competency examinations at both the preclinical and clinical levels.

In a similar manner, in an EBD curriculum, students first learn key concepts and skills in a classroom setting as part of a graded course (Figure 15.1). At UTHSCSA School of Dentistry, students further demonstrate competency of their newly acquired EBD skills through writing a CAT.[5,7] In the preclinical setting, a CAT is the EBD equivalent of a typodont crown preparation—that is, an application of skills in preparation for future patient care. Once in the clinic, students transfer their EBD skills to patient encounters, investigating clinical problems and using an evidence-based approach to inform the clinical decision-making process. Evidence-based formal case presentations are used to confirm mastery of EBD skills at the clinical level.

Within a curriculum, educational activities must communicate the desired outcomes and impart the knowledge and behaviors necessary to achieve these outcomes.

Figure 15.1. A Comparison of Curricula for Fixed Prosthodontics and Evidence-Based Dentistry

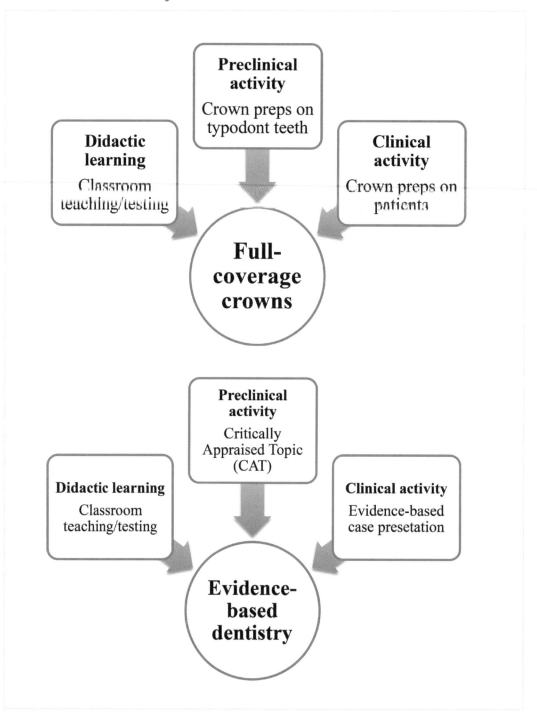

Obstacles and Strategies

Content, time, and methods for teaching EBD vary significantly among U.S. dental schools. Current educational strategies may not be efficient or optimal to develop EBD skills. Unfortunately, only limited evidence exists to inform faculty regarding the most effective methods of teaching evidence-based medicine.[16] Because of the complex and challenging nature of the knowledge, skills, and behaviors required for EBD competence, many obstacles and barriers to teaching and learning EBD in dental schools exist. Barriers to teaching are similar to those experienced in dental practices, including lack of time and limited EBD skills.[17,18] Faculty commonly lack formal EBD training and operational knowledge regarding the EBD process,[19] although training and educational opportunities exist through the ADA Center for EBD.[20]

Clinicians possess internal and external biases influencing their practice of EBD;[21] similarly, faculty may have personal barriers to teaching EBD. Dental faculty are from diverse backgrounds with differing experiences, perspectives, and opinions, which are introduced in both didactic and clinical education. Faculty may rely on dental school experiences or perceive EBD as rigid, time-consuming, or impractical, which can impact teaching efforts.[22]

The complexity of information can itself be a barrier because of the time required for comprehension and application in treatment planning and decision-making. Polk et al. reported that most dental schools are not implementing EBD guidelines effectively and efficiently, but some are, thus showing a positive trend.[23] EBD competency will be advanced as more educators begin to value the practice and as they become increasingly competent in the knowledge and skills needed to provide training to students. Thus, faculty training and standardization is essential to achieve a cohesive and effective EBD curriculum in U.S. dental schools.

Program Evaluation

Accreditation Standards

CODA creates standards to protect public welfare, promote an educational environment that fosters innovation, guide program development and evaluation, and ensure that predoctoral dental programs meet stated objectives for achieving minimum competencies. Competencies identify the knowledge and skill sets required for unsupervised dental practice. Curricula include a series of measurable objectives or outcomes that define competence and identify how learning objectives relate to competencies and CODA standards.[10]

For example, the syllabus for a predoctoral epidemiology course at Tufts University School of Dental Medicine (TUSDM) includes applicable CODA standards such as the previously mentioned CODA Accreditation Standard 2-21, as well as CODA Accreditation Standard 2-9, which states, "Graduates must be competent in the use of critical thinking and problem-solving, including their use in the comprehensive care of patients, scientific inquiry, and research methodology." The syllabus also states the objective "Explain what is meant by 'confidence interval,'" which is consistent with CODA standards. Students' understanding of confidence intervals may be assessed through exam questions, written papers, or oral presentations. Additionally, TUSDM has program competencies within courses.

Adaptations for Nonacademic Settings

This chapter emphasizes EBD instruction of predoctoral students with the objective of providing guidance to dental faculty seeking to implement or advance current EBD curricula. Conjointly, the content and strategies for EBD instruction are similar for other audiences, including peer faculty, clinicians pursuing CE, and journal clubs. In this section, we provide guidance for tailoring the content to specific audiences.

Depth of Instruction

Designing evidence-based instruction that is tailored to the knowledge and skills of the audience is key to engaging learners. If one considers a continuum from novice to expert in EBP instruction,[13] educational activities will be learner-centered (Table 15.1).

Table 15.1. Examples of Educational Objectives by Learner Skill Level

Learner	Instructional Objectives
Novice	Introduce learners to foundational knowledge, skills, and resources to initiate evidence-based practice (EBP).
Advanced beginner	Review foundational concepts in EBP through application to patient scenarios and critical appraisal of evidence-based resources.
Competent	Advance knowledge and skills through peer-to-peer EBP instruction.
Proficient	Guide participation in contributing evidence-based information (for example, critical summaries and critically appraised topics [CATs]).
Expert	Mentor participation in EBP panels.

Audiences beyond the Formal Educational Setting

Many practicing clinicians did not benefit from formal EBD training during dental school. After all, CODA standards relating to EBD became effective in 2013. Even so, many dentists recognize the value of integrating relevant scientific evidence at the point of care.

The educational aims and goals of practitioners are likely to differ from those of faculty in the academic arena. Practicing clinicians who seek EBD training likely desire improved knowledge and health care outcomes.

Although the curricular content—covered in this chapter—may be the same for both dental student and practicing clinician audiences, the presentation of content is likely to differ. Practitioners are often busy entrepreneurs with many demands on their time. While many practitioners set aside time for routine CE courses, some may lack the time to participate in EBD CE.

With that in mind, Table 15.2 offers some ideas on how EBD training in nonacademic settings can be tailored to the amount of time available.

Table 15.2. EBD Instruction in Nonacademic Settings with Considerations to Timing

One to Two Hours (Study Club, Local Dental Society Meeting)

Focus: very limited

How EBD can help the dentist/dental team provide optimum care, assess appropriate therapies, and evaluate emerging clinical approaches and tools

Plus a broad overview of one of the topics listed below

- Finding and using clinical practice guidelines
- Finding and using preappraised evidence (for example, critical summaries)
- Asking precise, structured clinical (PICO) questions and finding answers by searching PubMed

Half-Day Workshop

Focus: limited

How EBD can help the dentist/dental team provide optimum care, assess appropriate therapies, and evaluate emerging clinical approaches and tools

Plus one or more hands-on activities on the topics listed below

- Finding and using clinical practice guidelines
- Finding and using preappraised evidence (for example, critical summaries)
- Asking precise, structured clinical (PICO) questions and finding answers by searching PubMed
- Understanding clinical trial designs
- Judging the validity of a research article

Intensive Multiday Workshop

Focus: in-depth training with multiple hands-on activities on the topics listed below

- Implementing best evidence in clinical practice
- Asking precise, structured clinical (PICO) questions
- Finding the best evidence using PubMed and other search tools
- Critically reading and appraising evidence
- Finding and using preappraised evidence (for example, critical summaries), clinical practice guidelines, and systematic reviews
- Understanding clinical trial designs for therapy and diagnosis
- Calculating and using odds ratios, risk reduction, relative risk, and numbers needed to treat

Conclusion

EBP is a systematic approach guiding clinical decision-making using the best available scientific evidence. The rationale for teaching EBP in dental schools is evident. Unfortunately, few curricular guidelines exist. This chapter identifies necessary curricular content and outlines strategies for teaching EBD that can be adapted for audiences in a variety of learning environments.

References

1. "About EBD." American Dental Association Center for Evidence-Based Dentistry. 2013. *http://ebd.ADA.org/about. aspx.* Accessed 2-19-19.

2. ADEA House of Delegates. "Competencies for the new general dentist." *J Dent Edu.* 2008;72(7): 823-826.

3. Commission on Dental Accreditation. "Accreditation Standards for Dental Education Programs." Chicago: American Dental Association, 2018. *https://www.ADA.org/~/media/CODA/Files/pde.pdf?la=en.* Accessed 2-2-19.

4. "POGIL Implementation Guide." The POGIL Project. *https://pogil.org/uploads/attachments/ cjay281cc08qzw0x4ha9nt7wd-implementationguide.pdf.* Accessed 2-19-19.

5. Rugh JD, Hendricson WD, Hatch JP, Glass BJ. "The San Antonio initiative." *J Am Coll Dent.* 2010;77(2):16-21.

6. Rugh JD, Hendricson WD, Glass BJ, et al. "Teaching evidence-based practice at the University of Texas Health Science Center at San Antonio dental school." *Tex Dent J* 2011;128(2):187-190.

7. Suavé S, Lee HN, Meade MO, Lang JD, Farkouh M, Cook DJ, Sackett DL. "The critically appraised topic: a practical approach to learning critical appraisal." *Ann R Coll Physicians Surg Can.* 1995;28:396-398.

8. "Welcome to CATs Library." *cats.uthscsa.edu.* Accessed 3-27-19.

9. Rugh JD, Sever N, Glass BJ, Matteson SR. "Transferring evidence-based information from dental school to practitioners: a pilot 'academic detailing' program involving dental students." *J Dent Educ.* 2011;75(10):1316-1322.

10. Hendricson WD, Rugh JD, Hatch JP, Stark DL, Deahl T, Wallmann ER. "Validation of an instrument to assess evidence-based practice knowledge, attitudes, access, and confidence in the dental environment." *J Dent Educ.* 2011;75(2):131-144.

11. Marshall TA, Straub-Morarend CS, Handoo N, Solow CM, Cunningham-Ford CA, Finkelstein MW. "Integrating Critical Thinking and Evidence-Based Dentistry Across a Four-Year Dental Curriculum: A Model for Independent Learning." *J Dent Edu.* 2014;78(3):359-367.

12. Ilic D, Nordin RB, Glasziou B, Tilson JK, Villanueva E. "Development and validation of the ACE tool: assessing medical trainee's competency in evidence based medicine." *BMC Med Educ.* 2014;14:114.

13. Marshall TA, Straub-Morarend CL, Guzman-Armstrong S, McKernan SC, Marchini L, Handoo NQ, Cunningham MA. "An approach on defining competency in evidence-based dentistry." *Eur J Dent Edu.* 2018;22(1):e107-e115.

14. Marshall TA, McKernan SC, Straub-Morarend CL, Guzman-Armstrong S, Marchini L, Handoo NQ, Cunningham MA. "Evidence-based dentistry skill acquisition by second-year dental students." *Eur J Dent Educ.* 2018 doi:10.1111/ eje.12364.

15. Marshall TA, Straub-Morarend, Guzman-Armstrong S, Handoo N. "Evidence-based dentistry: assessment to document progression to proficiency." *Eur J Dent Edu.* 2016 doi:10.1111eje.12202.

16. Ilic D, Nordin R, Glasziou P, Tilson J, Villanueva E. "A randomized controlled trial of a blended learning education intervention for teaching evidence-based medicine." *BMC Med Edu.* 2015;15:39.

17. Marshall TA, Straub-Morarend CL, Qian F, Finkelstein MW. "Perceptions and practices of dental school faculty regarding evidence-based dentistry." *J Dent Educ.* 2013;77(2):146-151.

18. Spallek H, Song M, Polk DE, Bekhuis T, Frantsve-Hawley J, Aravamudhan K. "Barriers to implementing evidence-based clinical guidelines: a survey of early adopters." *J Evid Based Dent Pract.* 2010;10(4):195-206.

19. Werb SB, Matear DW. "Implementing evidence-based practice in undergraduate teaching clinics: a systematic review and recommendations." *J Dent Educ.* 2004;68(9):995-1003.

20. ADA Center for Evidence-Based Dentistry. *https://ebd.ADA.org/en* Accessed 3-27-19.

21. Coleman BG, Johnson TM, Erley KJ, Topolski R, Rethman M, Lancaster DD. "Preparing Dental Students and Residents to Overcome Internal and External Barriers to Evidence-Based Practice." *J Dent Educ.* 2016;80(10):1161-1169.

22. Guyatt G, Cairns J, Churchill D, et al. "Evidence-based medicine: a new approach to teaching the practice of medicine." *JAMA* 1992;268(17):2420-2425.

23. Polk DE, Nolan BA, Shah NH, Weyant RJ. "Policies and procedures that facilitate implementation of evidence-based clinical guidelines in U.S. dental schools." *J Dent Educ.* 2016;80(1):23-9.

Chapter 16. Implementing Evidence into Practice

Satish S. Kumar, D.M.D., M.D.Sc., M.S.; Ben Balevi, D.D.S., M.Sc.; Rebecca Schaffer, D.D.S.; Romesh Nalliah, D.D.S., M.H.C.M.; Martha Ann Keels, D.D.S., Ph.D.; Norman Tinanoff, D.D.S., M.S.; and Robert J. Weyant, D.M.D., Dr.P.H., M.S.

Defining the Scope of Implementation Science

The National Institutes of Health (NIH) defines implementation science as the "study of methods to promote the adoption and integration of evidence-based practices, interventions, and policies into routine health care and public health settings."[1] NIH acknowledges that the scope of implementation science is broad and by necessity includes understanding what motivates the behavior of health professionals, organizational change theory, how consumers and policymakers influence the adoption of new evidence, and how factors such as culture and health care financing impact program sustainability and improve health outcomes.

The empirical basis of implementation science is rapidly maturing and now provides a framework for the effective implementation of evidence-based practices. This chapter provides an overview of the current evidence of best practices in implementation science. At its most elemental, implementation research shows that mere dissemination of the best available evidence is insufficient to produce effective and sustainable change in routine care delivery in most clinical settings. Simply publishing clinical practice guidelines (CPGs), systematic reviews (SRs), and other types of evidence and hoping that it will be read and adopted into routine care is not supported by research. Producing and disseminating evidence is a necessary step but is far from enough for achieving adoption of an evidence-based practice into routine care. The adoption of evidence into routine practice requires that evidence be accompanied by an implementation plan that addresses the barriers to full implementation.

Even in its simplest form, implementation science focuses on system-level change, and that implies that barriers to implementation will exist and must be addressed at multiple levels. Changing the behavior of individual providers is without question needed for successful implementation, but achieving that in a sustainable manner requires higher level system interventions, as individual-level behavior is in large part determined by system-level forces. For example, adopting a new clinical process may require the development of staff training programs and deployment of monitoring processes to check and reward compliance. Changing clinical practice may impact clinical revenue or be counter to patient expectations. Such barriers must be anticipated and addressed, or the implementation will likely fail. Changes to clinical practice may also result in anxiety among staff if they feel that a new clinical care process is outside the current standard of care, triggering fear that can lead to staff noncompliance. In short, many systems (for example, dental clinics) are stable and inherently resistant to change.

When a new clinical practice is proposed, there are many factors that can work to resist the change. What implementation science attempts to do is determine where such resistance will likely occur and develop strategies to overcome it such that sustainable implementation is the result. Current implementation research can be a valuable guide when anticipating sources of resistance to change and selecting effective intervention strategies. But implementation research also clearly tells us that each clinical setting is unique, and any implementation plan will require local adaptions.

Provided below is an overview of the main issues that are salient for implementation of evidence-based practices into routine dental care settings. Examples of these settings are small private dental offices, large multiprovider group practices, and dental schools. The goal is to highlight important lessons from implementation science literature that would likely apply to these settings. This is not an implementation manual, but rather an attempt to sensitize the reader to the various, often complex issues that must be attended to for an implementation plan to succeed.

Even in its simplest form, implementation science focuses on system-level change, and that implies that barriers to implementation will exist and must be addressed at multiple levels.

Translation of Scientific Evidence to Clinical Practice

Clinical decision-making is often made under conditions of uncertainty. To quote Sir William Osler, clinical practice "is a science of uncertainty and an art of probability."[2] As such, the likelihood of a clinical decision resulting in a desired outcome is, in part, related to the certainty in the available information the decision is based on. The adoption of evidence-based dentistry (EBD) approaches to clinical practice aims to optimize oral health clinical decisions to individual patient care by integrating scientific research evidence with clinician expertise and patient values and preferences.[3] Patients rely on the oral health professional to be an expert in the oral health sciences and to be current in relevant scientific knowledge and its application to dental care. The degree to which oral health professionals maintain up-to-date expertise depends on several factors, such as the quality and availability of evidence, the mode of evidence dissemination, and the ability of clinicians to implement that evidence in routine patient care. Many CPGs are not effectively translated to clinical practice, and consequently, health outcomes may suffer. Several barriers make this translation challenging. It is the role of translational science researchers and the field of implementation science to identify these barriers to implementation and develop strategies to overcome them.

Pitts describes the process of translating scientific evidence to clinical practice as consisting of three phases.[4,5,6] The first phase is the synthesis of current evidence to answer a specific clinical question. This involves identifying, selecting, summarizing, and critically appraising relevant clinical research. This process results in an SR (see Chapter 6) that summarizes the desirable and undesirable consequences of an intervention (beneficial and harm outcomes) and assesses the certainty of the evidence (that is, an assessment of potential issues of risk of bias, imprecision, inconsistency, indirectness, and publication bias) (see Chapter 14).

Phase two is the dissemination of the evidence. Typically, for an SR, this is through publication and conference presentations as well as through the creation of synopsis documents in journals such as *Evidence-Based Dentistry,*[7] the *Journal of Evidence-Based Dental Practice,*[8] and the *Journal of the American Dental Association,*[9] which publishes synopses via its JADA+ Clinical Scans section[10] (see Chapter 2). In some cases, the evidence provided by the review is used by an expert panel as the basis for development of a CPG (see Chapter 7). The National Academy of Medicine (NAM, formerly the Institute of Medicine) defines a CPG as "recommendation statements intended to optimize patient care that are informed by an SR of evidence and an assessment of the benefits and harms of alternative care options."[11] Good CPGs are often consensus statements derived from a thorough assessment of the reviewed scientific evidence and generalization of this evidence to individual patient care after consultation with stakeholders.[12,13]

The final phase in translating evidence to clinical practice is implementation, which occurs when the best available evidence is brought into routine clinical practice.

Four Phases of Implementation

Implementation of evidence relevant to clinical practice is a complex process affected by several factors such as individual and organizational characteristics, leadership, and funding. After reviewing several published processes of implementation, Aarons et al.[14] proposed a four-phase implementation process where each phase contains several inner and outer contextual factors (that is, contexts). In brief, the four phases of implementation are exploration, adoption decision/preparation, active implementation, and sustainment. Within each phase, the authors list various inner and outer contexts that must be taken into consideration for a successful phase. Examples of outer contexts are sociopolitical context (such as legislation and policies), funding, advocacy, interorganizational networks, and public–academic collaboration. Examples of inner contexts are organizational characteristics, individual adopter characteristics, leadership, and staffing. This chapter will discuss some key contexts relevant to dentistry within these four phases of implementation.

1. Exploration

Assessing the Need and Readiness for Change

The first step in the implementation process is to determine the need for change. Implementing new patient care practices should be based on a carefully documented care gap or quality gap analysis. This means that it can be shown that the care currently being provided differs in some important dimension from the optimal care delivery suggested by the current best available evidence. Examples of simple and effective methods to identify gaps are systematic data collection through surveys and audits.[15] In conducting a gap analysis, several issues need to be addressed. One such issue is the degree to which the staff (that is, all individuals involved in the care delivery system) are aware of deficiencies in their care delivery and perceive that change would be desirable. Successful implementation also depends on staff's readiness for change.

Understanding Issues and Theories of Behavior Change

Implementation is fundamentally a system-level process that considers barriers and facilitators both at the individual and organizational level. For example, implementing a new CPG in a multiprovider dental clinic will generally require changes in the knowledge and attitudes of individual providers, staff training procedures, patient workflow, financial or reimbursement models, clinic culture, and metrics that measure the care delivery process and outcomes. This requires the support of senior clinic managers and buy-in from line staff. Because of the need to address barriers at multiple levels, effective implementation generally depends on using proven strategies for both individual-level (that is, staff-level) change and organizational-level change.

Considering the complex processes involved in implementation, scientists have utilized theories of behavior change to predict and plan for challenges ahead of time to help the implementation processes go smoothly. Grol et al.[16] explain in detail various theories on factors that are related to individual professionals, social interactions and context, organizational context, and economics. Some of these theories provide a framework to begin predicting barriers and planning for the steps in implementation. An example of such a framework for implementation is the Consolidated Framework for Implementation Research (CFIR), which was proposed by Damschroder et al. in 2009 and has five domains:

intervention, inner setting, outer setting, individuals, and the implementation process. CFIR emphasizes the need to understand individual characteristics (for example, knowledge and beliefs about the intervention) as well as system-level characteristics (for example, organizational culture) to be effective.[17]

2. Adoption Decision/Preparation

Defining the Challenges and Barriers of Translating Best Evidence to Practice in Different Practice Settings

Commonly reported reasons for the failure to adopt new evidence into clinical practice are lack of time to keep abreast of new scientific information, economic factors associated with changes in care delivery, and concerns over how new approaches comport with standards of practice.[18,19,20] A brief discussion of some of these reasons follows:

- *Financial.* Financial concerns exist at every level of the health care system and can undermine any implementation plan. Anticipating and addressing financial issues are important steps that cannot be ignored. Unanticipated costs, such as those associated with staff training (and retraining when staff turn over), must be included in the plan. The impact of cost on patient demand may also need to be explored. For example, informing patients that the optimal treatment (for example, dental sealants) may not be covered by their insurance may result in unanticipated changes in clinical revenue. There may be upsides in clinical revenue as well. If, for example, a clinic chooses to provide dental sealants applied by expanded-function hygienists rather than restorations that require a dentist for the treatment of early carious lesions, staff salary costs per patient may decline.

  It is likely that even the most thoughtful review of cost issues will not fully anticipate the financial impact of changes to care delivery processes. Thus, an organization may need to be prepared for this impact until the new process becomes fully integrated into the clinical workflow and the delivery system is adjusted to accommodate the change. Using the sealant scenario above, there may be short-term losses in clinic revenue as a result of current insurance reimbursement restrictions. But in the longer term, a large clinic might change its staff model to align with the changing care delivery requirements. Additionally, a clinic could document the improved patient outcomes over the long term and address this with payers as part of a renegotiation of the reimbursement model.

  Dental schools are mandated by the Commission on Dental Accreditation (CODA) to create and implement evidence-based practice into curricula. This requires a significant investment of time, revenue, and multiple other resources in hiring, training, and calibrating faculty.[21] Public health organizations (such as community and school clinics, federally qualified health care centers, hospital emergency rooms, and private nonprofits) struggle with limited financial resources as well as significant staff turnover. Creating a culture of evidence-based practice can face significant hurdles. "Safety net" clinics, however, provide an excellent laboratory for exploring and designing workable models. Primary care is often offered under one roof, creating opportunity for interprofessional collaboration and information sharing. Prioritizing treatment according to established CPGs for preventive care (for example, CPGs on sealants or fluoride application) is a common practice in these settings, and outcomes can be measured provided there is financial support for the measurement of outcomes. At the private/group practice level, financial barriers to implementing EBD ranked high among dentists surveyed.[20] Traditional methods of reimbursement present a major challenge to the private practitioner. Reimbursement as a function of procedure, rather than diagnosis, can be a disincentive to implementing best available evidence into practice. Third-party insurer coverage rules may not align with EBD and standards of care, and plans might be incentivized to disregard them to limit company exposure. An excellent example of coverage rules that may not align with EBD is the use of pit-and-fissure sealants. There is moderate-quality evidence that shows that placing a sealant over a noncavitated lesion will arrest progression of decay.[22] However, some insurance companies may not reimburse for this procedure for premolars and/or patients over an arbitrary age limit.[23]

Issues with Medicaid reimbursement are beyond the scope of this chapter. However, approximately 40 million children are insured through Medicaid and the Children's Health Insurance Program,[24] and these numbers should not be ignored when analyzing barriers to implementing EBD. Rewarding providers who prioritize evidence-based practice for this population is worth studying.[25] Reimbursement issues rank high as a barrier for private practice.

In creating an EBD-friendly environment, the cost of supplies and equipment, return on investment, and training for the entire team must be considered—including the cost of access to evidence. The American Dental Association (ADA) provides access to CPGs and SRs on its EBD webpage,[26] and ADA members can access additional scientific research (for example, Cochrane SRs) through the ADA Library and Archives.[27] For nonmember practitioners with no university affiliation, however, there may be additional costs to accessing primary and secondary research papers.[26]

Finally, the reality is that for the average private practitioner, evidence-based practice takes time. For example, it takes more time to explain to a patient that treating an incipient lesion medically rather than surgically is, in certain scenarios, a preferred option. Patients need to give informed consent, be educated on home fluoride application, be given appropriate oral hygiene instruction (OHI), and receive professional monitoring. These efforts might not be reimbursed. At the consumer level, insurance reimbursement can influence treatment decisions more than evidence-based advice. Proposing and implementing an evidence-based treatment plan depends on many factors, such as ethical considerations and the patient's perceived value of treatment and oral health. Addressing oral health literacy in many consumer segments demands an enormous investment in time, reframing practice philosophy, and appropriate continuing education for one's dental team. None of this can take place without a partnership among all stakeholders in oral health.

> Proposing and implementing an evidence-based treatment plan depends on many factors, such as ethical considerations and the patient's perceived value of treatment and oral health.

- *Clinical awareness.* There are approximately 2.5 million scientific papers being published each year.[28] In 2014, there were 28,100 peer-reviewed journals in print and online. The incredible growth in literature has advantages and disadvantages. The obvious advantages are that we have much more information on various processes and interventions regarding what works and what doesn't. However, there is some evidence that the growing pool of literature is leading to scientists citing fewer and fewer publications.[29] This may mean that highly relevant but older papers are not being read anymore.

  Practicing dentists do not have the time to wade through the thousands of new dental articles that are published each year. However, they could benefit significantly from better understanding current research. Materials, equipment, and processes improve over time. SRs critically analyze multiple research studies on the same topic to provide a broad summary of the current literature to a particular research question. Critical summaries succinctly describe the pertinent findings of an SR. Online databases such as Epistemonikos provide access to such SRs and critical summaries of current research in dentistry.[30] Referencing these resources as an EBD practitioner represents an alteration in the way some clinicians have been taught to diagnose and treat patients in the past, when there was not a step to check the latest scientific evidence.

- *Evidence-based dentistry skill.* EBD is an important skill set that requires training, as detailed in the previous chapters. Fortunately, implementing EBD in large dental practice or school settings does not need to rely on the evidence selection skills of individual providers. Large organizations might instead have in place a committee of well-trained individuals to periodically review the scientific literature and select current best evidence for implementation. The new evidence could then be driven by organizational-level policy and adopted through best practices of implementation, such as staff training and incentives.

- *Staff training.* Without proper staff training, implementation with high fidelity is impossible for many clinical procedures and innovations. Thus, an appropriate staff (professional and nonprofessional) training plan should be adopted for each clinical procedure and innovation being implemented. This training plan should be fully developed and consider costs (both direct and opportunity costs), retraining frequency, fidelity monitoring, and the management of staff turnover (for example, consideration of new hires who require timely training before engaging in patient care, and changes in clinic leadership). In some settings, such as large group practices, the use of coaches who are highly trained and supportive can be important in increasing compliance and fidelity among the staff.

  Monitoring adoption and fidelity should also be an element of the training plan. Compliance monitoring is typically done through audit and feedback, thus giving each provider the information needed to monitor and manage their own performance. Fidelity is assessed in various ways (such as clinical chart review), again as a means of alerting each provider as to how well they are providing the desired care. The training plan should make clear that such oversight is a regular part of the plan for everyone and is not intended to reflect distrust of any individual provider or result in punitive action.

- *Information technology issues.* An appropriate, well-developed information technology (IT) infrastructure can help support an implementation plan. For example, if dental sealants are to be applied to noncavitated carious lesions, then an electronic health record must be able to capture the diagnosis and treatment plan accordingly. Evidence from implementation research also suggests that monitoring for fidelity and compliance with new clinical processes is generally required until these processes become the "new normal." This is known as audit and feedback. Thus, IT infrastructure must support periodic report generation that allows for the monitoring of both fidelity and compliance at the provider level.

- *Diagnostic codes.* Diagnostic codes are defined by the ADA as "a unique, alphanumeric string of characters that represents a disorder or disease concept. Diagnostic coding is the translation of written descriptions of diseases, illnesses, and injuries into standardized codes."[31] When used in conjunction with dental claims, codes on dental procedures and nomenclature (CDT codes) allow for an improved assessment of the appropriateness of care provided and can become an important element in a quality management program. These codes are derived from the International Statistical Classification of Diseases and Related Health Problems, 10th revision, Clinical Modification (ICD-10-CM).[32] At present, there is no universal obligation to use an ICD-10-CM code on dental claims, but there is a growing emphasis from payers on their use.

  The appropriate use of diagnostic codes within an implementation plan is just now developing in dentistry. It seems clear that they can provide a valuable contribution to the audit and feedback process and allow for measurement of the degree to which the implementation plan is succeeding. They can also provide feedback on the oral health of a patient population, track trends in oral health status, document fidelity to best practices, permit analysis of patient care services, and analyze the cost-effectiveness and quality of care. The Systematized Nomenclature of Dentistry (SNODENT) is a clinical terminology designed for use in dentistry and is compatible with electronic health and dental records.[33] One of its intended purposes is to provide standardized terms for describing dental disease.

- *Peer influence.* Peer influence can be an important factor requiring careful management for certain implementation plans to succeed. It is understood that dentists often tend to behave in ways they believe are consistent with their peers.[34] In so doing, they are reassured about the appropriateness of the care they provide. This desire to conform creates what might be considered a culture of care in a clinic or community, which can substantially influence decisions about how care is delivered. Managing peer influences can be challenging. Best practices in implementation science suggest that compliance reporting or audit and feedback can be of value when it shows a dentist that peer behavior follows the desired evidence-based practices. Such information can help a dentist to feel confident in adopting a new clinical procedure.

Peer influence can be an important factor requiring careful management for certain implementation plans to succeed. It is understood that dentists often tend to behave in ways they believe are consistent with their peers.[34]

Beyond simple compliance reporting, the use of champions or coaches who are respected peers, can play an important role. Coaches can provide prompt assistance to coachees when, for instance, questions arise around appropriate application of a CPG. Champions are respected thought leaders who, by demonstrating their support of an evidence-based approach, can legitimize its use among others.

- *Policy issues.* Within a clinical setting, senior leadership (for example, clinic directors) plays an important role by setting policy around how care should be delivered and how quality and compliance will be assessed. Central to the success of any implementation plan is support from senior leadership for the plan. Through policy guidance, leadership should make clear the importance of the plan and provide details that describe how the plan will be supported (for example, training, workflow changes, and incentive plans) and how fidelity will be monitored (for example, audit and feedback).

- *Organizational barriers and facilitators.* Like most organizations, dental clinics are complex systems. They are made up of care providers and patients who are interacting and responding to clinical, financial, social, and other forces that structure their behavior. Systems are inherently stable and tend to continue to perform in a consistent manner until interventions alter that behavior. An implementation plan is designed to be such an intervention. Effective implementation plans must address in detail the system of care delivery and what barriers and facilitators of change exist within the system. Barriers that need to be addressed are context-specific, meaning that what barriers exist and how they can be removed will vary from clinic to clinic and, just as importantly, from innovation to innovation (for example, implementing a CPG). Although it is hard to generalize what a successful approach will look like, general categories of barriers exist within a clinical setting that need to be considered. Examples of such barriers are lack of knowledge, skill, and openness to change among the professional staff; lack of awareness of an innovation; lack of incentives to change; lack of outcome expectancy; and lack of self-efficacy. Examples of external barriers contributing to these issues are patient and CPG factors such as patient preferences and CPG characteristics, respectively. Multiple environmental factors can also play a role, such as lack of time, lack of resources, reimbursement issues, malpractice liability, and organizational constraints.[35,36]

3. Active Implementation

How to Implement a Clinical Practice Guideline in Various Dental Settings

Judgment is the process by which a conclusion or decision is reached after careful thought and reasoning. The stronger the rationale used to reach that conclusion or decision, the easier it will be to defend. Therefore, because each patient brings his or her own unique circumstances to a clinical problem, the decision to manage that patient's health must consider the context of the environment and be respectful of that patient's autonomy in making a decision in their best interest based on the evidence available to them. In other words, judgment is a shared decision between the clinician and the patient made on the pertinence of the relevant clinical research. The challenge here is figuring out how to apply data from clinical research articles to the needs and values of the individual patient.

The mission of every oral health care professional is to implement quality care for individual patients. The Agency for Healthcare Research and Quality defines quality health care as "the degree to which health care services for individuals and populations increase the likelihood of desired health outcomes and are consistent with current professional knowledge."[37] The phrase "current professional knowledge" implies EBD. In addition, the six aims for health care systems, according to the NAM, are that they are the following:

1. Safe
2. Effective
3. Patient-centered
4. Timely
5. Efficient
6. Equitable

In other words, the mission of every clinical practice is to get "the right care at the right time to the right patient."[38] Implementing such a mission requires not only the application of EBD to clinical decision-making but also the development of an implementation strategy, which often means a successful change in the culture and systems currently used to manage patient care.

The Institute for Healthcare Improvement (IHI) is an organization that promotes the advancement of better health outcomes.[39] It has many resources to help health care providers effectively implement best practices. For example, one approach it promotes is the Model for Improvement (MFI). For this model to be successful, it is important that a clinical practice has a willingness to change ideas and is committed to executing that change. The MFI is based on addressing three fundamental questions followed by engaging in an iterative system of executing and sustaining change in clinical practice. The three questions are as follows:

1. What are we trying to accomplish?
2. How will we know a change is an improvement?
3. What change can we make that will result in an improvement?

The application of the MFI in clinical practice is a five-step systematic approach to achieving sustainable change. As an example of such an application, the following section describes how the ADA CPG on the nonsurgical treatment of chronic periodontitis (CP) was used to implement the best available evidence to patient care in a private general dental practice (Table 16.1). The parameters discussed were selected by one of the authors (B.B.), a general practitioner, and customized to his patient population. Hence the discussion on MFI application is not a definitive recommendation. Instead, it is presented as an example of how one clinician used the MFI in clinical practice for the implementation of a CPG.

Table 16.1. The Institute for Healthcare Improvement's Five-Step Process for Implementing Change[38]

Step	Process	Description	Example
1	Set an aim.	A general statement (for example, "We will improve our infection rate") isn't good enough. The aim statement should be time-specific and measurable, stating exactly "How good?" "By when?" and "For whom?"	Ninety-five percent of patients diagnosed with chronic periodontitis (CP) will need only maintenance care six months after active treatment. OR The referral rate for patients with CP (active disease) will go from the current level of 25% to 5% in six months.
2	Establish metrics.	You need feedback to know if a specific change leads to an improvement, and quantitative measures can often provide the best feedback.	*Periodontal outcomes:* • Objective criteria of periodontal parameters such as bleeding on probing (BOP) and probing depth. *Patient-centered outcomes:* • Halitosis: Yes or No Patient-perceived status of their oral health: • Good: if score ≥7 on a visual analog scale • Not good: if score <7
3	Identify the change.	How are you going to achieve your aim? Where do new ideas come from? You can spark creative thinking in various ways, and there are tools that can help.	Implementation of the American Dental Association clinical practice guideline (CPG) on the nonsurgical treatment of CP
4	Test the change.	This is where the planning, doing, studying, and acting (PDSA) cycle portion of the Model for Improvement comes in. By planning a test of change, trying the plan, observing the results, and acting on what you learn, you will progressively move toward your aim.	During the PDSA cycle, at least five problems and barriers were identified and managed.
5	Implement the change.	After you have a change that results in an improvement under many conditions, the logical next step is to implement it—that is, make the change the new standard process in one defined setting.	The ADA CPG is adopted as a standard of care in the practice and regularly monitored.

- *Step 1: Set an aim.* Almost half of the U.S. adult population has periodontitis, and a majority of these cases involve the mild to moderate form of chronic periodontitis (CP).[40] As such, CP is a common diagnosis in clinical practice. The goal of the practice in this particular example was to improve the periodontal health of patients by initiating a periodontal treatment protocol that would achieve the delivery of safe, effective, accessible, and less costly care to patients. Considering the prevalence of severe periodontitis is about 5% to 15% of those with CP, it was determined that an achievable goal for the practice would be to have 85% of the practice's CP cases successfully maintained in the general practice setting. Success was defined as a patient with positive periodontal and patient-centered outcomes after three months of initiating care for active disease. Patients with successful outcomes were then transferred to periodontal maintenance care and remained in maintenance care if they continued to show positive periodontal and patient-centered outcomes during regularly scheduled hygiene appointments (that is, appointments occurring every three to 12 months, depending on the level of periodontal suffering and risk).

- *Step 2: Establish metrics.* CP is defined by the American Academy of Periodontology as "an infectious disease resulting in inflammation within the supporting tissues of the teeth [and] progressive attachment and bone loss"; it "is characterized by pocket formation and/or gingival recession" and "is recognized as the most frequently occurring form of periodontitis."[41] Patient periodontal status was a binary outcome. Either a patient was diagnosed with CP or they were not. The periodontal outcomes were binary: Observing gingival bleeding on probing (BOP) and an increased probing depth (PD) or gingival recession (GR) after treatment (compared with initial readings) constituted active disease. Patient-centered outcomes were whether a patient reported halitosis and a score of seven or greater on a visual analog scale asking how they felt about their periodontal health. A threshold of seven or greater was established after a preliminary survey of new patients in the practice with CP gave an average score between three and four.

- *Step 3: Identify the change.* The goal of the practice was to improve the periodontal health of patients and hence decrease the need for referrals of patients diagnosed with CP to a periodontal specialist from the current level of 25% to 5%. To achieve this aim, a two-pronged approach was conceived: delivering treatment to the patient in the clinic and then following up with the patient after at least three months to assess periodontal and patient-centered outcomes. Historically, the clinic's first line of treatment for CP was nonsurgical therapy (scaling and root planing) followed by OHI. However, the practice wondered if there were better therapies than the traditional nonsurgical therapy used to manage CP. In other words, the benefits of interventions such as antibiotics, mouthwashes, lasers, and interdental cleaning devices (for example, interdental brushes) for the management of CP needed to be better understood.

The PICO (population, intervention, comparison, outcomes) questions facing the clinic can be summarized as follows:

1. In patients with CP, do interventions such as antibiotics, lasers, and mouthwashes compared with nonsurgical scaling and root planing reduce gingival BOP and reduce or maintain healthy PD or GR?

2. In patients with CP, does the use of interdental cleaning devices compared with flossing alone reduce gingival BOP and reduce or maintain healthy PD or GR?

3. In patients with CP, does nonsurgical scaling and root planing compared with no treatment reduce halitosis?

4. Do patients with CP report that their mouths feel healthier after nonsurgical therapy (such as scaling and root planing) compared with no treatment?

To answer these questions, a search was conducted of the current scientific evidence. The first question was appropriately addressed by the ADA CPG on the nonsurgical treatment of CP.[42] This CPG was informed by an exhaustive SR of all the scientific literature up to the date of the CPG's publication.[43] This CPG strongly recommends nonsurgical therapy (scaling and root planing) as the first line of treatment for CP and states that there is limited evidence of the benefit of adjunctive therapies such as systemic or localized antibiotics and lasers and that these therapies come with a risk of harm and/or significant cost.

A Cochrane database of SRs contained an article that addressed the second question. Although the article was unable to find a difference in PD or GR between interdental cleaning devices and flossing alone, it did report interdental cleaning devices in conjunction with flossing improved gingivitis scores by half compared with flossing alone.[44,45] Unfortunately, there are no SRs that address the association between halitosis and CP. The Centers for Disease Control and Prevention reports halitosis as a possible sign of periodontitis.[46] Furthermore, this association appears to be supported through some scientific evidence published in primary studies and a narrative review.[47,48,49]

- *Step 4: Test the change.* Armed with the evidence and knowledge above, the practice developed the following preliminary protocol to pilot. The MFI describes the testing of change as an integrative process of planning, doing, studying, and acting (PDSA) (Figure 16.1). All patients were thoroughly examined, and baseline periodontal and patient-centered outcomes were recorded and followed by a health literacy session in which a dental health educator taught patients about general oral health, periodontal disease, and treatment options. Patients were initially diagnosed with CP based on the clinical finding of BOP and radiographic evidence of periodontal bone loss. If a patient consented to treatment, they were then referred to a dental hygienist for nonsurgical periodontal therapy and OHI.

Figure 16.1. Flowchart for Implementing ADA Clinical Practice Guideline on the Nonsurgical Treatment of Chronic Periodontitis

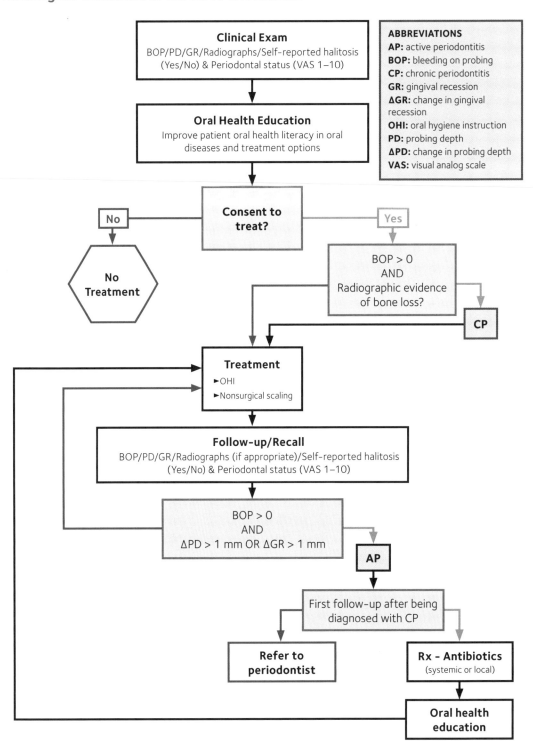

Clinical Exam
BOP/PD/GR/Radiographs/Self-reported halitosis (Yes/No) & Periodontal status (VAS 1–10)

Oral Health Education
Improve patient oral health literacy in oral diseases and treatment options

Consent to treat?

No

No Treatment

Yes

BOP > 0 AND Radiographic evidence of bone loss?

CP

Treatment
► OHI
► Nonsurgical scaling

Follow-up/Recall
BOP/PD/GR/Radiographs (if appropriate)/Self-reported halitosis (Yes/No) & Periodontal status (VAS 1–10)

BOP > 0 AND ΔPD > 1 mm OR ΔGR > 1 mm

AP

First follow-up after being diagnosed with CP

Refer to periodontist

Rx – Antibiotics
(systemic or local)

Oral health education

ABBREVIATIONS
AP: active periodontitis
BOP: bleeding on probing
CP: chronic periodontitis
GR: gingival recession
ΔGR: change in gingival recession
OHI: oral hygiene instruction
PD: probing depth
ΔPD: change in probing depth
VAS: visual analog scale

Patients were re-evaluated three months later. If their score met the minimum desired outcome, the patient was referred to the regular maintenance protocol. If the patient continued to show signs of BOP, the patient underwent another session of nonsurgical therapy and OHI. Also, if there was a less than 1 mm increase in the PD or GR, the patient underwent another session of nonsurgical scaling with adjunctive care (that is, systemic or localized antibiotic therapy). If the patient exhibited two consecutive follow-up sessions with an increase in PD, the patient was referred to a periodontal specialist for further assessment. In other words, if after the second session (that is, more than 6 months from the initiation of active treatment) the patient continued to show clinical evidence of periodontal disease progression (BOP and increased PD and GR), the patient was referred to a periodontal specialist.

Because there is limited evidence to establish the extent to which the benefits of using laser therapy outweigh the potential harms, the practice decided that it was not cost-effective for them to offer this service. The equipment is expensive, and because the prevalence of nonresponsive CP is low in the population of patients the practice serves, it was decided that the cost of acquiring this technology could not be justified. Nevertheless, the practice made all patients aware of this technology and the paucity of evidence supporting this technology.

The plan was evaluated after the first six months (that is, the studying step). After executing the plan over two sessions (that is, the doing step), the referral rate was down by about half. Although in 88% of patients, PD and GR were stable or decreased, about 12% continued to show BOP. At this point, a review of the protocol and an evaluation of the delivery of care was discussed with all members of the caring team to try to identify and resolve any barriers, problems, and deficiencies. For example, some patients were not given take-home instruction sheets because the office ran out of them. Also, many patients could not find or access the practice's webpage featuring videos on how to floss and maintain oral health. Adjustments within the system were made to eliminate these barriers.

During a second PDSA cycle, it was noted that some patients did not follow through with OHI or disclosed a systemic medical condition that may be associated with less-than-optimal outcomes (for example, a change in medication, cancer diagnosis, or recent period of stress that resulted in oral neglect). This was new information that was not considered when the initial protocol was developed. As such, rather than refer these patients to a specialist, the clinician addressed these specific risk factors by again educating and reviewing OHI with the patient as well as by consulting with a physician to adjust the patient's medication or to address a possible medical health issue. Please see the adjusted protocol in Figure 16.2.

Figure 16.2. Flowchart of Modified Planning, Doing, Studying, and Acting (PDSA) Cycle for Implementing ADA Clinical Practice Guideline on the Nonsurgical Treatment of Chronic Periodontitis

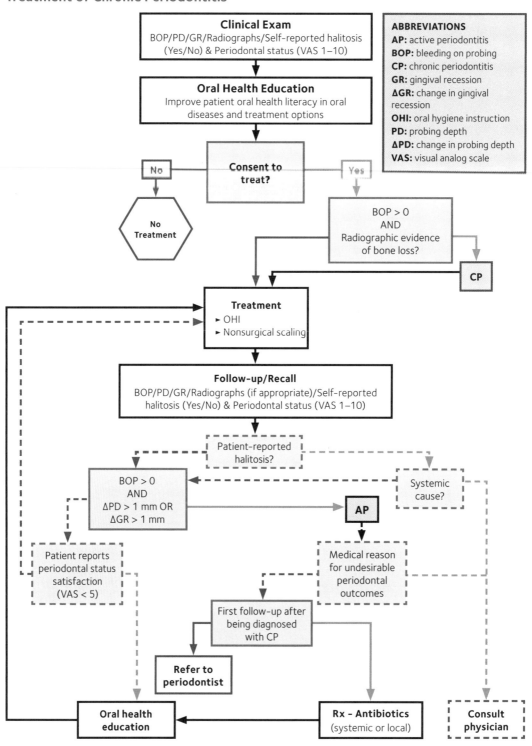

Clinical Exam
BOP/PD/GR/Radiographs/Self-reported halitosis
(Yes/No) & Periodontal status (VAS 1–10)

Oral Health Education
Improve patient oral health literacy in oral
diseases and treatment options

Consent to treat?

No → **No Treatment**

Yes →

BOP > 0
AND
Radiographic evidence
of bone loss?

CP

Treatment
➤ OHI
➤ Nonsurgical scaling

Follow-up/Recall
BOP/PD/GR/Radiographs (if appropriate)/Self-reported
halitosis (Yes/No) & Periodontal status (VAS 1–10)

Patient-reported
halitosis?

BOP > 0
AND
ΔPD > 1 mm OR
ΔGR > 1 mm

Systemic
cause?

AP

Patient reports
periodontal status
satisfaction
(VAS < 5)

Medical reason
for undesirable
periodontal
outcomes

First follow-up after
being diagnosed
with CP

**Refer to
periodontist**

**Oral health
education**

Rx – Antibiotics
(systemic or local)

**Consult
physician**

ABBREVIATIONS
AP: active periodontitis
BOP: bleeding on probing
CP: chronic periodontitis
GR: gingival recession
ΔGR: change in gingival recession
OHI: oral hygiene instruction
PD: probing depth
ΔPD: change in probing depth
VAS: visual analog scale

Another problem that was identified after a few PDSA iterations was that some patients who showed improvement in periodontal outcomes were still complaining of halitosis or did not see value in the care they were receiving. To test the suspicions of patients who believed that their halitosis was not improving, a hygienist conducted a smell test. If this test proved that a patient's halitosis had not improved, the patient was referred to their physician for an assessment of other systemic etiology. And the few patients who showed improved periodontal outcomes but did not feel any value in it were referred to a health care educator to reinforce the benefit of the care to overall health.

Other patient-centered barriers to implementation were noted. For example, health care educators were not reimbursed by Medicaid, thus making them reluctant to provide the service. Also, some third-party private insurers would not adequately reimburse patients for OHI or would limit the number of times periodontal scaling and root planing could be provided per year to fewer times than what was deemed necessary. This made patients reluctant to follow through with the proposed treatment.

To overcome these barriers, the clinic offered oral hygiene and health literacy sessions to groups of patients at a nominal fee. It was deemed that the number of patients who were not fully subsidized was small and most of them felt that education was valuable enough that they were willing to pay the out-of-pocket difference. This cycle of PDSA continued with the aim of seamlessly achieving the predictable change desired (Figure 16.2).

- *Step 5: Implement the change.* The above PDSA cycle of testing change went through many iterations before the goal of a 95% retention rate was achieved. Once the protocol was perfected, constant clinical evaluation was then required to monitor how well implementation was working. It is critical to regularly and continuously monitor the implementation protocol because changing behavior is difficult and it is human nature to want to revert to old ways. Also, it is important that dental practices are prepared to make adjustments as new evidence becomes available.

In summary, the example mentioned above demonstrates how to implement an EBD CPG into clinical practice using a well-established and validated implementation approach. A continued commitment to implementation will ensure that the quality of care delivered by the clinic meets the six aims of health care quality established by the NAM that were previously mentioned in this chapter.

4. Sustainment

Establishing an Ongoing Process for Finding the Latest Evidence

As discussed earlier in this chapter, one of the main barriers to implementing the latest evidence in clinical practice is a lack of awareness of the latest evidence. Establishing an ongoing process for finding the best available evidence will be valuable for any practice. As discussed earlier, there are numerous online resources that provide direct links to the latest evidence. Some examples are the ADA Center for EBD,[3] Cochrane,[50] JADA+ Clinical Scans,[10] and Epistemonikos[30] (see Chapter 2). Automatic e-mail reminders and updates can be set up from these resources to ensure that clinicians stay up-to-date on the latest evidence.

Issues in Program Sustainability

Successful implementation plans require strategies to sustain the plan over the long term. Once initial implementation has achieved the goal of widespread adoption with fidelity, ongoing monitoring must be maintained. There are many forces that could ultimately derail a plan over the long term. A change in clinic leadership could alter support for an innovation such as the implementation of a CPG. Similarly, staff transitions will result in the need to train new hires. Changes in reimbursement for the innovation could impact clinic revenue. Of course, many other factors, which are often unanticipated, can impact the sustainability of a clinical innovation. Successful and sustainable implementation depends on the ability to adapt to these changing factors.

Conclusion

The goal of implementing EBD into clinical practice is to optimize patient care by integrating scientific evidence with clinician expertise and patient values and preferences. There are many barriers to this implementation. For instance, it can be difficult to stay abreast of the ever-expanding scientific evidence while at the same time managing the economic and regulatory challenges of a busy clinic and focusing on the delivery of patient care. To combat this difficulty, there are many resources available to dental practices that can bring relevant scientific evidence to the optimization of patient care. However, access to these resources alone is likely not enough to change clinical practice. A validated approach to implementing the best available scientific evidence created by the entire oral health care team is necessary to achieve quality patient care. The MFI protocol based on the PDSA cycle described by IHI is one such approach to executing and sustaining change in clinical practice. Successfully implementing change through this approach will help ensure that the quality of care delivered by the clinic meets the six aims of health care quality established by the NAM.

References

1. National Institutes of Health Fogarty International Center. "Implementation Science Information and Resources." *https://www.fic.nih.gov/ResearchTopics/Pages/ImplementationScience.aspx*. Accessed on February 5, 2018.

2. Sir William Osler, Mark E. Silverman, T. J. Murray, Charles S. Bryan, American College of Physicians—American Society of Internal Medicine (2008). *The Quotable Osler* Revised Paperback edition, p.46, ACP Press.

3. American Dental Association Center for Evidence-Based Dentistry *http://www.ebd.ADA.org*.

4. Pitts N. "Understanding the jigsaw of evidence-based dentistry: 1. Introduction, research and synthesis." *Evid Based Dent*. 2004; 5:2-4.

5. Pitts N. "Understanding the jigsaw of evidence-based dentistry. 2. Dissemination of research results." *Evid Based Dent*. 2004; 5(2):33-5.

6. Pitts N. "Understanding the jigsaw of evidence-based dentistry. 3. Implementation of research findings in clinical practice." *Evid Based Dent*. 2004; 5(3):60-4.

7. *Evidence-Based Dentistry. https://www.nature.com/ebd.*

8. *Journal of Evidence-Based Dental Practice. https://www.sciencedirect.com/journal/journal-of-evidence-based-dental-practice.*

9. *Journal of the American Dental Association. https://jada.ADA.org .*

10. *Journal of the American Dental Association* (JADA) Clinical Scans. *http://jada.ADA.org/clinicalscans*.

11. Institute of Medicine. 2011. *Clinical Practice Guidelines We Can Trust*. Washington, DC: The National Academies Press.

12. Appraisal of Guidelines and Research Evaluation (AGREE). *http://www.agreetrust.org*.

13. Richards D. "Appraising guidelines: the AGREE Instrument." *Evid Based Dent*. 2002;3:109-110.

14. Aarons GA, Hurlburt M, Horwitz SM. "Advancing a conceptual model of evidence-based practice implementation in public service sectors." *Adm Policy Ment Health*. 2011 Jan; 38(1):4-23.

15. McCluskey A. "Implementing Evidence into Practice." In: *Evidence-Based Practice across the Health Professions*. Edited by Hoffmann T, Bennett S, Del Mar C. Second Ed. 2013.

16. Grol R, Wensing M, Bosch M, Hulscher M, Eccles M. "Theories of Implementation of Change in Healthcare." In: *Improving Patient Care: The Implementation of Change in Health Care*. Edited by Grol R, Wensing M, Eccles M. 2013. John Wiley & Sons, Ltd.

17. Damschroder LJ, Aron DC, Keith RE, Kirsh SR, Alexander JA, Lowery JC. "Fostering implementation of health services research findings into practice: a consolidated framework for advancing implementation science." *Implement Sci*. 2009 Aug 7;4:50.

18. Isham A, et al. "A Systematic Literature Review of the Information-Seeking Behavior of Dentists in Developed Countries." *J Dent Ed* (2016) 80:569-577.

19. Fox C, et al. "Evidence-based dentistry – overcoming the challenges for the UK's dental practitioners." *BDJ* (2014) 217, 191-94.

20. Spallek H, et al. "Barriers to implementing evidence-based clinical guidelines: A survey of early adopters." *J Evid Based Dent Pract*. 2010 December; 10(4): 195-206.

21. Accreditation Standards for Dental Education Programs; Standards for Predoctoral Dental Education: Commission on Dental Accreditation: *www.ADA.org/coda*.

22. Wright JT, Crall JJ, Fontana M, Gillette EJ, Novy BB Dhar V, Donly K, Hewlett ER, Quinonez RB, et al. "Evidence-based clinical practice guideline for the use of pit-and-fissure sealants: A report of the American Dental Association and the American Academy of Pediatric Dentistry." (2016) *J Am Dent Assoc*, 147(8) 672-682e12.

23. Kao RT. "The challenges of transferring evidence-based dentistry into practice." *J Evid Based Dent Pract* 2006;6(1):125-8.

24. *Medicaid.gov: www.medicaid.gov/chap/download/fy-2016-childrens-enrollment-report.pdf*; accessed July 14, 2017.

25. Committee on Redesigning Health Insurance Performance Measures PaPIP, Board on Health Care Services. *Rewarding provider performance: aligning incentives in Medicare*. Washington, DC: National Academies Press; 2007.

26. Richards D. "American Dental Association evidence-based dentistry website." *Evid Based Dent* 2009;10:59-60.

27. ADA Library & Archives. *www.ADA.org/en/member-center/ada-library*.

28. *www.stm-assoc.org/2015_02_20_STM_Report_2015.pdf.*

29. Evans JA. "Electronic publication and the narrowing of science and scholarship." *Science*. 2008 Jul 18; 321(5887):395-9.

30. *www.epistemonikos.org.*

31. *www.ADA.org/en/member-center/member-benefits/practice-resources/dental-informatics/standard-terminologies-and-codes/faq-icd-10-cm.*

32. *International Classification of Diseases,* Tenth Revision, Clinical Modification (ICD-10-CM). *www.cdc.gov/nchs/icd/icd10cm.htm.*

33. SNODENT User Guide, March, 2014, Available at: *http://www.ADA.org/~/media/ADA/Member%20Center/FIles/SNODENT_User_Guide_Final.pdf?la=en.* Accessed on Oct. 25, 2017.

34. Matthews DC, McNeil K, Brillant M, Tax C, Maillet P, McCulloch CA, Glogauer M. "Factors Influencing Adoption of New Technologies into Dental Practice: A Qualitative Study." *JDR Clin Trans Res*. 2016 Apr;1(1):77-85.

35. Yamalik, N., et al. (2015). "Implementation of evidence-based dentistry into practice: analysis of awareness, perceptions and attitudes of dentists in the World Dental Federation—European Regional Organization zone." *Int Dent J*, 65. 127–145.

36. Cabana MD, Rand CS, Powe NR, Wu AW, Wilson MH, Abboud PA, Rubin HR. "Why don't physicians follow clinical practice guidelines? A framework for improvement." *JAMA*. 1999 Oct 20;282(15):1458-65.

37. Agency for Healthcare Research and Quality *www.ahrq.gov.*

38. *Crossing the Quality Chasm: A New Health System for the 21st Century Committee on Quality of Health Care in America, Institute of Medicine.* Washington, DC, USA: National Academies Press; 2001.

39. Institute for Healthcare Improvement *www.ihi.org.*

40. Eke P et al. "Prevalence of periodontitis in adults in the United States: 2009 and 2010." *J Dent Res*. (2012) 91:914-20.

41. American Academy of Periodontology *www.perio.org.*

42. Smiley CJ et al. "Evidence-based clinical practice guideline on the nonsurgical treatment of chronic periodontitis by means of scaling and root planing with or without adjuncts." *J Am Dent Assoc*. (2015) 146:525-35.

43. Smiley CJ et al. "Systematic review and meta-analysis on the nonsurgical treatment of chronic periodontitis by means of scaling and root planing with or without adjuncts." *J Am Dent Assoc*. (2015) 146:508-24.e5.

44. Sambunjak D et al. "Flossing for the management of periodontal diseases and dental caries in adults." *Cochrane Database Syst Rev*. 2011 Dec 7;(12):CD008829. DOI: 10.1002/14651858.CD008829.

45. Poklepovic T et al. "Interdental brushing for the prevention and control of periodontal diseases and dental caries in adults." Cochrane Database Syst Rev. 2013 Dec 18;(12):CD009857. DOI: 10.1002/14651858.CD009857.

46. Oral Health: Periodontal Disease; U.S. Centers for Disease Control and Prevention. *www.cdc.gov/oralhealth/periodontal_disease/index.htm.*

47. De Geest S et al. "Periodontal diseases as a source of halitosis: a review of the evidence and treatment approaches for dentists and dental hygienists." *Periodontol* 2000. (2016)71 :213-27.

48. Ademovski E, et al. "The effect of periodontal therapy on intra-oral halitosis: a case series." *J Clin Periodontol*. (2016) 43:445-452.

49. Iatropoulos A, et al. "Changes of volatile sulphur compounds during therapy of a case series of patients with chronic periodontitis and halitosis." *J Clin Periodontol*. (2016) 43:359-65.

50. Cochrane Reviews. *www.cochranelibrary.com.*

Chapter 17. Health Policymaking Informed by Evidence

Jane Gillette, D.D.S., M.P.H.; Romesh Nalliah, D.D.S., M.H.C.M.; and Robert J. Weyant, D.M.D., Dr.P.H., M.S.

Introduction

Efficiently translating complex science into effective policy, as defined by the triple aim (that is, an improved patient experience in terms of satisfaction and quality, better population health, and reduced per capita cost of health care) is a central responsibility of the biomedical research and health care delivery community.[1] This responsibility is implied in the social contract underlying publicly supported research and care delivery as well as in the core values of health care professionals. Evidence-informed policy is the essential mechanism required for the conversion of scarce biomedical resources into improved population health outcomes. The challenge, in general, is engaging the relevant stakeholders in this process. Historically, because of a lack of resources devoted to the task, little attention was paid to the process of translating basic and clinical science research into broadly applied health-related policy. The so-called bench-to-bedside process was primarily reserved for pharmaceuticals with commercial potential. Fortunately, the focus on translational research was substantially broadened by the launch of the National Institutes of Health (NIH) Clinical and Translational Science Awards (CTSA) Program in 2006 and the subsequent creation of the NIH National Center for Advancing Translational Sciences in 2011,[2] resulting in more than 60 universities now supported to engage in the full range of translational research. CTSA supports the training of translational researchers, educating all researchers on their role in the translational process, and addresses policy barriers that impede efficient implementation of new discoveries into routine clinical practice.

As the primary purveyor of oral health care services, dentistry must rise to the challenge of supporting the profession's evidence base. The American Dental Association (ADA) has responded to this challenge through a variety of interconnected mechanisms aimed at supporting and advancing evidence-based practice and informing oral health policy in support of population health. These mechanisms include supporting policy decisions through development of high-quality systematic reviews and clinical practice guidelines. But much more work needs to be done.

Below we explore the process of how high-quality evidence can and should be used as the foundation for effective health policy, and we emphasize its importance within the oral health care system. In addition, we explore barriers and strategies relevant to the translational process. It is our goal to make the reader aware of the vital importance of bringing high-quality evidence to bear on the policy process and how that can most effectively be accomplished.

What Is Policy?

The challenge (and opportunity) in evidence-based health care is translating the science that we have into the decisions that we need to make. Organizations, institutions, and all levels of government use policies to define issues of significance and to formulate guidance and plans to address those issues. Science advocates such as academics, researchers, students, practicing dental professionals, and those working in government and public health can use the policymaking process to promote the uptake of science by those who oversee the health and opportunities of the public, communities, and patients.

The Centers for Disease Control and Prevention (CDC) defines policy "as a law, regulation, procedure, administrative action, incentive, or voluntary practice of governments and other institutions."[3] Policy in public health and health care is important because policy directs the parameters and actions that will be used to achieve the desired patient and population outcomes (Box 17.1).

> **Box 17.1. Evidence-Informed Policy in Action**
>
> In a 1967 address to Congress, President Lyndon Johnson used scientific evidence to advocate that all Medicaid-insured children have access to early health screenings and prevention:[4]
>
> > *"Recent studies confirm what we have long suspected: In education, in health, in all of human development, the early years are the critical years. Ignorance, ill health, personality disorder—these are disabilities often contracted in childhood: afflictions which linger to cripple the man and damage the next generation."*
>
> Through President Johnson's science advocacy, the Early and Periodic Screening, Diagnostic, and Treatment (EPSDT) benefit in Medicaid became policy.[5] EPSDT services are those services that are medically necessary to correct or ameliorate identified health conditions. There are many services that, if delivered early in life, can prevent or reduce disease and suffering in adulthood. All state Medicaid programs are required, according to federal policy, to cover these services, including immunization, vision, hearing, and dental services.[6]

There are five domains of the policy development process, each of which represents an opportunity for the integration of scientific evidence:[7]

- *Problem definition and identification.* Clarify the scope of the issue and its impact on population health. Multiple sources and types of data must be analyzed before coming to any conclusion. Proper identification of scope will facilitate successful implementation of change.

- *Policy analysis.* Identify different policy options to address the issue, and utilize quantitative and qualitative methods to comprehend the impact on health of each approach. Accurate analysis will help enable selection of the most efficient or suitable option.

- *Strategy and policy development.* Determine the strategy for effective adoption of policy and operational factors. Effective evaluation during the development process helps ensure successful enactment and implementation.

- *Policy enactment.* Define and enact internal and/or external processes. This step includes evaluation of the enactment process by identifying barriers that may impact implementation.

- *Policy implementation.* Translate the enacted policy into action, monitor adherence to the new policy, and ensure full implementation. The impact of the policy must be closely monitored to help ensure ongoing effectiveness.

Fundamental processes, such as stakeholder engagement and evaluation, provide additional opportunities to translate science. Policymakers gather input from partners, content experts, and target communities through a process called stakeholder engagement, which provides science advocates with the opportunity to participate in and provide input into the policymaking process. Evaluation, the formal assessment of a program's impact and outcomes, is another fundamental component of the policy process and a natural entry point for science; however, every step of the policy process should be informed by data and/or science when it exists. The interface between the evaluation process and science translation is discussed later in this chapter.

Responsible Policy Development

Policymakers have been urged, with good reason, to make evidence-informed decisions, as they are directly responsible for many high-stakes decisions that impact the well-being, productivity, and health of many.[8,9] Because of the heaviness of this responsibility, leaders in evidence-based health care have advocated that decision-making based on science should be the norm and not the exception. As noted by Chalmers:[10]

"Professional good intentions and plausible theories are insufficient for selecting policies and practices for protecting, promoting, and restoring health. Humility and uncertainty are preconditions for unbiased assessments of the effects of the prescriptions and proscriptions of policymakers and practitioners for other people. We will serve the public more responsibly and ethically when research designed to reduce the likelihood that we will be misled by bias and the play of chance has become an expected element of professional and policymaking practice, not an optional add-on."

The U.S. government spends about $30 billion per year on health care research, with the overall goal of improving the health outcomes of Americans and reducing health care costs.[11] Unfortunately, much of that research fails to find its way into policy decisions, and as a result, optimal health outcomes are not realized. It is not always clear why this translation fails, but a common reason is that high-quality evidence is not fully considered by policymakers. Failing to consider such things as the presentation of evidence that is in opposition to political philosophy, the influence of donors and advocacy groups, concerns over cost, lack of awareness of the evidence, and insufficient scientific literacy can hinder policymakers' ability to objectively evaluate evidence quality.

A study conducted in the U.K. found that policymakers had a broad definition of what constituted "evidence" and that they tended to rely on anecdotal stories and local data, even in the face of contradicting national data or research-based literature.[12] Another study conducted in the U.S. confirmed the tendency of policymakers to rely on constituent stories instead of scientific evidence.[13] For instance, one legislator interviewed in the study noted:

> "The other important source of information is certainly not an evidence-based approach, but there are a growing number of anecdotal reports coming really across the gamut from parents."

Another legislator said:

> "My experience has been . . . that these decisions [about what is important] are seldom made on a study or review of the studies that's out there, on evidence that may be provided. It's based on a much simpler approach of gut or something someone read in an article or something like that."

However, in general, policymakers acknowledged the importance of evidence-informed policymaking (EIPM):

> "[There is] overall interest in evidence-based practice that's floating around now. There's a lot of general discussion, both in some of the journals as well as in the government's view of how to move forward some of their programs."

"Moving forward programs" is likely the key benefit of EIPM. Similar to using evidence in patient care, the EIPM process systematically minimizes bias and maximizes objectivity, which results in many impacts that can "move forward programs," including:

- Improved outcomes by choosing policy options that work;
- Reduced waste by choosing policy options with a high return on investment and by retiring programs with poor results per dollars spent; and
- Greater accountability through more accurate and meaningful program monitoring and evaluation.

EIPM can be powerful as an advocacy tool when combined with individual stories to paint a picture of the perceived need more clearly and bring it down to the individual level. The practice of EIPM has direct benefits for policymakers as well. Inherent to evidence-based decision-making is an acknowledgment of one's level of confidence in the science and noted research gaps. This acknowledgment of the uncertainty in the science reduces political risk when programs do not achieve their intended outcomes; further, it sets the expectation that the course can be corrected (Box 17.2).[14]

> ## Box 17.2. What Is Evidence-Informed Policymaking?
>
> Evidence-informed policymaking is the systematic and transparent process by which policymakers access, appraise, and explicitly make judgments about the implications of policy options.[14] "Evidence-informed" is a more reflective term than "evidence-based" because policymakers must also consider other factors in their decision-making process. Often, these factors are equally compelling or in competition with one another. Such factors include community and society values, availability of required resources, degree of need, the priorities of the constituents or organizations involved, and, of course, cost.

Types of Evidence Used in Health Policy

Policymakers must consider a variety of evidence types when developing programs and making policy decisions (Box 17.3). Systematic reviews (see Chapter 6) and evidence-based clinical practice guidelines (see Chapter 7) are some of the fundamental types of scientific evidence employed in the EIPM process, and use of these resources helps policymakers answer focused questions and rate their level of confidence in the findings. However, the decisions that policymakers face almost always have economic and/or resource impacts, either for government entities or the public. As such, policymakers additionally rely on economic evaluations and health technology assessments. An economic evaluation systematically appraises the expected costs and effectiveness of a program or care approach and involves different outcome measures depending on the level of evaluation needed. Cost-of-illness analysis and program cost analysis measure the net costs of a disease or program, respectively. Program cost analysis is the first step to a more comprehensive set of analyses, including cost-benefit analysis (monetary value of costs compared with monetary value of benefits), cost-effectiveness analysis (costs compared with a health outcome), and cost-utility analysis (cost per quality-adjusted life-year [QALY] gained).[15]

> ## Box 17.3. Evidence Resources for Health Policy
> - The Guide to Community Preventive Services (guidelines for community health)
> - ECRI Guidelines Trust (guidelines)
> - U.S. Preventive Services Task Force (guidelines)
> - Effective Health Care Program (systematic reviews)
> - The Centre for Reviews and Dissemination (economic evaluations and health technology assessments)
> - Cochrane (systematic reviews and health technology assessments)
> - American Dental Association Center for Evidence-Based Dentistry (systematic reviews and guidelines)
> - Dental Quality Alliance
> - National Quality Forum

One step beyond an economic evaluation is an even more thorough evaluation of the implication of a health care investment called a health technology assessment. Health technology assessments not only include economic evaluations but also include considerations as to the social, ethical, and even legal aspects of a technology or care approach.

Evidence is not the only consideration in making policy judgments. Policymakers must consider whether the evidence and policy being considered will translate to the community of interest and have a similar expected impact. Details related to local context are critical to consider and can vary greatly depending on the magnitude of the problem, resources, health care delivery infrastructure, financing, and even values and preferences. Types of evidence that are referenced when examining local factors include epidemiological data, population health surveillance survey data, and community needs assessments.[16]

Barriers to and Facilitators of Evidence-Informed Policymaking (EIPM)

The policymaking process is dynamic, complex, and sometimes frenzied. Particularly with respect to quickly emerging critical issues, decisions of great significance may be made with limited time to consider even the simplest and most concise forms of evidence. Studies that have examined the uptake of science in policymaking have identified key barriers and facilitators to this process.[13,17–19] Like clinicians, policymakers report accessibility of timely, reliable, and relevant research findings as a key barrier to (or facilitator of) using evidence in the policymaking process. Because policymakers often do not have scientific backgrounds, the production of short, concise study findings, free of jargon, assists in uptake, as does building relationships with science advocates.

In fact, building relationships between policymakers and science advocates is beneficial on many levels. Mutual mistrust between policymakers and science advocates can be a significant barrier as policymakers may perceive science advocates to have political naivety, and science advocates may perceive policymakers to be naive of science.[18] Collaborative relationships can increase trust and facilitate timely communication. Furthermore, policymakers report they lack the skills needed to find and interpret research and that supportive training in this area by science advocates can be constructive. Having established partnerships not only improves the efficiency of the EIPM process but also helps scientists better understand the policy research gaps that require future study. Lastly, although not unique to public health and health care policy, all policymaking is subject to power and budget struggles and political instability, which can compete with or undermine the objectives of EIPM.

Strategies for Science Advocates in Promoting EIPM

Science advocates, including academics, researchers, students, public health practitioners, and practicing clinicians, have an important role in promoting the EIPM process. Upon evaluation of the barriers and facilitators of EIPM, it becomes clear that there are sensible and manageable approaches that science advocates can use to promote the translation of science into policy. Best practices for science advocates to consider include the following:

- *Producing relevant and concise rapid-response briefs.*[20-22] As critical issues swiftly emerge, there is a need for policymakers to make decisions quickly. Producing systematic reviews on a particular topic of interest often takes many more months than are available. Accordingly, science advocates can best support the EIPM process by producing rapid-response briefs based on evidence-based dentistry (EBD) guidelines or systematic reviews when possible. When developing rapid-response briefs, it is important that the methods are transparent, limitations in the science are noted, and, if applicable, the need for future systematic reviews is noted. Rapid-response briefs should be short (that is, no longer than one page) and free from technical jargon.

- *Inviting policymakers to participate in committees and workgroups.* Coalitions, community-based programs, and research studies all require broad partner engagement and participation. This provides the ideal opportunity for policymakers to participate in addressing topics important to science advocates and to give input with respect to their own interests and research needs. Additionally, these venues for collaboration assist in establishing trusting relationships, which can provide benefits into the future.

- *Providing educational skill-building opportunities in searching for and appraising evidence.* Policymakers and their advisers rarely have science backgrounds. Science advocates can provide a multitude of learning opportunities to assist policymakers and their advisers in gaining skills in the process of searching for and appraising evidence. Such learning opportunities could include webinars, lunch-and-learns, and hands-on learning sessions.

- *Advocating for legislation that defines in statute the term "evidence-based" along with its application in the public programming management process.* Simply having common definitions for terms such as "evidence-based program" versus "promising practice" and directing how evidence will be used and incorporated in state government can drive significant change in science uptake and achieving quality outcomes. Articulating these concepts in a statute has the benefit of helping to ensure that these approaches endure despite changes in administration. Washington State and Mississippi represent successful examples of this approach. With respect to social programming, both states passed statutes that require selected portions of state government to categorize new and existing programs by the level of quality of supporting evidence.[23,24] These statutes further require the development of evidence-based cost-benefit ratios, which are then used in the state budgeting process.

Strategies for Organizations Engaging in EIPM

There is a diverse compilation of entities that develop policies and/or administer policy-directed programs, including policymakers, their advisers, charitable and philanthropic organizations, and, of course, local, state, and federal governments. Those working in these organizations are ideally positioned to promote sound science, as the discrete phases of the policymaking process already use the inclusion of data as a key variable in policy development and evaluation. For organizations that make a commitment to EIPM, the biggest hurdles will be ensuring that all related staff have sufficient competency in evidence-informed decision-making and that EIPM is systematically embedded into work processes and organizational culture.

The first and most fundamental step for an organization in the EIPM engagement process is to conduct a self-assessment to evaluate the organization's level of commitment and capacity to engage in EIPM.[25,26] To meet this need, the Canadian Foundation for Healthcare Improvement developed a four-part tool to assist in the evaluation of an organization's capacity to use research. The four assessment domains of this tool include the following:

- *Acquire.* Can the entity find and obtain scientific studies?

- *Assess.* Can the entity critically appraise and assess the relevancy of the scientific studies?

- *Adapt.* Does the entity share study findings in a way that is clear and helpful to decision-makers?

- *Apply.* To what level does the entity have the skills, institutional framework, processes, and culture needed for science-based decision-making?

Identifying skill and capacity gaps in the self-assessment can spur organizations to either make improvements on their own or reach out to partners, such as researchers and science translation organizations who have the technical skill and expertise to support the organization in evidence-informed decision-making throughout the many phases of policymaking.

The first phase of policymaking that presents the opportunity to use systematically reviewed and critically appraised science is the issue-defining phase.[27] Defining an issue is a fundamental first step in the policymaking process. Similar to establishing a PICO (population, intervention, comparison, outcomes) question, how an issue is framed dramatically influences the outcome. Policymakers and their advisers should use evidence to clarify the exact issue (for example, a health disparity or an issue with publicly funded health care) and determine if the issue actually warrants attention or if it is an isolated problem. The magnitude of the problem can then be assessed by using scientific studies, epidemiological data (for example, CDC Oral Health Data and Healthy People 2020 data), and even health services data (for example, Medical Expenditure Panel Survey and Uniform Data System data). Finally, to the extent that it is relevant or feasible, evidence should be used to make comparisons within a group and also between reference groups to better understand the magnitude of the problem. For example, caries rates in a regional group of children can be evaluated over time and through subgroup analysis (for example, according to race or socioeconomic status), and it can also be evaluated by comparisons to national caries rates or even national health improvement initiative goals, such as Healthy People 2020.

In the spirit of EIPM, organizations should be explicit in the methods used to search for and appraise evidence, so as to minimize bias and maximize transparency. Evaluation methods should be developed and made available to stakeholders before the evaluation begins, as well as clearly stated in all documents. An added benefit to having clearly stated methods is that other organizations with overlapping interests can use the developed methods in approaching the same or similar issues.[28]

The second opportunity for integrating evidence occurs when assessing the effectiveness of current or proposed programs.[3,29] This process begins with the development of standardized definitions for the terms "evidence-based" and "promising practice" programs. Entities should use these definitions consistently and accurately to catalog and categorize programs according to their evidence of effectiveness.

Proposed programs demand a more involved level of scrutiny before an investment of valuable funds and resources is made. As with existing programs, proposed programs should be evaluated and categorized according to their evidence of effectiveness (that is, "evidence-based" versus "promising practice"). However, consideration should also be given to other factors and forms of evidence, such as the following:

- *Assess the transferability of the research results to the population of interest.* Are there important differences in the environment or constraints? Is the health system dramatically different? Is the underlying disease/condition/issue different?

- *Identify a program's real or potential harms or negative consequences.* This may include consequences such as risk of death, drug interactions, postoperative infections, or retreatment and failure rates.

- *Determine which stakeholder views might influence an option's acceptability.* Stakeholders may be patients, providers, or even employers. To the extent that these stakeholders' views might impact the acceptability of the proposed program, studies that qualitatively examine the views and experiences of such stakeholders should be considered.

- *Identify a program's real or potential cost-effectiveness (that is, outcomes achieved per dollars invested).* This is particularly important when comparing and considering two different approaches to solving a problem.

Assessing a program's cost-effectiveness can be particularly challenging in dentistry because of the lack of recognized and validated quality health outcome measures. Nevertheless, incorporating evidence of program effectiveness into the budgeting phase of policymaking is a critical third opportunity. Given the ever-increasing constraints put on budgets, this aspect of EIPM becomes particularly significant as it helps decision makers give priority funding to those programs with the highest return on investment. It additionally helps policymakers to identify which programs are not cost-effective and should perhaps be discontinued.

To promote EIPM in the budgeting and management process, organizations should do the following:

- *Report program performance during the budgeting development process.* This activity demands that an organization develop evidence-based performance measures and benchmarks. The developed measures should be meaningful to the population that the program serves. For example, "number of caries averted" is a more patient-centric outcome than "number of clients served." The performance measures, along with the cost to administer the program, can be used to determine the cost-effectiveness of the program (that is, caries averted per dollars spent). Results should be expected to be similar to those predicted by research, and policymakers should examine programs that are underperforming.

- *Develop and share program performance data in plain language summaries with decision-makers.* To assist in knowledge transfer, program divisions should be required to regularly report program performance in a standardized format. The standardized format, which should include a plain language evidence synopsis, can be shared during committee and budget hearings.

- *Ensure grants and contracts have evidence-based performance requirements.* Agencies should consider performance-based contracts instead of a fee-for-service model, which pays for the volume of services delivered. As an example, a school's dental health improvement program to reduce six-year molar decay rates by 10% in target children could be paid for by a state Medicaid agency instead of through individual service payments.

Finally, embedding evidence into the outcome evaluation process is arguably one of the most essential opportunities in the policymaking process, as the evidence-informed performance measures used in the evaluation process are utilized throughout all of the previously discussed phases of policymaking. Program outcome evaluation has similar parallels to clinical dentistry. There are many times in clinical care when dentists evaluate patient outcomes—for example, during postoperative checks, evaluations of crown margin quality, and the monitoring of periodontal status throughout periodontitis treatment. Similarly, those working in public health programming and government agencies routinely measure and report outcome data to determine whether programs are achieving the desired results. As discussed earlier, when programs do this, they should report evidence-based performance measures in a standardized plain language format. Additionally, they should maintain program evaluations in a centralized repository.

Putting It All Together

Systematically reviewed and critically appraised evidence, including EBD guidelines, can be used by science advocates to support policymakers in developing evidence-informed policies and programs. Through disciplined commitment, policymakers can use evidence to ensure that valuable resources are prioritized for those activities that deliver the highest results at the lowest cost. As the scientific knowledge base and partner networks in dentistry become more extensive, so does EIPM in dentistry. As an example, the ADA convened a multi-stakeholder group called the Dental Quality Alliance (DQA) that consists of dental scientists, government agencies, insurers, and dental care providers. Through the work of these stakeholders, the DQA successfully utilized high-quality synthesized dental sealant science to develop quality performance measures in dentistry. Multiple government agencies then used these measures to inform policy to promote the use of caries-preventing sealants in children (Box 17.4).

Below, we consider how science-informed policy can help oral health care progress toward the triple aim. To accomplish this, effective collaboration and consensus is required between those stakeholders who create high-quality evidence and advocate for its incorporation into policy decisions (for example, scientists, academics, and clinicians) and those responsible for making and implementing policy decisions (for example, government officials and health care administrators).

Box 17.4. Case Study: Incorporating Evidence in Quality Measure Development

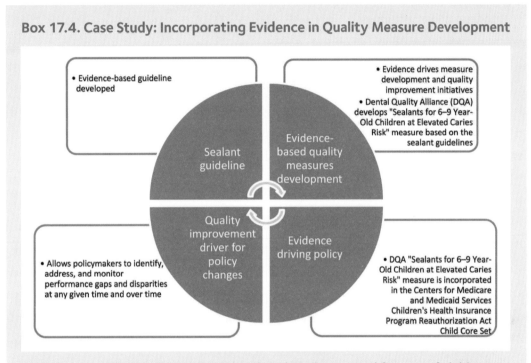

- Evidence-based guideline developed

Sealant guideline

Evidence-based quality measures development

- Evidence drives measure development and quality improvement initiatives
- Dental Quality Alliance (DQA) develops "Sealants for 6–9 Year-Old Children at Elevated Caries Risk" measure based on the sealant guidelines

Quality improvement driver for policy changes

Evidence driving policy

- Allows policymakers to identify, address, and monitor performance gaps and disparities at any given time and over time

- DQA "Sealants for 6–9 Year-Old Children at Elevated Caries Risk" measure is incorporated in the Centers for Medicare and Medicaid Services Children's Health Insurance Program Reauthorization Act Child Core Set

Evidence recommends that sealants be placed on the pits and fissures of children's primary and permanent teeth when it is determined that the tooth, or the patient, is at risk of experiencing caries.[30] The evidence for sealant effectiveness in permanent molars is stronger than the evidence for sealant effectiveness in primary molars.[30] Sealants benefit children across a wide age range; however, for the greatest effectiveness in caries prevention, it is recommended that sealants be placed on teeth soon after they erupt.[31,32] The Dental Quality Alliance (DQA) "Sealants for 6–9 Year-Old Children at Elevated Caries Risk" measure captures whether children at moderate or high caries risk received a sealant on a permanent first molar. Permanent first molars usually erupt between the ages of six and seven years. Thus, this measure addresses both the tooth type on which sealants are placed and the timeliness of the care provision. The measure allows an assessment of whether children at risk for caries are receiving evidence-based prevention and facilitates targeting performance improvement initiatives accordingly.

The DQA convened by the American Dental Association is a multi-stakeholder quality measure developer that creates measures for the appropriate assessment of state and federal programs such as Medicaid agencies, dental plans, and dental practices. Measures developed by the DQA are endorsed by the National Quality Forum[33] and are incorporated in both public and private programs. The DQA "Sealants for 6–9 Year-Old Children at Elevated Caries Risk" measure is part of the Core Set of Children's Health Care Quality Measures for Medicaid and CHIP (the Children's Health Insurance Program). A parallel measure, the DQA "Sealants for 6–9 Year-Olds eMeasure," is incorporated by the Health Resources and Services Administration for reporting by Federally Qualified Health Centers into their Uniform Data System.

Incorporation of an evidence-based quality measure into a public reporting system allows policymakers to identify, address, and monitor performance gaps and disparities at any given time and over time. A balanced measurement approach that evaluates multiple aspects of care is essential to promoting improved outcomes, understanding disparities, and planning for improved performance. Performance improvement is an ongoing process, and iterative measurement is essential for identifying, implementing, evaluating, monitoring, and sustaining quality improvement initiatives. Using evidence-based quality measures for performance improvement advances oral health outcomes and the overall health and well-being of children in the U.S.

Conclusion

Trusting collaborations among science advocates, policymakers, and administrators, along with purposeful policy processes that utilize high-quality evidence, can support the translation of complex science into effective policy. Health policies, aligned with evidence, work to achieve the triple aim: an improved patient experience (satisfaction and quality), better population health, and reduced per capita cost of health care.

References

1. Berwick DM, Nolan TW, Whittington J. "The Triple Aim: Care, Health, And Cost." *Health Affairs.* 2008;27(3):759-769.

2. Reis SE, Berglund L, Bernard GR, et al. "Reengineering the national clinical and translational research enterprise: the strategic plan of the National Clinical and Translational Science Awards Consortium." *Acad Med* 2010;85(3):463-9.

3. "CDC Policy Process." Atlanta, GA.: U.S. Department of Health and Human Services, Centers for Disease Control and Prevention, Office of the Associate Director for Policy; 2015. *https://www.cdc.gov/policy/analysis/process/index. html.* Accessed Sep 15, 2017.

4. Lyndon B. Johnson: "Special Message to the Congress Recommending a 12-Point Program for America's Children and Youth," February 8, 1967. Online by Gerhard Peters and John T. Woolley, The American Presidency Project. *http:// www.presidency.ucsb.edu/ws/?pid=28438.* Accessed Sep 15, 2017.

5. "Early and Periodic Screening, Diagnostic and Treatment." Baltimore, Md.: U.S. Department of Health and Human Services, Center for Medicare & Medicaid Services. *https://www.medicaid.gov/medicaid/benefits/epsdt/index.html.* Accessed Sep 15, 2017.

6. "Dental Care." Baltimore, Md.: U.S. Department of Health and Human Services, Center for Medicare & Medicaid Services. *https://www.medicaid.gov/medicaid/benefits/dental/index.html.* Accessed Sep 15, 2017.

7. "Using Evaluation to Inform CDC's Policy Process." Atlanta, GA.: U.S. Department of Health and Human Services, Centers for Disease Control and Prevention; 2015.

8. "Evidence-Based Policymaking: A Guide for Effective Government." Philadelphia, PA.: Pew-MacArthur Results First Initiative. The Pew Charitable Trusts; 2014.

9. "State Policy Guide: Using Research in Public Health Policymaking." Lexington, KY.: The Council of State Governments; 2008.

10. Chalmers I. "If Evidence-Informed Policy Works in Practice, Does It Matter If It Doesn't Work in Theory?" *Evidence & Policy: A Journal of Research, Debate and Practice.* 2005;1(2):227-242.

11. Brownson RC, Chriqui JF, Stamatakis KA. "Understanding Evidence-Based Public Health Policy." *Am J Public Health.* 2009;99(9):1576-1583.

12. Wye L, Brangan E, Cameron A, Gabbay J, Klein JH, Pope C. "Evidence Based Policy Making and the 'Art' of Commissioning – How English Healthcare Commissioners Access and Use Information and Academic Research in 'Real Life' Decision-making: an Empirical Qualitative Study." *BMC Health Services Research.* 2015;15:430.

13. Apollonio DE, Bero LA. "Interpretation and Use of Evidence in State Policymaking: a Qualitative Analysis." *BMJ Open.* 2017;7(2):e012738.

14. Oxman AD, Lavis JN, Lewin S, Fretheim A. "SUPPORT Tools for Evidence-Informed Health Policymaking (STP) 1: What Is Evidence-Informed Policymaking?" *Health Research Policy and Systems.* 2009;7(1):S1.

15. Rabarison KM, Bish CL, Massoudi MS, Giles WH. "Economic Evaluation Enhances Public Health Decision Making." *Front Public Health.* 2015;3.

16. Lewin S, Oxman AD, Lavis JN, Fretheim A, Marti SG, Munabi-Babigumira S. "SUPPORT Tools for Evidence-Informed Policymaking in Health 11: Finding and Using Evidence about Local Conditions." *Health Research Policy and Systems.* 2009;7(1):S11.

17. Oliver K, Innvar S, Lorenc T, Woodman J, Thomas J. "A Systematic Review of Barriers to and Facilitators of the Use of Evidence by Policymakers." *BMC Health Services Research.* 2014;14:2.

18. Murthy L, Shepperd S, Clarke MJ, et al. "Interventions to Improve the Use of Systematic Reviews in Decision-making by Health System Managers, Policy Makers and Clinicians." *Cochrane Database Syst Rev.* 2012;(9):CD009401.

19. Innvaer S, Vist G, Trommald M, Oxman A. "Health Policy-makers' Perceptions of Their Use of Evidence: a Systematic Review." *J Health Serv Res Policy.* 2002;7(4):239-244.

20. Lavis J, Davies H, Oxman A, Denis J-L, Golden-Biddle K, Ferlie E. "Towards Systematic Reviews that Inform Health Care Management and Policy-making." *J Health Serv Res Policy.* 2005;10 Suppl 1:35-48.

21. Oxman AD, Schünemann HJ, Fretheim A. "Improving the Use of Research Evidence in Guideline Development: 8. Synthesis and Presentation of Evidence." *Health Research Policy and Systems.* 2006;4:20.

22. Lavis JN. "How Can We Support the Use of Systematic Reviews in Policymaking?" *PLOS Medicine.* 2009;6(11):e1000141.

23. House Bill 2536. Olympia, WA.: Washington State 62nd Legislature; 2012. *http://lawfilesext.leg.wa.gov/ biennium/2011-12/Pdf/Bills/House%20Passed%20Legislature/2536-S2.PL.pdf.* Accessed Sep 15, 2017.

24. House Bill 677. Jackson, MS.: State of Mississippi Legislature; 2014. *http://billstatus.ls.state.ms.us/documents/2014/ html/HB/0600-0699/HB0677SG.htm.* Accessed Sep 15, 2017.

25. Oxman AD, Vandvik PO, Lavis JN, Fretheim A, Lewin S. "SUPPORT Tools for Evidence-Informed Health Policymaking (STP) 2: Improving How Your Organisation Supports the Use of Research Evidence to Inform Policymaking." *Health Research Policy and Systems.* 2009;7(1):S2.

26. National Collaborating Centre for Methods and Tools (2009). "Tool: Is Research Working for You?" Hamilton, ON: McMaster University. (Updated 30 August, 2017) Retrieved from *http://www.nccmt.ca/knowledge-repositories/ search/35.*

27. Lavis JN, Oxman AD, Lewin S, Fretheim A. "SUPPORT Tools for Evidence-Informed Health Policymaking (STP) 3: Setting Priorities for Supporting Evidence-Informed Policymaking." *Health Research Policy and Systems.* 2009;7(Suppl 1):S3.

28. Schünemann HJ, Fretheim A, Oxman AD. "Improving the Use of Research Evidence in Guideline Development: 1. Guidelines for Guidelines." *Health Research Policy and Systems.* 2006;4:13.

29. Lavis JN, Wilson MG, Oxman AD, Grimshaw J, Lewin S, Fretheim A. "SUPPORT Tools for Evidence-Informed Health Policymaking (STP) 5: Using Research Evidence to Frame Options to Address a Problem." *Health Research Policy and Systems.* 2009;7(1):S5.

30. Wright JT, Crall JJ, Fontana M, et al. "Evidence-Based Clinical Practice Guideline for the Use of Pit-and-Fissure Sealants: A Report of the American Dental Association and the American Academy of Pediatric Dentistry." *J Am Dent Assoc.* 2016;147(8):672-682.e12.

31. "Dental Sealants." Atlanta, GA.: U.S. Department of Health and Human Services, Centers for Disease Control and Prevention; 2013. *http://www.cdc.gov/OralHealth/publications/faqs/sealants.htm.* Accessed Sept. 15, 2017.

32. U.S. Dept. of Health and Human Services, National Institute of Dental and Craniofacial Research. "Oral Health in America: a Report of the Surgeon General." Rockville, Md.: U.S. Public Health Service, Dept. of Health and Human Services; 2000.

33. National Quality Forum. "Health and Well-Being Measures." Washington, DC: National Quality Forum; 2015. *http://www.qualityforum.org/Health_and_Well-Being_Measures.aspx.* Accessed Sept. 15, 2017.

Index

observational studies, 187–188
odds ratio, 192
CBA (cost-benefit analysis), 147, 279
CDT codes, 262
CEA (cost-effectiveness analysis), 146, 147, 150, 279
CEAC (cost-effectiveness acceptability curve), 156
Center for EBD, 23
certainty of evidence, 227–238
CIs. *See* confidence intervals
citation managers, 37
Clinical and Translational Science Awards (CTSA) Program, 275
clinical decisions
appraising randomized controlled trials for, 44–52
informing with diagnostic tests, 74, 76–85
informing with economic analysis, 149–159
informing with observational studies, 62–68
informing with qualitative studies, 131–132
informing with randomized control trials, 44–52
informing with systematic reviews, 93–100
using economic analyses, 149–159
using systematic reviews, 93–100
clinical expertise, 5
clinical guidelines, 12, 112–115
clinical interpretation, 186–188
clinical observations, 4
clinical practice guidelines, 263–271
clinical procedures, 5, 261
Clinical Queries, 13, 30
clinical questions
components, 5, 10, 11
EBD process, 5–6
examples, 7, 10, 11
PICO framework, 10–14
related to diagnosis, 11, 74–76
related to etiology, 11
related to harm, 11, 58–61
related to prevention, 11
related to prognosis, 11, 14
related to systematic reviews, 91, 93, 101–103
related to therapy, 11, 41–42, 43
clinical significance, 175, 180–181
clinical studies. *See also* research; studies
bias issues in, 209–226

clinical significance, 175, 180–181
considerations, 4
misleading results, 165–174
statistical significance, 175, 176–179
subgroup analyses, 171–172
clinical trials. *See also* randomized control trials; trials
bias in. *See* bias
considerations, 7, 171
controlled, 17
in gray literature, 38, 94
resources, 20, 23–25, 32, 38
unpublished, 94
ClinicalKey, 20
Cochrane Library, 23–25
Cochrane Oral Health, 1
cohort studies
bias, 61, 62, 64
clinical research, 186
considerations, 59, 61, 193
described, 59
example of, 60
observational studies, 187–188
odds ratio, 192
prognostic studies, 217
risk and, 66
committees, 281
communication, 242
comparison groups, 186
compliance monitoring, 257
confidence coefficient, 206
confidence intervals (CIs)
considerations, 206
interpreting, 199–201
meta-analysis and, 101–104
overview, 198
population and, 182, 198, 206
research findings, 182
risk and, 67, 71, 199–200
sample size and, 199–200
treatment effect, 50–51
width of, 182, 199–200, 204, 206
conflicts of interest, 123, 124, 128, 165, 166
confounder, 187
confounding, 209, 210–211, 218, 224
contracts, 284
control groups
absolute risk and, 199–200
economic analysis, 163, 182–183

exposure vs. outcome, 66
  hazard ratio and, 195
  prognosis factors, 46
  treatment effect, 50
cost analysis, 146, 147, 279
cost components, 151–152, 158
cost-benefit analysis (CBA), 147, 279
cost-effectiveness acceptability curve (CEAC), 156
cost-effectiveness analysis (CEA), 146, 147, 150, 279
cost-effectiveness plane, 154
cost-of-illness analysis, 279
costs. *See also* economic analysis
  vs. benefits, 52, 105, 158–159, 164
  incremental cost, 153, 155–157, 159, 163
  of interventions, 146–147, 154, 159
  long-term cost, 148
  recording, 150
  treatment cost, 146–147, 152
costs and consequences, 148, 149–152, 163
costs and effects, 153, 155–156, 163, 164
cost-utility analysis (CUA), 146–147, 279
CPG factors, 263
cross-sectional studies
  considerations, 61, 75
  described, 59, 61
  diagnostic tests, 75
  example of, 60
  observational studies, 187, 188
crude result, 211
CTSA (Clinical and Translational Science Awards) Program, 275
CUA (cost-utility analysis), 146–147, 279

D
data
  analyzing, 48, 90, 132, 138, 176
  collection of, 99, 132–135, 137
  errors, 97
  interval data, 204
  ratio data, 204
databases
  gray literature and, 38, 94
  searching, 8–14, 96, 114
decision models, 148
decision tree, 148
decision-making, 5, 105, 112. *See also*
  recommendations

demographic data, 134, 137
dental clinics, 263
Dental Quality Alliance (DQA), 284–285
dental recall examinations, 156
dental schools, 259
descriptive statistics, 195
descriptive studies, 188
detection bias, 214
diagnosis, 78–88
  appraising/using articles on, 73–88
  clinical questions related to, 11, 74–76
  clinical scenario, 73
  cross-sectional studies, 75
  PICO framework, 74
  randomized control trials, 75
  study designs for, 75–76
diagnostic codes, 262
diagnostic dilemma, 77, 79, 87
diagnostic studies, 75, 222–223
diagnostic tests
  applying results to patient care, 84–85
  appraising results of, 81–83
  bias and, 76–81, 220–224
  considerations, 85
  described, 74
  reference standard, 74–83, 87
  reproducibility of, 84, 88
  using to inform clinical decisions, 74, 76–85
dichotomous outcomes, 99
didactic learning, 243
differential statistics, 195
discounting, 152
disease severity, 222
distribution, 201
double blinding, 187
double-blind trials, 47
DQA (Dental Quality Alliance), 284–285

E
EBD (evidence-based dentistry)
  articles about. *See* articles
  clinical practice guidelines, 263–271
  components, 4
  definition of, 1, 3, 4
  history of, 3
  learning about. *See* training/education
  overview, 3–5
  personalization, 3
  principles of, 4–5

ADA, 112, 122, 128
AHA, 112, 119–120, 211
appraising recommendations, 114–123,
127–128
bias, 229
conflicts of interest, 123, 124
considerations, 228–229, 231, 233
developing/updating guidelines, 112–113
NICE, 112, 118, 119
strength of recommendations, 119–123
guidelines. *See* clinical guidelines

H
harm
benefits vs. harm, 52, 68, 105, 159, 171
clinical questions related to, 11, 58–61
clinical scenario, 57
considerations, 58
exposure/outcome, 65–67
observational studies, 58–69
PICO framework, 58
risk of, 58, 66–67, 68, 71
study designs for, 58–61
using articles on, 57–72
hazard ratio (HR), 66, 189, 195
health care interventions. *See* interventions
health outcomes. *See* outcomes
health policymaking, 275–288
health technology assessments, 279, 280
heterogeneity, 99, 101, 103, 229, 230
homogenous sampling, 132
HR (hazard ratio), 66, 189, 195
hypotheses, 195–198, 203, 206
hypothesis testing, 177, 179, 195–198, 206.
See also P values

I
ICER (incremental cost-effectiveness ratio),
154, 155
IHI (Institute for Healthcare Improvement),
264
implementation science, 255–274
active implementation phase, 263–371
adoption decision/preparation phase,
259–263
considerations, 256, 272
defining scope of, 255–256
exploration phase, 258–259

overview, 255–256
sustainment phase, 272
translating evidence into practice, 257–272
imprecision, 231
incremental cost-effectiveness ratio (ICER),
154, 155
index tests. *See* diagnostic tests
indirectness, 233
inferential statistics, 195
information technology (IT), 262
input variables, 211
Institute for Healthcare Improvement (IHI),
264
intention-to-treat (ITT) principle, 47–48, 215
Internet search engines, 36–37
interval data, 204
interventions
in clinical research, 176
considerations, 168, 170
cost of, 146–147, 154, 159
diagnostic tests as, 75
effectivity of, 154
local, 92
success of, 5
interviews, 133, 134, 137
IT (information technology), 262
ITT (intention-to-treat) principle, 47–48, 215

J
*JADA (Journal of the American Dental
Association)*, 1, 26
*JEBDP (Journal of Evidence-Based Dental
Practice)*, 26
*Journal of Evidence-Based Dental Practice
(JEBDP)*, 26
*Journal of the American Dental Association
(JADA)*, 1, 26
journals, 1, 26

K
Kappa statistic, 222
keyword searches, 8, 25, 32
knowledge synthesis, 90

L
lag bias, 234
legislation, 281
level of power, 204

patient care
  applying diagnostic test results to, 84–85, 88
  applying economic analysis to, 158–159, 164
  applying observational study results to, 67–68
  applying qualitative study results to, 139, 140–141
  applying RCT results to, 51–52
  applying systematic review results, 104–105, 110
  prognosis of patient. *See* prognosis
patient information resources, 39
patient-important outcome, 51, 104, 116, 117, 229
patient-reported outcome measures (PROMs), 181
patients
  care of. *See* patient care
  diagnostic dilemma, 77, 79, 87
  evaluating in RCTs, 51
  personalized treatment, 3
  study patients, 51, 56, 67, 72
  subgroups, 151, 156
PDSA cycle, 271
peer influences, 262–263
performance bias, 214
performance, program, 284
PICO components, 5
PICO framework, 10–14
  diagnosis questions, 74
  harm questions, 58
  therapy questions, 41, 42
placebos, 47
point estimates, 99, 100, 101, 199
point-of-care resources, 19–20
policies, 276–280
policy development process, 277
policy issues, 263
policymakers, 277–286
policymaking process, 280–284
pooled estimates, 99–100, 101
population
  characteristics of, 221–222
  confidence intervals and, 182, 198, 206
  considerations, 72, 74, 187
  described, 42
  hypothesis testing and, 195
  selection bias, 218
  true population, 198, 204, 207
population health outcomes, 275

population, intervention, comparison, outcomes. *See* PICO
population mean, 198, 204
population of interest, 67, 91, 283
positive studies, 234
prevention, 11, 147, 285
primary studies, 75, 98–100
priori hypotheses, 230
probability
  diagnostic tests, 79, 81–83
  of intervention, 157, 159
  normal curve and, 201–204
  overview, 81–83
  risk and, 189–190, 191, 195
  sample size and, 204–205
  significance testing and, 197–198
  statistical significance, 176–177, 179
probability values. *See* P values
professionalism, 242
prognosis
  clinical questions related to, 11, 14
  considerations, 46, 90
  risk of bias and, 44, 55
prognosis balance, 46–48, 55
prognostic factor measurement, 218
prognostic factors, 44, 46, 62–63, 217, 218
prognostic imbalance, 48, 62, 63
prognostic studies, 217–220
program cost analysis, 279
program outcome evaluation, 284
program performance, 284
PROMs (patient-reported outcome measures), 181
publication bias, 215, 234–236
PubMed, 27–37
purposeful sampling, 132

Q

QALYs (quality-adjusted life-years), 146–147
QAPY (quality-adjusted prosthesis-years), 155
qualitative research, 129–144
  considerations, 131
  credibility of results, 132–139
  critically appraising, 131–132
  demographic data, 134, 137
  ethical considerations, 133
  overview, 19
  purposeful sampling, 132
  relevance of, 130, 136

Transparency and Rigor Using Standards of Trustworthiness (TRUST) Scorecard, 22
treatment benefits
  vs. costs/risks, 158–159, 164
  vs. harms/costs, 52, 68, 105, 159, 171
  intention-to-treat principle, 47–48, 215
treatment decisions, 2, 146–147, 260
treatment effects
  appraising, 49–51
  long-term consequences of, 148
  measuring with CIs, 199, 200
  pros/cons of, 52
  randomized control trials, 46, 49–51
  sample size and, 204, 205
trial-based economic analysis, 148
trials. See also randomized control trials; studies
  bias in. See bias
  clinical. See clinical trials
  considerations, 7, 171
  double-blind, 47
  experimental, 187
  unpublished, 94
Trip database, 17–18
TRUST (Transparency and Rigor Using Standards of Trustworthiness) Scorecard, 22
type I errors, 176
type II errors, 177

U

UI COD (University of Iowa College of Dentistry) EBD instructional track, 247–248
University of Iowa College of Dentistry (UI COD) EBD instructional track, 247–248
University of Texas Health Science Center San Antonio (UTHSCSA) School of Dentistry, 245–247
UpToDate database, 19–20
U.S. Preventive Services Task Force (USPSTF), 119–120
USPSTF (U.S. Preventive Services Task Force), 119–120
UTHSCSA (University of Texas Health Science Center San Antonio) School of Dentistry, 245–247

V

VCU (Virginia Commonwealth University) School of Dentistry, 244–245
verification bias, 222
vertical line of no effect, 101
Virginia Commonwealth University (VCU) School of Dentistry, 244–245

W

Web of Science, 34–35
weight, 101
workgroups, 281

Z

zero, true, 204